Intracerebral Hemorrhage

Intracerebral Hemorrhage

Edited by

J. R. Carhuapoma
Johns Hopkins University Hospital, Baltimore, MD, USA

S. A. Mayer
Columbia University Medical Center, New York, NY, USA

D. F. Hanley
Johns Hopkins University Hospital, Baltimore, MD, USA

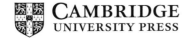

CAMBRIDGE UNIVERSITY PRESS

Cambridge, New York, Melbourne, Madrid, Cape Town, Singapore, São Paulo, Delhi

Cambridge University Press
The Edinburgh Building, Cambridge CB2 8RU, UK

Published in the United States of America by
Cambridge University Press, New York

www.cambridge.org
Information on this title: www.cambridge.org/9780521873314

First published 2010

Printed in the United Kingdom at the University Press, Cambridge

A catalog record for this publication is available from the British Library

Library of Congress Cataloging-in-Publication Data

Intracerebral hemorrhage / edited by J. R. Carhuapoma, S. A. Mayer,
D. F. Hanley.
    p. ; cm.
    Includes bibliographical references and index.
    ISBN 978-0-521-87331-4 (hardback)
    1.   Brain–Hemorrhage.   I. Carhuapoma, J. R. (J. Ricardo)   II.   Mayer,
Stephan A.   III.   Hanley, D. F. (Daniel F.), 1949–   IV.   Title
    [DNLM: 1.   Cerebral Hemorrhage. WL 355 I6083 2009]
    RC394.H37I372 2009
    616.8′1–dc22

                                                                    2009034806

ISBN 978-0-521-87331-4 Hardback

Additional resources for this publication at www.cambridge.org/
9780521873314

To my son Ethan and my family for their unconditional support JRC
To Catherine, Philip and Elizabeth SAM
To my wife and family who have supported my career DFH

Contents

Contributors

Marie-Germaine Bousser MD
Department of Neurology,
Lariboisière Hospital, Paris, France

Joseph P. Broderick MD
Department of Neurology,
University of Cincinnati,
Cincinnati, OH, USA

Ken Butcher MD PhD FRCPC
Division of Neurology,
University of Alberta,
Edmonton, Alberta, Canada

Louis R. Caplan MD
Department of Neurology,
Beth Israel Deaconess Medical Center,
Boston, MA, USA

J. Ricardo Carhuapoma MD FAHA
Departments of Neurology, Neurosurgery,
and Anesthesiology & Critical Care Medicine,
Division of Neurosciences Critical Care,
The Johns Hopkins Medical Institutions,
Baltimore, MD, USA

José Castillo MD PhD
Department of Neurology,
Hospital Clínico Universitario,
University of Santiago de Compostela,
Santiago de Compostela, Spain

Michael Chen MD
Departments of Neurology and Radiology,
Rush University Medical Center,
Chicago, IL, USA

Rush H. Chewning BA
Department of Radiology,
The Johns Hopkins Hospital,
Baltimore, MD, USA

Frederick Colbourne PhD
Department of Psychology,
University of Alberta, Edmonton, Alberta,
Canada

Isabelle Crassard MD
Department of Neurology,
Lariboisière Hospital, Paris, France

Antoni Dávalos MD PhD
Department of Neurosciences,
Hospital Germans Trias i Pujol,
Barcelona, Spain

Stephen M. Davis MD FRACP
Department of Neurology,
Royal Melbourne Hospital,
Melbourne, Victoria, Australia

Lisa M. DeAngelis MD
Department of Neurology,
Memorial Sloan-Kettering Cancer Center,
New York, NY, USA

Matthew L. Flaherty MD
Department of Neurology,
University of Cincinnati, Cincinnati, OH, USA

Steven M. Greenberg MD PhD
Neurology Stroke Service,
Massachusetts General Hospital,
Boston, MA, USA

Daniel F. Hanley MD
Departments of Neurology, Neurosurgery,
and Anesthesiology & Critical Care Medicine,
Division of Brain Injury Outcomes Research,
The Johns Hopkins Hospital,
Baltimore, MD, USA

Ameer E. Hassan DO
Department of Neurology,

University of Minnesota Medical Center,
Minneapolis, MN, USA

Julian T. Hoff MD
Formerly Department of Neurosurgery,
University of Michigan,
Ann Arbor, MI, USA

Andreas F. Hottinger
Department of Neurology,
Memorial Sloan-Kettering Cancer Center,
New York, NY, USA

Hagen B. Huttner MD
Department of Neurology,
University of Heidelberg, Heidelberg,
Germany

Carlos S. Kase MD
Department of Neurology,
Boston Medical Center, Boston, MA, USA

Richard F. Keep PhD
Department of Neurosurgery,
University of Michigan,
Ann Arbor, MI, USA

Crystal MacLellan PhD
Department of Psychology,
University of Alberta, Edmonton, Alberta, Canada

Stephan A. Mayer MD
Department of Neurology,
Columbia University Medical Center,
New York, NY, USA

A. David Mendelow PhD FRCSEd
Department of Neurosurgery,
Newcastle General Hospital,
Newcastle upon Tyne, UK

J. P. Mohr MD PhD
Department of Neurology,
Columbia University Medical Center,
New York, NY, USA

Kieran P. Murphy MD
Department of Radiology,
The Johns Hopkins Hospital,
Baltimore, MD, USA

Neeraj S. Naval MD
Department of Neurology, Neurosurgery,
and Anesthesia Critical Care Medicine,
Neurosciences Critical Care Division,
Oregon Health Sciences University School of Medicine,
Oregon, USA

Paul A. Nyquist MD
Department of Neurology, Neurosurgery,
and Anesthesiology & Critical Care Medicine,
Division of Neurosciences Critical Care,
Johns Hopkins Medical Institutions,
Baltimore, MD, USA

James Peeling PhD
Department of Chemistry,
University of Winnipeg, Winnipeg,
Manitoba, Canada

Adnan I. Qureshi MD
Department of Neurology,
University of Minnesota Medical Center,
Minneapolis, MN, USA

Manuel Rodriguez-Yáñez MD
Department of Neurology,
Hospital Clínico Universitario,
University of Santiago de Compostela,
Santiago de Compostela, Spain

Christian Stapf MD
Department of Neurology,
Lariboisière Hospital, Paris, France

Thorsten Steiner MD
Department of Neurology,
University of Heidelberg, Heidelberg, Germany

Stanley Tuhrim MD
Department of Neurology,
Mt Sinai Medical Center, New York, NY, USA

Kenneth R. Wagner PhD
Department of Neurology,
University of Cincinnati, Cincinnati,
OH, USA

Daniel Woo MD
Department of Neurology,
University of Cincinnati, Cincinnati,
OH, USA

Guohua Xi MD
Department of Neurosurgery,
University of Michigan,
Ann Arbor, MI, USA

Haralabos Zacharatos DO
Department of Neurology,
University of Minnesota Medical Center,
Minneapolis, MN, USA

Wendy C. Ziai MD
Department of Neurology,
The Johns Hopkins Hospital,
Baltimore, MD, USA

Mario Zuccarello MD
Department of Neurology,
University of Cincinnati, Cincinnati,
OH, USA

Foreword

Intracerebral Hemorrhage is the first major text devoted to non-traumatic intracerebral hemorrhage (ICH) to appear in almost 20 years. The 21 chapters detail a generation of progress since the introduction of brain computerized tomography (CT) in 1973. At that time, and for the first time, the phenotype of non-traumatic ICH could be clarified. The Polaroid-print images of ICH pasted into patient medical records were understandable in all languages. The distinction between ICH and territorial cerebral infarction was no longer fuzzy, to await the final verdict at the autopsy table. Testable hypotheses replaced speculation.

During the next two decades, faster and more accurate CT scanning and then magnetic resonance imaging (MRI) allowed rigorous clinical-radiographic studies (Chapters 8–10). Publications related to ICH sky-rocketed in number. In 1991, the National Institutes of Health funded the first investigator-initiated R01 research grant to study ICH in emergency departments. The US federal funding of additional studies of ICH surged. Worldwide, CT-based clinical studies described the dynamic profile of ICH. The pivotal role of ICH volume growth in clinical deterioration during the first minutes and hours after symptom onset was established. In parallel with the studies of ICH in the emergency department setting, experimental (Chapters 17, 18) and clinical studies proceeded (Chapters 1–8). Subtypes of ICH were identified with greater precision, facilitating epidemiological studies, mechanistic experimental studies, and, more recently, genetic studies by subtype.

Outcomes research has clearly shown that survival and recovery after ICH is improved when patients are cared for in specialized neurological intensive care units, with a focus on aggressive medical support and best medical practices. The search for a "magic bullet" has been more elusive. In 1995, recombinant tissue plasminogen activator (rt-PA) was shown to be safe and effective as treatment for ischemic stroke, if administered intravenously within 3 hours of symptom onset. Medical centers engaged in administration of rt-PA as urgent treatment geared-up for a similar emergency approach to ICH. Complex multi-departmental systems for urgent patient transport, diagnosis, and treatment were already in place at these centers. Active bleeding during the first minutes and hours after ICH onset provides a logical therapeutic target. The 40%-plus major morbidity and mortality following ICH has provided opportunity for firm clinical end points to evaluate treatment outcomes. Accordingly, attempts at very early surgery via craniotomy or endoscopic techniques were initiated (Section 5). Thrombolytic agents including instillation of rt-PA were utilized in several trials. Unfortunately, these attempts at treatment within 3–12 hours suffered from slow enrollment and from disappointing therapeutic results. Surgical evacuation of ICH within 90 minutes, or even 3 hours, was not an achievable goal, and complete surgical evacuation has been difficult to achieve. Fortunately, encouraging technical results were observed following catheter-based techniques for clot removal in the setting of intraventricular hemorrhage, particularly when employed in combination with locally instilled thrombolytic drugs. Controlled studies of these techniques for parenchymal and intraventricular hemorrhage are currently underway (Chapter 15).

In 2005, the long-awaited results of the International Surgical Trial in Intracerebral Haemorrhage (STICH) were published, the results of which are discussed in Chapter 14 by the principal investigator, David Mendelow. The STICH trial was a major accomplishment as 1033 patients were randomized at 83 centers from 27 countries. Overall, the operated patients did not benefit, though subgroup analysis suggested that early surgery may improve outcomes for patients with lobar ICH. The STICH II trial, designed to answer that question, is also described by Dr. Mendelow in Chapter 14.

Medical treatments for ICH are detailed in Sections 5, 6, and 7. General supportive treatments in intensive care units and rehabilitation treatments in dedicated units have improved outcomes. For specific medical treatment, ongoing bleeding following onset of ICH is the logical target for intervention. Optimal management of blood pressure, and perhaps even acute lowering of blood pressure, may be shown to influence outcome (Chapter 13). Of particular interest, the recent randomized trials of procoagulant therapy have shown promise in slowing bleeding (Chapter 21). Both the phase II and phase III studies of recombinant factor VIIa as very early treatment for ICH demonstrated lower ICH volumes in the actively treated patients compared to those treated with placebo. Clinical outcomes were improved in the phase II trial but not in the phase III trial. In the future, initiation of procoagulant treatment even earlier and with improved patient selection may be shown to enhance clinical outcomes after ICH.

Perhaps most importantly, the biggest transformation over the past 20 years has been widespread acceptance of the concept that ICH is a treatable medical illness. Historically ICH was viewed as a hopeless, life-negating event for which caregivers had nothing to offer other than prayers and compassion. What has become dramatically clear, however, is that many ICH patients die as a result of self-fulfilling prophecies of doom. As caregivers have been more aggressive with their interventions and persistent with their support, the biggest surprise has been how often functional recovery far exceeds what we once thought was possible. This is the key insight that has served as the ultimate motivation for the contributors to this book, who have devoted their careers to finding effective treatments for this devastating disease.

Thomas Brott, MD
Mayo Clinic
Jacksonville, FL

The epidemiology of intracerebral hemorrhage

Matthew L. Flaherty, Daniel Woo, and Joseph P. Broderick

Introduction

Advances in brain imaging have dramatically changed our understanding of intracerebral hemorrhage (ICH). In the pre-CT era, many small ICHs were misclassified as ischemic strokes and patients with massive ICH or subarachnoid hemorrhage (SAH) were often difficult to correctly classify. This chapter reviews the epidemiology of non-traumatic ICH in light of modern neuroimaging and includes discussions of the incidence, etiology, clinical presentation, and natural history of this condition.

Incidence of intracerebral hemorrhage

Intracerebral hemorrhage accounts for 10–15% of all strokes in Western populations and is defined as the non-traumatic, abrupt onset of severe headache, altered level of consciousness, or focal neurological deficit associated with a focal collection of blood within the brain parenchyma on neuroimaging or at autopsy which is not due to trauma or hemorrhagic conversion of a cerebral infarction [1].

The incidence of ICH is defined as the percentage of a population experiencing a first ICH in a given time period (usually a year). When reviewing studies of ICH incidence it is important to consider the criteria utilized, as investigators may include or exclude hemorrhages associated with vascular malformations, anticoagulants, thrombolytic agents, or illicit drugs. Comparisons of incidence rates are further complicated by methodological differences in case ascertainment, imaging rates, variations in population structure, and the range of ages reported.

Given these limitations, incidence rates of ICH in the Western hemisphere during the CT era have generally ranged from 10 to 30 cases per 100 000 persons [2–11]. Intracerebral hemorrhage incidence rates are higher in eastern Asia, where ICH has historically accounted for a larger percentage of all strokes than in Western populations [12–14]. This balance may be changing due to declining rates of ICH in the East [12,15,16].

The incidence of ICH declined between the 1950s and the 1980s [17–19]. Studies of incidence trends in subsequent years have produced mixed results. There was a trend toward a reduction in ICH incidence in Oxfordshire, England between 1981 and 2006 [20]. Intracerebral hemorrhage incidence also declined during the 1990s in several Chinese cities [12]. However, similar declines have not been seen in other studies [2,8,21,22]. The stabilization of ICH incidence in the last two decades is at least partially attributable to the detection and proper classification of small hemorrhages with modern neuroimaging [8,23,24].

Risk for ICH appears to be marginally greater in men than in women, driven by an excess of deep hemorrhages [11,25,26]. In the United States blacks and Hispanics have significantly higher rates of ICH than whites [11,27]. Among blacks and Hispanics, the excess risk of ICH is most notable in young and middle-aged persons (Table 1.1) [11,27,28].

The predominant location of ICH within the brain varies in different populations (Table 1.2). In the United States, Europe, and Australia, deep cerebral ICH (hemorrhage originating in the periventricular white matter, caudate nucleus, internal capsule, putamen, globus pallidus, or thalamus) is most common, followed closely by lobar hemorrhages originating in the gray matter or subcortical white matter. In a large population-based study in Japan, however, lobar hemorrhage accounted for only 15% of ICHs [13].

Intracerebral Hemorrhage, ed. J. R. Carhuapoma, S. A. Mayer, and D. F. Hanley. Published by Cambridge University Press.
© J. R. Carhuapoma, S. A. Mayer, and D. F. Hanley 2010.

Table 1.1. Age-specific risk ratios for ICH defined by location in the Greater Cincinnati Area, black vs. white*

Age	Lobar		Deep		Brainstem		Cerebellum	
	RR	95% CI	RR	95% CI	RR	95% CI	RR	95% CI
20–34	2.1	0.5–9.3	2.1	0.5–9.3	0	0–20.1	0	0.67
35–54	3.7	2.1–6.7	4.5	3.0–6.8	9.8	4.2–23.0	4.0	1.5–10.8
55–74	1.7	1.1–2.7	2.3	1.7–3.3	3.0	1.2–7.4	0.8	0.2–2.4
75–84	1.2	0.7–2.0	1.1	0.7–1.8	3.6	1.2–11.1	0.7	0.2–2.1
85+	1.0	0.4–2.2	0.9	0.4–1.9	0	0–3.3	0.6	0.1–3.7
All	1.4	1.0–1.8	1.7	1.4–2.1	3.3	2.0–5.5	0.9	0.5–1.6

Notes: *Risk ratio calculated from unadjusted incidence rates.
RR = risk ratio, RR > 1 indicates greater risk among blacks.
Source: From [11].

Table 1.2. Proportional distribution of ICH in different studies

	Total ICH	Lobar (%)	Deep (%)	Brainstem (%)	Cerebellum (%)
Greater Cincinnati [11]	1038	359 (35)	512 (49)	65 (6)	102 (10)
Izumo City, Japan [13]	350	53 (15)	242 (69)	30 (9)	25 (7)
Southern Sweden [148]	341	176 (52)	121 (36)	15 (4)	29 (9)
Jyvaskyla region, Finland [9]	158†	53 (34)	77 (49)	11 (7)	17 (11)
Dijon, France [149]	87	16 (18)	58 (67)	5 (6)	8 (9)
Perth, Australia [150]	60*	19 (32)	31 (52)	4 (7)	6 (10)

Notes: †Includes 9 intraventricular hemorrhages, here included in the deep group.
*Includes 13 "massive cortical" hemorrhages, here included in the deep group.
Source: From [11].

In most populations, cerebellar hemorrhage accounts for approximately 10% of ICH and brainstem hemorrhage for 5–10% of ICH (Table 1.2). In the United States, the greatest excess risk of ICH in blacks and Hispanics as compared to whites occurs in deep cerebral and brainstem locations (Table 1.1) [11,28].

Risk factors for intracerebral hemorrhage

Age and race

Age is the greatest risk factor for ICH. Incidence rates increase dramatically among persons older than 60 (Fig. 1.1). As discussed previously, there are geographic and racial variations in ICH incidence. Studies to date have not determined whether these variations can be explained entirely by known risk factors or whether there are additional factors, possibly genetic, which remain undiscovered.

Hypertension

Hypertension is the most important and prevalent modifiable risk factor for ICH. In the biracial population of Greater Cincinnati during 1988, the presence of hypertension among patients with ICH was remarkably similar for whites (73%), African-Americans (71%), men (72%), and women (73%) [29]. Untreated hypertension is a greater risk factor than treated hypertension, and hypertensive patients who discontinue their medications have greater risk than those who continue them [30,31].

Among modifiable risk factors for ICH, hypertension accounts for the greatest attributable risk for hemorrhage in deep hemispheric and brainstem locations [32]. The role of hypertension in lobar ICH is less clear, but accumulating evidence suggests hypertension is also a risk factor for hemorrhage in this location (albeit less potent) [31,33]. The relative effect of hypertension as a risk factor for ICH is greater in younger patients than the elderly [31,34]. In one case-control study the odds ratio for hypertension in ICH fell from 7.7 among patients age 15–54 years to 1.3 among those aged 65–74 years [31]. Treatment trials for hypertension have shown reduced ICH risk with improved blood pressure control [35,36].

The use of illicit sympathomimetic drugs, particularly cocaine and amphetamines, has been associated with hemorrhagic stroke in some (but not all) studies [37–39]. This relationship may be due to drug-induced hypertension or drug-induced cerebral vasculitis.

Cerebral amyloid angiopathy

Once thought to be a rare cause of ICH, cerebral amyloid angiopathy (CAA) is now considered an important cause of lobar hemorrhage in the elderly (Fig. 1.2) [40–42]. Its principal pathological feature is the deposition of amyloid protein in the media and adventitia of leptomeningeal arteries, arterioles, capillaries, and, less often, veins [40–44]. The hypothesized pathogenesis of ICH due to CAA involves destruction of the normal vascular structure by deposition of amyloid in the media and adventitia and subsequent miliary aneurysm formation or double barreling and fibrinoid necrosis [40–42]. The brittle blood vessels and microaneurysms may then be prone to rupture in response to minor trauma or sudden changes in blood pressure [19]. Cerebral amyloid angiopathy may also be responsible for transient neurological symptoms and dementia with leukoencephalopathy [45].

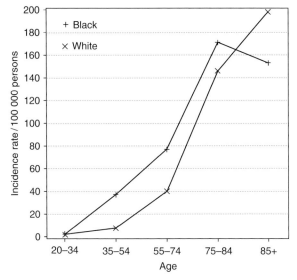

Fig. 1.1 Annual age-specific, race-stratified incidence rates of ICH per 100 000 persons in the Greater Cincinnati/Northern Kentucky region, 1998–2003 (author's unpublished data).

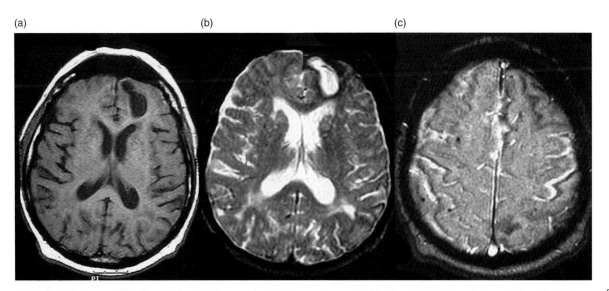

Fig. 1.2 Gradient echo MRI of a patient with previous microhemorrhages in multifocal regions typical of cerebral amyloid angiopathy. (a) T1-weighted image demonstrating an old lesion in the left frontal lobe. (b) T2-weighted image demonstrates a hemosiderin ring around the left frontal lesion. (c) Gradient echo imaging reveals microbleeds in the right frontal and parietal lobes.

Amyloid protein becomes increasingly frequent in cortical blood vessels with advancing age, affecting only 5–8% of persons age 60–69 years but 57–58% of those age 90 years or older [46, 47]. The deposition of amyloid is most prominent in the parieto-occipital regions and is rarely found in the basal ganglia or brainstem [40–43]. Cerebral amyloid angiopathy equally affects men and women [41].

Apolipoprotein E and CAA

The relationshiop of Apolipoprotein E and CAA is discussed in more detail in Chapter 4. Several studies have examined the relationship of Apolipoprotein E $\epsilon2$ and $\epsilon4$ with lobar ICH and CAA [32,33,48–51].

In a population-based, case-control study of hemorrhagic stroke in Greater Cincinnati/Northern Kentucky (the Genetic and Environmental Risk Factors for Hemorrhagic Stroke, or GERFHS, study), cases of lobar ICH were age-, race-, and gender-matched to controls from the same population, allowing investigators to control for putative ICH risk factors and determine the prevalence of Apolipoprotein E genotype in the population from which cases were identified. After controlling for the presence of hypertension, hypercholesterolemia, frequent alcohol use, smoking history, and other risk factors, Apolipoprotein E $\epsilon4$ was found to be an independent risk factor for lobar ICH but not non-lobar ICH. In addition, haplotypes inferred using 12 markers over the $5'$ untranslated region, promoter region, and exons of the Apolipoprotein E gene identified significant association with lobar ICH, which suggests that regulation of the gene may affect the risk of disease [33].

Aneurysms and vascular malformations

Although ruptured berry aneurysms typically cause SAH, on occasion bleeding is directed into the brain parenchyma without significant subarachnoid extension [52]. Vascular malformations associated with ICH include arteriovenous malformations (AVMs), cavernous malformations, dural arteriovenous fistulae, venous malformations, and capillary telangiectasias [53]. Reports of ICH mechanism suggest that aneurysms and vascular malformations are particularly important as a cause of ICH among young people [52,54–56]. In a prospective autopsy series, 4% of all brains were found to have vascular malformations, of which 63% were venous malformations. This

Table 1.3. Comparison of the frequency of vascular malformations in autopsy series vs. series of symptomatic ICH patients

	Population-based autopsy [151]	ICH patients autopsy [152]
Venous	105 (63%)	2 (1.3%)
Telangiectasia	28 (17%)	1 (0.6%)
Arteriovenous	24 (14%)	159 (88%)
Cavernous	16 (10%)	6 (3%)
Mixed type	N/A	11 (6%)

Note: Some patients had more than one type of malformation. N/A = not reported.

contrasts starkly with lesions that cause hemorrhage as reported by autopsy (Table 1.3). While venous malformations are the most common lesions in the general population, they are associated with only a small percentage of ICH cases. Similarly, cerebral telangiectasias are more common at autopsy than AVMs or cavernous malformations but rarely hemorrhage. The natural history, clinical evaluation, and management options for intracranial vascular malformations have been recently reviewed [53].

Anticoagulant- and thrombolytic-associated ICH

The use of warfarin for prevention of ischemic stroke among patients with atrial fibrillation increased significantly during the late 1980s and 1990s following publication of the Stroke Prevention in Atrial Fibrillation (SPAF) trials, European Atrial Fibrillation Trial, and other important studies on this topic [57–60]. Warfarin distribution in the United States quadrupled on a per-capita basis during the 1990s [61]. During the same period, the incidence of anticoagulant-associated intracerebral hemorrhage (AAICH) quintupled in the Greater Cincinnati region [61]. Studies from other regions have shown similar trends [62,63].

In most trials of warfarin for treatment of atrial fibrillation or myocardial infarction the risk of AAICH has ranged from 0.3% to 1.0% per patient-year, with risk on the lower end of this spectrum in more recent studies [64,65]. Several trials have tested warfarin for secondary stroke prevention in patients with cerebral ischemia of non-cardiac origin. The Warfarin-Aspirin Recurrent Stroke Study (WARSS) compared aspirin to warfarin (goal INR 1.4–2.8), and found no difference between groups in effectiveness or risk of major hemorrhage (including ICH) [66]. The Stroke Prevention in Reversible Ischemia Trial (SPIRIT) compared aspirin to high intensity warfarin (goal INR 3.0–4.5) [67]. It was stopped before completion because of a 7.0% annual risk of major hemorrhage in the warfarin group, including a 3.7% annual risk of intracranial bleeding [68].

Studies of anticoagulation outside of clinical trials show that well-managed warfarin at conventional INRs can produce acceptable rates of ICH (similar to or slightly higher than in trials); however, the hemorrhage risk must be balanced against the benefit of anticoagulation for each patient [64,69–72]. The relative risk of ICH in anticoagulated patients as compared to the general population is approximately 7–10 [64,69]. Data from clinical trials and community surveillance suggest that clinical factors that increase the risk of AAICH are advanced age, prior ischemic stroke, hypertension, leukoaraiosis, and higher intensity of anticoagulation [64,65,68]. The addition of antiplatelet agents to warfarin probably increases the risk compared to warfarin alone [64,65,73]. Strict management of blood pressure and INR in anticoagulated patients reduces the risk of hemorrhage [65].

Thrombolysis for myocardial infarction carries a small but definite risk of intracranial hemorrhage. Rates of intracranial hemorrhage in this setting have generally ranged from 0.4% to 1.5% of patients treated with various regimens of thrombolytic agents and anticoagulants [74–76]. Risk factors for hemorrhage after thrombolysis for myocardial infarction include older age, female sex, black race, hypertension, prior stroke, excessive anticoagulation, and lower body weight [74,76,77]. In the large GUSTO-1 trial, the majority of such hemorrhages were intraparenchymal (81%) or intraparenchymal plus subdural (15%), with relatively few pure subdural (3%) or pure intraventricular (1%) bleeds [75]. Among intraparenchymal hemorrhages, the majority (77%) occurred in lobar regions of the brain [75]. Intraventricular (49%) and subarachnoid (11%) extension of bleeding was relatively common [75].

Thrombolytic treatment of ischemic stroke carries a greater risk of intracranial hemorrhage than thrombolysis for myocardial infarction, but discussion of this matter is beyond the scope of this chapter [78].

Antiplatelet drugs

Antiplatelet drugs probably increase the risk of ICH by a small amount [79]. The absolute risk of intracranial hemorrhage among elderly persons taking aspirin has been estimated at 0.2–0.3% annually (vs. 0.15% in similar persons not taking antiplatelets or anticoagulants) [65]. This risk increases with age and aspirin doses > 325 mg daily [79,80]. In trials comparing the antiplatelet agents clopidogrel or ticlopidine to aspirin among patients at high risk of vascular events, rates of intracranial hemorrhage were similar between groups [81]. However, the combination of aspirin plus clopidogrel led to more intracranial hemorrhages than clopidogrel alone when used for secondary stroke prevention in the MATCH trial [65,82]. A meta-analysis of trials using dipyridamole for secondary stroke prevention found the combination of aspirin and dipyridamole did not cause more bleeding than aspirin alone, although specific rates for intracranial hemorrhage were not reported [83].

Cerebral microbleeds

The use of gradient echo MRI to detect small, asymptomatic hemorrhages in the brain parenchyma ("microbleeds") has received considerable recent attention. Gradient echo MRI accentuates signal dropout from chronic blood products and is more sensitive at detecting small hemorrhages than standard T2 sequences [84,85]. The prevalence of microbleeds in the general population is best estimated from two studies of middle-aged and elderly adults without known cerebrovascular disease or dementia, in which microbleeds were found in 6.4% and 4.7% of the respective populations [86,87]. Microbleeds are associated with both ischemic (especially lacunar) and hemorrhagic cerebrovascular disease as well as hypertension, leukoaraiosis, advancing age, and male gender [86–89]. Microbleeds are common in hemorrhagic stroke, occurring in 54–71% of ICH patients (Fig. 1.2) [90]. They appear to be equally prevalent in cases of deep cerebral and lobar hemorrhage, and are therefore not specific for amyloid angiopathy or hypertensive ICH; however, in some studies the location of microbleeds has correlated with the site of symptomatic hemorrhage (i.e., deep cerebral microbleeds are associated with deep cerebral ICH while lobar microbleeds are associated with lobar ICH) [91,92]. Many clinicians consider microbleeds to be markers of small-vessel disease and a hemorrhage-prone state.

Although microbleeds have been associated with a variety of demographic variables and disease states, their practical value in predicting hemorrhage risk is less clear. A small, prospective Chinese study scanned 121 acute stroke patients with gradient echo MRI and found that 35.5% had microbleeds. Over a mean follow-up of 27.2 months, 4 patients (9.3%) with microbleeds had a subsequent ICH, compared to 1 patient (1.3%) without microbleeds (p = 0.053) [93]. Additionally, in a referral-based study of lobar ICH patients, increasing burden of microbleeds was shown to predict recurrent hemorrhage [94]. However, these studies are too small to guide patient management at present. The power of microbleeds to predict subsequent hemorrhagic and ischemic cerebrovascular disease and the value they might add to risk–benefit analyses for antiplatelet or anticoagulant use are important questions which remain unanswered.

Prior cerebral infarction

Prior cerebral infarction is associated with a 5- to 22-fold increased risk of ICH [32,95,96]. The strong relationship between ICH and cerebral infarction is not surprising since hemorrhage and infarction share similar risk factors, such as hypertension. In the GERFHS case-control study in Greater Cincinnati 15% of ICH patients had a history of previous ischemic stroke; the multivariate odds ratio for ICH in patients with prior stroke compared to controls was 7.0 [32].

Hypocholesterolemia

While hypercholesterolemia is a risk factor for cardiac disease and ischemic stroke, hypocholesterolemia appears to increase risk of ICH. Data from case-control studies have been mixed, but the preponderance of evidence supports an inverse relationship between cholesterol levels and ICH risk [26,97–102]. This relationship is also supported by several cohort studies [26]. Potential explanations for the association of low cholesterol and ICH include reduced platelet aggregation, increased fragility of the cerebral vasculature, and confounding by medical illness or nutritional deficiencies [98]. Given these findings, there is theoretical concern that widespread use of cholesterol lowering medications may increase rates of ICH. Analysis of the GERFHS study showed that hypercholesterolemia was protective for ICH, but that statin use was not associated with increased ICH risk [97].

Large randomized trials of statin drugs for primary and secondary prevention of cardiovascular disease have not shown increased ICH rates [103,104]. However, a randomized trial of high-dose atorvastatin versus placebo for patients with transient ischemic attack or stroke did find a trend toward more hemorrhagic strokes among the atorvastatin group during follow-up [105].

Heavy alcohol use

Numerous studies have identified a relationship between alcohol use and the risk of hemorrhagic stroke [26,37,106,107]. There is probably a dose–response relationship with increased risk among heavy but not light drinkers [26,107]. Heavy alcohol use has also been implicated in early hematoma expansion, possibly due to adverse effects upon platelet and liver function [108].

Tobacco use

There may be a weak association between tobacco use and ICH but data have been conflicting [26,37]. Several recent studies suggest that current smoking (as opposed to past smoking or never smoking) increases the risk of ICH in a dose-dependent manner [38,109,110].

Diabetes

Diabetes is associated with greater risk of ICH in some case-control studies. A review of available data produced an overall risk ratio of 1.3 with borderline statistical significance [26]. The association of diabetes and ICH may vary by age group and location of hemorrhage [38]. Clarification of the role of diabetes as a "minor risk factor" for ICH will require larger studies [111].

Heritability

There is a genetic component to ICH risk but its absolute value is small. Among probands in the GERFHS case-control study, 6% of patients had an affected first-degree relative and 6% an affected second-degree relative. Among cases the odds ratio for an affected first-degree relative was high (6.3) but the population attributable risk was low (0.05) [32]. The association of apolipoprotein genotypes with lobar ICH was previously discussed.

Clinical presentation and natural history of intracerebral hemorrhage

The Harvard Cooperative Stroke Registry reported on the clinical findings associated with stroke [112]. The clinical features used to define ICH were presentation with a gradual progression (over minutes or days) or sudden onset of focal neurological deficit, usually accompanied by signs of increased intracranial pressure such as vomiting or diminished consciousness. As many as 91% of patients were hypertensive (blood pressure 160/100 mmHg or higher) at the onset of their stroke.

Vomiting was far more common in ICH and SAH (51% and 47% respectively) than for ischemic stroke (4–10% of cases). While SAH presented with headache at onset in 78% of cases, 33% of cases of ICH also had a headache at onset compared to 3–12% of ischemic stroke subtypes. Finally, SAH and ICH both presented with coma in 24% of cases compared to 0–4% of ischemic stroke subtypes. A particular characteristic of ICH was the smooth or gradual progression of stroke in 63% of cases, with sudden onset in 34% of cases (Table 1.4). A smooth or gradual onset of stroke was seen in only 5–20% of ischemic stroke subtypes and 14% of SAH. Thus, ICH is the stroke subtype most likely to worsen significantly in the first 24 hours.

Hematoma growth

Intracerebral hemorrhage was traditionally viewed as a monophasic event with a brief episode of bleeding followed by increasing edema and clinical deterioration. This view is no longer accepted. A prospective, population-based study of spontaneous ICH in 1993 showed that among hemorrhages imaged within 3 hours of onset 26% increased by > 33% in volume in the next hour and 38% increased by > 33% volume within the first day (Fig. 1.3) [113]. The importance of ICH expansion has been confirmed by other studies which demonstrate that most hematoma growth occurs within six hours of onset, and that growth is associated with worse outcomes [108,114–116]. Based upon these findings, the use of ultra-early hemostatic therapy to reduce hematoma growth and potentially improve outcome following ICH has become an active area of research [117]. Clinical predictors of early hematoma growth have been difficult to consistently identify. In one retrospective study hypertension (systolic blood pressure ≥ 160) was associated with enlargement [116]. This finding has

Table 1.4. Clinical presentation of symptoms by subtype of stroke

	Thrombosis	Lacune	Embolus	ICH	SAH
Maximal at onset	40%	38%	79%	34%	80%
Stepwise	34%	32%	11%	3%	3%
Gradual	13%	20%	5%	63%	14%
Fluctuating	13%	10%	5%	0%	3%

Source: From [112].

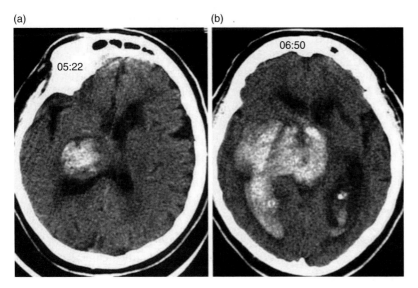

(a)　　　　　　(b)

05:22　　　　06:50

Fig. 1.3 Increase in hemorrhage size. A thalamic ICH (a) is seen in this patient with a history of hypertension. The patient's condition deteriorated over the next hour and repeat imaging (b) demonstrates enlargement of the hematoma and rupture into the ventricles.

(a)   (b)

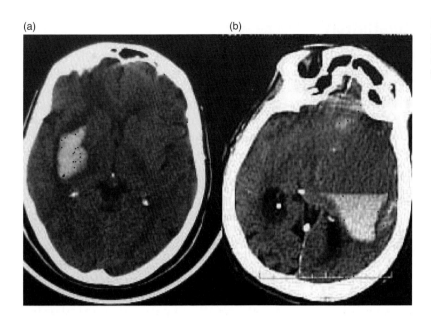

Fig. 1.4 (a) Spontaneous ICH with perihematomal edema. (b) Coagulopathy-associated ICH with minimal perihematomal edema despite greater hemorrhage size.

not been prospectively confirmed [113,118]. Another retrospective study identified earlier patient presentation, heavy alcohol consumption, reduced level of consciousness, and an irregularly shaped hematoma as predictors of enlargement [108]. The authors did not include hypertension after admission in their multivariate model because of concern that hypertension was an effect rather than a cause of hematoma growth [108]. Serum factors associated with hematoma growth have included low fibrinogen levels and elevated levels of interleukin-6 and cellular fibronectin [108,119].

Conflicting reports have compared the size of AAICH and bland ICH at presentation to medical care; some find no difference in size and some find larger hemorrhages in anticoagulated patients [120–122]. After presentation, hematoma enlargement and clinical deterioration are more common in anticoagulated patients [64,120,123]. Failure to promptly correct elevated INRs has been associated with hematoma enlargement [124].

Perihematomal edema

With the advent of CT technology, much has been learned about perihematomal edema. When whole blood is infused into the cerebral lobes of pigs, perihematomal edema develops within one hour of infusion [125]. Yet when packed red blood cells (no serum) are injected, edema does not develop for nearly 72 hours. This suggests that factors within serum are responsible for acute perihematomal

edema, while lysis of red blood cells contributes to edema at approximately 72 hours [125,126]. Studies have subsequently demonstrated that edema formation can occur when clotting factors alone (without serum or red blood cells) are injected into animal brains [127,128]. Thrombin and the fibrinogen cascade have been implicated in edema formation [127].

In humans, most hemorrhages due to thrombolysis are large and have little perihematomal edema [75]. Thrombolysis-related ICH has visible perihematoma less often than spontaneous ICH and has lower absolute and relative volumes of edema [129]. Figure 1.4 compares a case of spontaneous ICH to a case of ICH with coagulopathy.

Among patients not receiving anticoagulants, absolute edema volume generally doubles within the first day, while relative edema volume (defined as absolute edema volume divided by hematoma size) increases by a lesser amount [130]. One study found that greater relative edema volume in the hyperacute period paradoxically predicted better clinical outcomes, possibly because such edema resulted from successful hematoma clotting, but this finding has not been replicated [115,131]. Significant delayed edema may occur days to a week after initial bleeding and has been associated with neurological deterioration [132].

Morbidity and mortality

Intracerebral hemorrhage is often clinically devastating. Thirty-day case fatality rates in most studies

Table 1.5. Mortality of ICH based on volume and location of hematoma

	Overall 30-day mortality (n = 188)	≤ 30 cm³ ICH	30–60 cm³ ICH	≥ 60 cm³ ICH
Lobar (n = 66)	39%	23%	60%	71%
Deep (n = 76)	48%	7%	64%	93%
Pontine (n = 9)	44%	43%	100%	N/A
Cerebellum (n = 11)	64%	57%	75%	N/A

Note: N/A = not applicable.
Source: From [137].

range from 40% to 50%, with approximately half of deaths occurring within two days of onset [133–135]. Patients with ICH fare worse than those with ischemic stroke, and few are left without disability [133, 134]. Mortality after ICH was reportedly as high as 90% in the pre-CT area [17]. The lower mortality in more recent studies likely reflect a combination of identification bias in the pre-CT era (with mild hemorrhages misclassified as ischemic infarcts) and improved supportive care [23,135]. A study comparing mortality after ICH in 1988 and the late 1990s found no improvement in outcomes during that period [135].

Prognostic indicators

A variety of reports have examined clinical and radiographic factors associated with prognosis after ICH. Predictors of poor outcome include advanced age, poor neurological status at presentation (as measured by Glasgow Coma Scale [GCS] score), larger hematoma size, early hematoma growth, intraventricular extension of hemorrhage, anticoagulant use, and brainstem location of hemorrhage [13,121,135–138].

In a population-based study in Greater Cincinnati, the volume of ICH in combination with the GCS predicted overall 30-day mortality with 96% sensitivity and 98% specificity (Table 1.5). Patients with a volume of 60 cm³ and a GCS score ≤ 8 had a predicted mortality of 91% while those with a volume of ≤ 30 cm³ and a GCS score ≥ 9 had a predicted mortality rate of 19%. For ICH with a volume of ≥ 60 cm³, the 30-day mortality for deep hemorrhages was 93% and for lobar hemorrhages was 71% (Table 1.5) [137]. Several prediction models for outcome after ICH have been developed but have not gained widespread clinical use [136,138]. Nonetheless, in a recent study more deaths caused by ICH were associated with withdrawal of care or a "comfort care"

approach (68%) than progression to brain death (29%) or medical complications (3%) [139]. The "self-fulfilling prophecy" in neurological catastrophes like ICH has been described as the preconceived notion that medical care is futile, followed by withdrawal of care and death of the patient [140]. The complicated determinants of morbidity and mortality following ICH, together with expectations of the patient, family, and physicians require careful consideration in each case.

Risk of ICH recurrence

Because ICH is less common and more deadly than ischemic stroke, studies estimating ICH recurrence risk have been more difficult to perform. A review of studies tracking ICH recurrence found an aggregate risk of 2.4% per patient-year [141]. The studies selected excluded patients with "secondary" causes of ICH such as vascular malformations or anticoagulation. Most studies have found ICH recurrence is more common following lobar ICH than non-lobar ICH. In the cited review, risk of recurrence among patients presenting with lobar ICH was 4.4% per year, compared to 2.1% annually for those with non-lobar hemorrhage [141]. Risk of new cerebral ischemia (1.1% per year) was lower than the risk of recurrent ICH [141]. One study found that Apolipoprotein $\epsilon 2$ or $\epsilon 4$ genotypes increase the risk of recurrence following lobar ICH, presumably because of their association with amyloid angiopathy [142]. The 21% two-year recurrence risk after lobar ICH in this study was greater than other reports and likely reflects the highly selected patient cohort [142]. A recent population-based study of ICH in Izumo City, Japan, documented an annual recurrence risk of 2.3% among 279 patients [143]. Location of ICH did not predict recurrence in this population, consistent with epidemiological data showing that lobar hemorrhage (and presumably amyloid angiopathy) is less prominent in Asian populations than in the United States or Europe.

Primary intraventricular hemorrhage

Primary intraventricular hemorrhage (IVH) is rare among adults, comprising 2–3% of ICH admissions [144–147]. Study of this subject has been limited to small case series [144–147]. Signs and symptoms of IVH frequently include headache, vomiting, and altered level of consciousness. Many patients are hypertensive or coagulopathic and some have vascular malformations defined by angiography. Hydrocephalus and elevated intracranial pressure are frequent and potentially fatal complications.

References

1. National Institute of Neurological Disorders and Stroke. Classification of cerebrovascular diseases III. *Stroke* 1990; **21**: 637–676.

2. Kleindorfer D, Broderick J, Khoury J, *et al.* The unchanging incidence and case-fatality of stroke in the 1990s: a population-based study. *Stroke* 2006; **37**: 2473–2478.

3. Kissela B, Schneider A, Kleindorfer D, *et al.* Stroke in a biracial population: the excess burden of stroke among blacks. *Stroke* 2004; **35**: 426–431.

4. Rothwell PM, Coull AJ, Giles MF, *et al.* for the Oxford Vascular Study. Change in stroke incidence, mortality, case-fatality, severity, and risk factors in Oxfordshire, UK from 1981 to 2004 (Oxford Vascular Study). *Lancet* 2004; **363**: 1925–1933.

5. Thrift AG, Dewey HM, Macdonell AL, McNeil JJ, Donnan GA. Incidence of the major stroke subtypes: initial findings from the North East Melbourne Stroke Incidence Study (NEMESIS). *Stroke* 2001; **32**: 1732–1738.

6. Syme PD, Byrne AW, Chen R, Devenny R, Forbes JF. Community-based stroke incidence in a Scottish population: the Scottish Borders Stroke Study. *Stroke* 2005; **36**: 1837–1843.

7. Wolfe CDA, Giroud M, Kolominsky-Rabas P, *et al.* Variations in stroke incidence and survival in three areas of Europe. *Stroke* 2000; **31**: 2074–2079.

8. Brown RD Jr, Whisnant JP, Sicks JD, O'Fallon WM, Wiebers DO. Stroke incidence, prevalence, and survival: secular trends in Rochester, Minnesota, through 1989. *Stroke* 1996; **27**: 373–380.

9. Fogelholm R, Nuutila M, Vuorela A-L. Primary intracerebral haemorrhage in the Jyväskylä region, central Finland, 1985–89: incidence, case fatality rate, and functional outcome. *J Neurol Neurosurg Psychiatry* 1992; **55**: 546–552.

10. D'Alessandro G, Bottacchi E, Di Giovanni M, *et al.* Temporal trends of stroke in Valle d'Aosta, Italy. Incidence and 30-day fatality rates. *Neurol Sci* 2000; **21**: 13–18.

11. Flaherty ML, Woo D, Haverbusch M, *et al.* Racial variations in location and risk of intracerebral hemorrhage. *Stroke* 2005; **36**: 934–937.

12. Jiang B, Wang W, Chen H, *et al.* Incidence and trends of stroke and its subtypes in China: results from three large cities. *Stroke* 2006; **37**: 63–65.

13. Inagawa T, Ohbayashi N, Takechi A, Shibukawa M, Yahara K. Primary intracerebral hemorrhage in Izumo City, Japan: incidence rates and outcome in relation to the site of hemorrhage. *Neurosurgery* 2003; **53**: 1283–1298.

14. Tanaka H, Ueda Y, Date C, *et al.* Incidence of stroke in Shibata, Japan: 1976–1978. *Stroke* 1981; **12**: 460–466.

15. Zhang L-F, Yang J, Hong Z, *et al.* for the Collaborative Group of China Multicenter Study of Cardiovascular Epidemiology. Proportion of different subtypes of stroke in China. *Stroke* 2003; **34**: 2091–2096.

16. The Korean Neurological Association. Epidemiology of cerebrovascular disease in Korea. *J Korean Med Sci* 1993; **8**: 281–289.

17. Broderick JP, Phillips SJ, Whisnant JP, O'Fallon WM, Bergstralh EJ. Incidence rates of stroke in the eighties: the end of the decline in stroke? *Stroke* 1989; **20**: 577–582.

18. Ueda K, Omae T, Hirota Y, *et al.* Decreasing trend in incidence and mortality from stroke in Hisayama residents, Japan. *Stroke* 1981; **12**: 154–160.

19. Ueda K, Hasuo Y, Kiyohara Y, *et al.* Intracerebral hemorrhage in a Japanese community, Hisayama: incidence, changing pattern during long-term follow-up, and related factors. *Stroke* 1988; **19**: 48–52.

20. Lovelock CE, Molyneux AJ, Rothwell PM, on behalf of the Oxford Vascular Study. Change in incidence and aetiology of intracerebral haemorrhage in Oxfordshire, UK, between 1981 and 2006: a population-based study. *Lancet Neurol* 2007; **6**: 487–493.

21. Sivenius J, Tuomilehto J, Immonen-Raiha P, *et al.* Continuous 15-year decrease in incidence and mortality of stroke in Finland: the Finstroke study. *Stroke* 2004; **35**: 420–425.

22. Kubo M, Kiyohara Y, Kato I, *et al.* Trends in the incidence, mortality, and survival rate of cardiovascular disease in a Japanese community: the Hisayama study. *Stroke* 2003; **34**: 2349–2354.

23. Drury I, Whisnant JP, Garraway WM. Primary intracerebral hemorrhage: impact of CT on incidence. *Neurology* 1984; **34**: 653–657.

24. Rowe CC, Donnan GA, Bladin PF. Intracerebral haemorrhage: impact of CT on incidence. *BMJ* 1988; **297**: 1177–1178.

25. Labovitz DL, Halim A, Boden-Albala B, Hauser WA, Sacco RL. The incidence of deep and lobar intracerebral hemorrhage in whites, blacks, and Hispanics. *Neurology* 2005; **65**: 518–522.

26. Ariesen MJ, Claus SP, Rinkel G JE, Algra A. Risk factors for intracerebral hemorrhage in the general population. A systematic review. *Stroke* 2003; **34**: 2060–2066.

27. Morgenstern LB, Smith MA, Lisabeth LD, et al. Excess stroke in Mexican Americans compared with non-Hispanic whites: the Brain Attack Surveillance in Corpus Christi project. *Am J Epidemiol* 2004; **160**: 376–383.

28. Zahuranec DB, Brown DL, Lisabeth LD, et al. Differences in intracerebral hemorrhage between Mexican Americans and non-Hispanic whites. *Neurology* 2006; **66**: 30–34.

29. Broderick JP, Brott T, Tomsick T, Huster G, Miller R. The risk of subarachnoid and intracerebral hemorrhages in blacks as compared with whites. *N Engl J Med* 1992; **326**: 733–736.

30. Woo D, Haverbusch M, Sekar P, et al. The effect of untreated hypertension on hemorrhagic stroke. *Stroke* 2004; **35**: 1703–1708.

31. Thrift AG, McNeil JJ, Forbes A, Donnan GA, for the Melbourne Risk Factor Study Group. Three important subgroups of hypertensive persons at greater risk of intracerebral hemorrhage. *Hypertension* 1998; **31**: 1223–1229.

32. Woo D, Sauerbeck LR, Kissela BM, et al. Genetic and environmental risk factors for intracerebral hemorrhage: preliminary results of a population-based study. *Stroke* 2002; **33**: 1190–1196.

33. Woo D, Kaushal R, Chakraborty R, et al. Association of apolipoprotein e4 and haplotypes of the apolipoprotein e gene with lobar intracerebral hemorrhage. *Stroke* 2005; **36**: 1874–1880.

34. Curb JD, Abbott RD, MacLean CJ, et al. Age-related changes in stroke risk in men with hypertension and normal blood pressure. *Stroke* 1996; **27**: 819–824.

35. Chapman N, Huxley R, Anderson C, et al. Effects of a perindopril-based blood pressure-lowering regimen on the risk of recurrent stroke according to stroke subtype and medical history: the PROGRESS Trial. *Stroke* 2004; **35**: 116–121.

36. Perry HMJ, Davis BR, Price TR, et al. for the Systolic Hypertension in the Elderly Program (SHEP) Cooperative Research Group. Effect of treating isolated systolic hypertension on the risk of developing various types and subtypes of stroke: the Systolic Hypertension in the Elderly Program (SHEP). *JAMA* 2000; **284**: 465–471.

37. Thrift AG, Donnan GA, McNeil JJ. Epidemiology of intracerebral hemorrhage. *Epidemiol Rev.* 1995; **17**: 361–381.

38. Feldmann E, Broderick JP, Kernan WN, et al. Major risk factors for intracerebral hemorrhage in the young are modifiable. *Stroke* 2005; **36**: 1881–1885.

39. Qureshi A, Mohammad Y, Suri MF, et al. Cocaine use and hypertension are major risk factors for intracerebral hemorrhage in young African Americans. *Ethn Dis* 2001; **11**: 311–319.

40. Okazaki H, Whisnant JP. Clinical pathology of hypertensive intracerebral hemorrhage. In: Mizukami M, Kogure K, Kanaya H, Yamori Y, eds. *Hypertensive Intracerebral Hemorrhage.* New York, Raven Press. 1983; 177–180.

41. Vinters H. Cerebral amyloid angiography: a critical review. *Stroke* 1987; **18**: 311–324.

42. Vonsattel JP, Myers RH, Hedley-Whyte ET, et al. Cerebral amyloid angiopathy without and with cerebral hemorrhages: a comparative histological study. *Ann Neurol.* 1991; **30**: 637–649.

43. Mandybur T, Bates S. Fatal massive ICH complicating cerebral amyloid angiopathy. *Arch Neurol* 1978; **35**: 246–248.

44. Maruyama K, Ikeda S, Ishihara T, Allsop D, Yanagisawa N. Immunohistochemical characterization of cerebrovascular amyloid in 46 autopsied cases using antibodies to protein and cystatin c. *Stroke* 1990; **21**: 397–403.

45. Greenberg SM, Vonsattel JP, Stakes JW, Gruber M, Finklestein SP. The clinical spectrum of cerebral amyloid angiopathy: presentations without lobar hemorrhage. *Neurology* 1993; **43**: 2073–2079.

46. Vinters H, Gilbert J. Cerebral amyloid angiography: incidence and complications in the aging brain. Ii. The distribution of amyloid vascular changes. *Stroke* 1983; **14**: 924–928.

47. Tomonaga M. Cerebral amyloid angiopathy in the elderly. *J Am Geriat Soc* 1981; **29**: 151–157.

48. Greenberg SM, Vonsattel JP, Segal AZ, et al. Association of apolipoprotein e epsilon2 and vasculopathy in cerebral amyloid angiopathy. *Neurology* 1998; **50**: 961–965.

49. Greenberg SM, Rebeck GW, Vonsattel JP, Gomez-Isla T, Hyman BT. Apolipoprotein e epsilon 4

and cerebral hemorrhage associated with amyloid angiopathy. *Ann Neurol* 1995; **38**: 254–259.

50. Greenberg S, Briggs M, Hyman B, *et al.* Apolipoprotein e 4 is associated with the presence and earlier onset of hemorrhage in cerebral amyloid angiopathy. *Stroke* 1996; **27**: 1333–1337.

51. Nicoll J, Burnett C, Love S, *et al.* High frequency of apolipoprotein E epsilon 2 in patients with cerebral hemorrhage due to cerebral amyloid angiopathy. *Ann of Neurology* 1996; **39**: 682–683.

52. Zhu XL, Chan MSY, Poon WS. Spontaneous intracranial hemorrhage: which patients need diagnostic cerebral angiography? A prospective study of 206 cases and review of the literature. *Stroke* 1997; **28**: 1406–1409.

53. Brown RDJ, Flemming KD, Meyer FB, *et al.* Natural history, evaluation, and management of intracranial vascular malformations. *Mayo Clin Proc* 2005; **80**: 269–281.

54. Bevan H, Sharma K, Bradley W. Stroke in young adults. *Stroke* 1990; **21**: 382–386.

55. Toffol GJ, Biller J, Adams HPJ. Non-traumatic intracerebral hemorrhage in young adults. *Arch Neurol* 1987; **44**: 483–485.

56. Ruiz-Sandoval JL, Cantu C, Barinagarrementeria F. Intracerebral hemorrhage in young people: analysis of risk factors, location, causes, and prognosis. *Stroke* 1999; **30**: 537–541.

57. Stafford RS, Singer DE. National patterns of warfarin use in atrial fibrillation. *Arch Intern Med* 1996; **156**: 2537–2541.

58. Fang MC, Stafford RS, Ruskin JN, Singer DE. National trends in antiarrhythmic and antithrombotic medication use in atrial fibrillation. *Arch Intern Med* 2004; **164**: 55–60.

59. Osseby GV, Benatru I, Sochurkova D, *et al.* Trends in utilization of antithrombotic therapy in patients with atrial fibrillation before stroke onset in a community-based study, from 1985 through 1997. From scientific evidence to practice. *Prev Med* 2004; **38**: 121–128.

60. European Atrial Fibrillation Trial Study Group. Secondary prevention in non-rheumatic atrial fibrillation after transient ischemic attack or minor stroke. *Lancet* 1993; **342**: 1255–1262.

61. Flaherty ML, Kissela B, Woo D, *et al.* The increasing incidence of anticoagulant-associated intracerebral hemorrhage. *Neurology* 2007; **68**: 116–121.

62. Kucher N, Castellanos LR, Quiroz R, *et al.* Time trends in warfarin-associated hemorrhage. *Am J Cardiol* 2004; **94**: 403–406.

63. Lawrentschuk N, Kariappa S, Kaye AH. Spontaneous intracerebral hemorrhages-warfarin as a risk factor. *J Clin Neurosci* 2003; **10**: 550–552.

64. Hart RG, Boop BS, Anderson DC. Oral anticoagulants and intracranial hemorrhage. Facts and hypotheses. *Stroke* 1995; **26**: 1471–1477.

65. Hart RG, Tonarelli SB, Pearce LA. Avoiding central nervous system bleeding during antithrombotic therapy. *Stroke* 2005; **36**: 1588–1593.

66. Mohr JP, Thompson JLP, Lazar RM, *et al.* for the Warfarin-Aspirin Recurrent Stroke Study Group. A comparison of warfarin and aspirin for the prevention of recurrent ischemic stroke. *N Engl J Med.* 2001; **345**: 1444–1451.

67. Stroke Prevention in Reversible Ischemia Trial (SPIRIT) Study Group. A randomized trial of anticoagulants versus aspirin after cerebral ischemia of presumed arterial origin. *Ann Neurol* 1997; **42**: 857–865.

68. Gorter JW, for the Stroke Prevention in Reversible Ischemia Trial (SPIRIT) and European Atrial Fibrillation Trial (EAFT) Study Groups. Major bleeding during anticoagulation after cerebral ischemia: patterns and risk factors. *Neurology* 1999; **53**: 1319–1327.

69. Sjalander A, Engstrom G, Berntorp E, Svensson P. Risk of haemorrhagic stroke in patients with oral anticoagulation compared with the general population. *J Intern Med* 2003; **254**: 434–438.

70. Petty GW, Brown RD Jr, Whisnant JP, *et al.* Frequency of major complications of aspirin, warfarin, and intravenous heparin for secondary stroke prevention: a population-based study. *Ann Intern Med* 1999; **130**: 14–22.

71. Caro JJ, Flegel KM, Orejuela ME, *et al.* Anticoagulant prophylaxis against stroke in atrial fibrillation: effectiveness in actual practice. *CMAJ* 1999; **161**: 493–497.

72. Go AS, Hylek EM, Chang Y, *et al.* Anticoagulant therapy for stroke prevention in atrial fibrillation: how well do randomized trials translate into clinical practice? *JAMA* 2003; **290**: 2685–2692.

73. Hart RG, Senavente O, Pearce LA. Increased risk of intracranial hemorrhage when aspirin is combined with warfarin: a meta-analysis and hypothesis. *Cerebrovasc Dis* 1999; **9**: 215–217.

74. Gurwitz JH, Gore JM, Goldberg RJ, *et al.* Risk for intracranial hemorrhage after tissue plasminogen activator treatment for acute myocardial infarction. *Ann Intern Med* 1998; **129**: 597–604.

75. Gebel JM, Sila CA, Sloan MA, *et al.* for the GUSTO-1 Investigators. Thrombolysis-related intracranial

hemorrhage: a radiographic analysis of 244 cases from the GUSTO-1 trial with clinical correlation. *Stroke* 1998; **29**: 563–569.

76. Menon V, Harrington RA, Hochman JS, *et al.* Thrombolysis and adjunctive therapy in acute myocardial infarction: the Seventh ACCP Conference on Antithrombotic and Thrombolytic Therapy. *Chest* 2004; **126**(3 Suppl): 549S–575S.

77. Brass LM, Lichtman JH, Wang Y, *et al.* Intracranial hemorrhage associated with thrombolytic therapy for elderly patients with myocardial infarction. *Stroke* 2000; **31**: 1802–1811.

78. NINDS rt-PA Stroke Study Group. Tissue plasminogen activator for acute ischemic stroke. *N Engl J Med* 1995; **333**: 1581–1587.

79. Gorelick PB, Weisman SM. Risk of hemorrhagic stroke with aspirin use: an update. *Stroke* 2005; **36**: 1801–1807.

80. Thrift AG, McNeil JJ, Forbes A, Donnan GA. Risk of primary intracerebral hemorrhage associated with aspirin and non-steroidal anti-inflammatory drugs: case-control study. *BMJ* 1999; **318**: 759–764.

81. Hankey GJ, Sudlow C LM, Dunbabin DW. Thienopyridines or aspirin to prevent stroke and other serious vascular events in patients at high risk of vascular disease? A systematic review of the evidence from randomized trials. *Stroke* 2000; **31**: 1779–1784.

82. Diener H-C, Bogousslavsky J, Brass LM, *et al.* on behalf of the MATCH investigators. Aspirin and clopidogrel compared with clopidogrel alone after recent ischaemic stroke or transient ischaemic attack in high-risk patients (MATCH): randomised, double-blind, placebo-controlled trial. *Lancet* 2004; **364**: 331–337.

83. Leonardi-Bee J, Bath PMW, Bousser M-G, *et al.* on behalf of the Dipyridamole in Stroke Collaboration. Dipyridamole for preventing recurrent ischemic stroke and other vascular events: a meta-analysis of individual patient data from randomized controlled trials. *Stroke* 2005; **36**: 162–168.

84. Roob G, Fazekas F. Magnetic resonance imaging of cerebral microbleeds. *Curr Opin Neurol* 2000; **13**: 69–73.

85. Tanaka A, Yasushi U, Nakayama Y, Takano K, Takebayashi S. Small chronic hemorrhages and ischemic lesions in association with spontaneous intracerebral hematomas. *Stroke* 1999; **30**: 1637–1642.

86. Roob G, Schmidt R, Kapeller P, *et al.* MRI evidence of past cerebral microbleeds in a healthy elderly population. *Neurology* 1999; **52**: 991–994.

87. Jeerakathil T, Wolf PA, Beiser A, *et al.* Cerebral microbleeds: prevalence and associations with cardiovascular risk factors in the Framingham Study. *Stroke* 2004; **35**: 1831–1835.

88. Naka H, Nomura E, Wakabayashi S, *et al.* Frequency of asymptomatic microbleeds on T2*-weighted MR images of patients with recurrent stroke: association with combination of stroke subtypes and leukoaraiosis. *AJNR Am J Neuroradiol* 2004; **25**: 714–719.

89. Greenberg SM, Finklestein SP, Schaefer PW. Petechial hemorrhages accompanying lobar hemorrhage: detection by gradient echo MRI. *Neurology* 1996; **46**: 1751–1754.

90. Jeong SW, Jung KH, Chu K, Bae HJ, Lee SH, Roh JK. Clinical and radiologic differences between primary intracerebral hemorrhage with and without microbleeds on gradient echo magnetic resonance images. *Arch Neurol* 2004; **61**: 905–909.

91. Lee SH, Bae HJ, Kwon SJ, *et al.* Cerebral microbleeds are regionally associated with intracerebral hemorrhage. *Neurology* 2004; **62**: 72–76.

92. Roob G, Lechner A, Schmidt R, *et al.* Frequency and location of microbleeds in patients with primary intracerebral hemorrhage. *Stroke* 2000; **31**: 2665–2669.

93. Fan YH, Zhang L, Lam WWM, Mok V CT, Wong KS. Cerebral microbleeds as a risk factor for subsequent intracerebral hemorrhages among patients with acute ischemic stroke. *Stroke* 2003; **34**: 2459–2462.

94. Greenberg SM, Eng JA, Ning M, Smith EE, Rosand J. Hemorrhage burden predicts recurrent intracerebral hemorrhage after lobar hemorrhage. *Stroke* 2004; **35**: 1415–1420.

95. Okada H, Horibe H, Yoshiyuki O, Hayakawa N, Aoki N. A prospective study of cerebrovascular disease in Japanese rural communities, Akabane and Asahi. Part 1: Evaluation of risk factors in the occurrence of cerebral hemorrhage and thrombosis. *Stroke* 1976; **7**: 599–607.

96. Brott T, Thalinger K, Hertzberg V. Hypertension as a risk factor for spontaneous intracerebral hemorrhage. *Stroke* 1986; **17**: 1078–1083.

97. Woo D, Kissela B, Khoury JC, *et al.* Hypercholesterolemia, HMG-CoA reductase inhibitors, and risk of intracerebral hemorrhage. A case-control study. *Stroke* 2004; **35**: 1360–1364.

98. Tirschwell DL, Smith NL, Heckbert SR, *et al.* Association of cholesterol with stroke risk varies in stroke subtypes and patient subgroups. *Neurology* 2004; **63**: 1868–1875.

99. Segal AZ, Chiu RI, Eggleston-Sexton PM, Beiser A, Greenberg SM. Low cholesterol as a risk factor for primary intracerebral hemorrhage: a case-control study. *Neuroepidemiology* 1999; **18**: 185–193.

13

100. Giroud M, Creisson E, Fayolle H, *et al.* Risk factors for primary cerebral hemorrhage: a population-based study–the stroke registry of Dijon. *Neuroepidemiology* 1995; **14**: 20–26.

101. Thrift AG, McNeil JJ, Forbes A, Donnan GA, for the Melbourne Risk Factor Study (MERFS) Group. Risk factors for cerebral hemorrhage in the era of well-controlled hypertension. *Stroke* 1996; **27**: 2020–2025.

102. Zodpey SP, Tiwari RR, Kulkarni HR. Risk factors for haemorrhagic stroke: a case-control study. *Public Health* 2000; **114**: 177–182.

103. Byington RP, Davis BR, Plehn JF, *et al.* for the Prospective Pravastatin Pooling (PPP) Project Investigators. Reduction of stroke events with pravastatin. *Circulation* 2001; **103**: 387–392.

104. Heart Protection Collaborative Group. Effects of cholesterol-lowering with simvastatin on stroke and other major vascular events in 20,536 people with cerebrovascular disease or other high-risk conditions. *Lancet* 2004; **363**: 757–767.

105. Stroke Prevention by Aggressive Reduction in Cholesterol Levels (SPARCL) Investigators. High dose atorvastatin after stroke or transient ischemic attack. *N Engl J Med* 2004; **355**: 549–559.

106. Reynolds K, Lewis LB, Nolen JDL, *et al.* Alcohol consumption and risk of stroke. A meta-analysis. *JAMA* 2003; **289**: 579–588.

107. Thrift AG, Donnan GA, McNeil JJ. Heavy drinking, but not moderate or intermediate drinking, increases the risk of intracerebral hemorrhage. *Epidemiology* 1999; **10**: 307–312.

108. Fujii Y, Takeuchi S, Sasaki O, Minakawa T, Tanaka R. Multivariate analysis of predictors of hematoma enlargement in spontaneous intracerebral hemorrhage. *Stroke* 1998; **29**: 1160–1166.

109. Kurth T, Kase CS, Berger K, *et al.* Smoking and the risk of hemorrhagic stroke in men. *Stroke* 2003; **34**: 1151–1155.

110. Kurth T, Kase CS, Berger K, *et al.* Smoking and risk of hemorrhagic stroke in women. *Stroke* 2003; **34**: 2792–2795.

111. Thrift AG. Minor risk factors for intracerebral hemorrhage: the jury is still out. *Stroke* 2003; **34**: 2065–2066.

112. Mohr JP, Caplan LR, Melski JW, *et al.* The Harvard Cooperative Stroke Registry: a prospective registry. *Neurology* 1978; **28**: 754–762

113. Brott T, Broderick J, Kothari R, *et al.* Early hemorrhage growth in patients with intracerebral hemorrhage. *Stroke* 1997; **28**: 1–5.

114. Kazui S, Naritomi H, Yamamoto H, Sawada T, Yamaguchi T. Enlargement of spontaneous intracerebral hemorrhage. Incidence and time course. *Stroke* 1996; **27**: 1783–1787.

115. Leira R, Davalos A, Silva Y, *et al.* for the Stroke Project Cerebrovascular Diseases Group of the Spanish Neurological Society. Early neurologic deterioration in intracerebral hemorrhage: predictors and associated factors. *Neurology* 2004; **63**: 461–467.

116. Ohwaki K, Yano E, Nagashima H, *et al.* Blood pressure management in acute intracerebral hemorrhage: relationship between elevated blood pressure and hematoma enlargement. *Stroke* 2004; **35**: 1364–1367.

117. Mayer SA. Ultra-early hemostatic therapy for intracerebral hemorrhage. *Stroke* 2003; **34**: 224–229.

118. Jauch EC, Lindsell CJ, Adeoye O, *et al.* Lack of evidence for an association between hemodynamic variables and hematoma growth in spontaneous intracerebral hemorrhage. *Stroke* 2006; **37**: 2061–2065.

119. Silva Y, Leira R, Tejada J, *et al.* Molecular signatures of vascular injury are associated with early growth of intracerebral hemorrhage. *Stroke* 2005; **36**: 86–91.

120. Flibotte JJ, Hagan N, O'Donnell J, Greenberg SM, Rosand J. Warfarin, hematoma expansion, and outcome of intracerebral hemorrhage. *Neurology* 2004; **63**: 1059–1064.

121. Rosand J, Eckman MH, Knudsen KA, Singer DE, Greenberg SM. The effect of warfarin and intensity of anticoagulation on outcome of intracerebral hemorrhage. *Arch Intern Med* 2004; **164**: 880–884.

122. Radberg JA, Olsson JE, Radberg CT. Prognostic parameters in spontaneous intracerebral hematomas with special reference to anticoagulant treatment. *Stroke* 1991; **22**: 571–576.

123. Sjoblom L, Hardemark H-G, Lindgren A, *et al.* Management and prognostic features of intracerebral hemorrhage during anticoagulant therapy: a Swedish multicenter study. *Stroke* 2001; **32**: 2567–2574.

124. Yasaka M, Minematsu K, Naritomi H, Sakata T, Yamaguchi T. Predisposing factors for enlargement of intracerebral hemorrhage in patients treated with warfarin. *Thromb Haemost* 2003; **89**: 278–283.

125. Wagner KR, Xi G, Hua Y, *et al.* Lobar intracerebral hemorrhage model in pigs: rapid edema development in perihematomal white matter. *Stroke* 1996; **27**: 490–497.

126. Xi G, Keep RF, Hoff JT. Erythrocytes and delayed brain edema formation following intracerebral hemorrhage in rats. *J Neurosurg.* 1998; **89**: 991–996.

127. Lee KR, Betz AL, Kim S, Keep RF, Hoff JT. The role of the coagulation cascade in brain edema formation after intracerebral hemorrhage. *Acta Neurochir (Wien)* 1996; **138**: 396–400.

128. Lee KR, Betz AL, Keep RF, *et al.* Intracerebral infusion of thrombin as a cause of brain edema. *J Neurosurg.* 1995; **83**: 1045–1050.

129. Gebel JM, Brott TG, Sila CA, *et al.* Decreased perihematomal edema in thrombolysis-related intracerebral hemorrhage compared with spontaneous intracerebral hemorrhage. *Stroke* 2000; **31**: 596–600.

130. Gebel JM, Jauch EC, Brott TG, *et al.* Natural history of perihematomal edema in patients with hyperacute spontaneous intracerebral hemorrhage. *Stroke* 2002; **33**: 2631–2635.

131. Gebel JM, Jauch EC, Brott TG, *et al.* Relative edema volume is a predictor of outcome in patients with hyperacute spontaneous intracerebral hemorrhage. *Stroke* 2002; **33**: 2636–2641.

132. Zazulia AR, Diringer MN, Derdeyn CP, Powers WJ. Progression of mass effect after intracerebral hemorrhage. *Stroke* 1999; **30**: 1167–1173.

133. Broderick J, Brott T, Tomsick T, *et al.* Management of intracerebral hemorrhage in a large metropolitan population. *Neurosurgery* 1994; **34**: 882–887.

134. Dennis MS. Outcome after brain hemorrhage. *Cerebrovasc Dis* 2003; **16**(Suppl 1): 9–13.

135. Flaherty ML, Haverbusch M, Sekar P, *et al.* Long-term mortality after intracerebral hemorrhage. *Neurology* 2006; **66**: 1182–1186.

136. Hemphill JC 3rd, Bonovich DC, Besmertis L, Manley GT, Johnston SC. The ICH score: a simple, reliable grading scale for intracerebral hemorrhage. *Stroke* 2001; **32**: 891–897.

137. Broderick J, Brott T, Duldner J, Tomsick T, Huster G. Volume of intracerebral hemorrhage. A powerful and easy-to-use predictor of 30-day mortality. *Stroke* 1993; **24**: 987–993.

138. Cheung RT, Zou LY. Use of the original, modified, or new intracerebral hemorrhage score to predict mortality and morbidity after intracerebral hemorrhage. *Stroke* 2003; **34**: 1717–1722.

139. Zurasky JA, Aiyagari V, Zazulia AR, Shackelford A, Diringer MN. Early mortality following spontaneous intracerebral hemorrhage. *Neurology* 2005; **64**: 725–727.

140. Becker KJ, Baxter AB, Cohen WA, *et al.* Withdrawal of support in intracerebral hemorrhage may lead to self-fulfilling prophecies. *Neurology* 2001; **56**: 766–772.

141. Bailey RD, Hart RG, Benavente O, Pearce LA. Recurrent brain hemorrhage is more frequent than ischemic stroke after intracranial hemorrhage. *Neurology* 2001; **56**: 773–777.

142. O'Donnell HC, Rosand J, Knudsen KA, *et al.* Apolipoprotein e genotype and the risk of recurrent lobar intracerebral hemorrhage. *N Engl J Med* 2000; **342**: 240–245.

143. Inagawa T. Recurrent primary intracerebral hemorrhage in Izumo City, Japan. *Surg Neurol* 2005; **64**: 28–36.

144. Hameed B, Khealani BA, Mozzafar T, Wasay M. Prognostic indicators in patients with primary intraventricular hemorrhage. *J Pak Med Assoc* 2005; **55**: 315–317.

145. Marti-Fabregas J, Piles S, Guardia E, Marti-Vilalta JL. Spontaneous primary intraventricular hemorrhage: clinical data, etiology and outcome. *J Neurol* 1999; **246**: 287–291.

146. Darby DG, Donnan GA, Saling MA, Walsh KW, Bladin PF. Primary intraventricular hemorrhage: clinical and neuropsychological findings in a prospective stroke series. *Neurology* 1988; **38**: 68–75.

147. Passero S, Ulivelli M, Reale F. Primary intraventricular haemorrhage in adults. *Acta Neurol Scand* 2002; **105**: 115–119.

148. Nilsson OG, Lindgren A, Stahl N, Brandt L, Saveland H. Incidence of intracerebral and subarachnoid haemorrhage in southern Sweden. *J Neurol Neurosurg Psychiatry* 2000; **69**: 601–607.

149. Giroud M, Gras P, Chadab N, *et al.* Cerebral haemorrhage in a French prospective population study. *J Neurol Neurosurg Psychiatry* 1991; **54**: 595–598.

150. Anderson CS, Chakera TMH, Stewart-Wynne EG, Jamrozik KD. Spectrum of primary intracerebral haemorrhage in Perth, Western Australia, 1989–90: incidence and outcome. *J Neurol Neurosurg Psychiatry* 1994; **57**: 936–940.

151. Sarwar M, McCormick WF. Intracerebral venous angioma. Case report and review. *Arch Neurol* 1978; **35**: 323–325.

152. Hang Z, Shi Y, Wei Y. A pathological analysis of 180 cases of vascular malformation of brain. *Chung-Hua Ping Li Hsueh Tsa Chih [Chinese Journal of Pathology]* 1996; **25**: 135–138.

2 Acute hypertensive response in intracerebral hemorrhage

Ameer E. Hassan, Haralabos Zacharatos, and Adnan I. Qureshi

Acute hypertensive response is the elevation of blood pressure above normal and premorbid values that initially occurs within the first 24 hours of symptom onset in patients with intracerebral hemorrhage (ICH). We reviewed the existing data pertinent to acute hypertensive response derived from scientific guidelines, randomized trials, non-randomized controlled studies, and selected observational studies.

Chronic hypertension and intracerebral hemorrhage

Incidence of intracerebral hemorrhage and hypertension

Spontaneous, non-traumatic ICH from intraparenchymal blood vessels makes up approximately 8–15% of all strokes. Approximately 80–85% are primary spontaneous ICH which are either secondary to arterial hypertension or cerebral amyloid angiopathy [1]. It is estimated that 70% of the primary spontaneous ICH cases are attributed to arterial hypertension while roughly 5–20% are secondary to cerebral amyloid angiopathy. A total of 15–20% of stroke cases are attributed to secondary spontaneous ICH, related to oral anticoagulation (~ 4–20%), tumors (~ 5%), vascular malformations (~ 1–2%) and more uncommon reasons, such as sinus venous thrombosis, cerebral vasculitis, drugs, eclampsia, and others (~1 %) [2–6].

Risk factors for intracerebral hemorrhage

Hypertension is the most frequent and most important risk factor for ICH [1]. A rigorous identification of modifiable (hypertension, smoking, low cholesterol levels, diabetes, increased alcohol consumption, and drugs) and un-modifiable (increased age, male gender, and cerebral amyloid angiopathy) risk factors that contribute to ICH and its recurrence must be carried out due to the high morbidity and mortality associated with it. Other risk factors include gender (3.7- to 4.6-fold increase in men), age (almost twofold increase every ten years), smoking (2.1- to 2.7-fold increase), low cholesterol levels (< 150 mg/dl; increased twofold), diabetes (1.3-fold), increased alcohol consumption (moderate, 36–56 g/day: twofold increase; excessive, > 56 g/day: fourfold increase), drugs (i.e., cocaine and amphetamines) and coagulopathies [7–12].

The risk of ICH in one study showed that it doubled every decade, in-line with the results of other studies [7,13–15]. Age, > 65 years old, and non-white ethnicity have both been consistently positively associated with ICH [16,17]. In young patients in whom other causes such as arteriovenous malformation or trauma have been excluded illicit drug use, which leads to elevated systolic blood pressure, such as amphetamines, cocaine, and phenylpropanolamine should be excluded [18,19].

There are large racial variations with increased rates of intracerebral hemorrhage in Hispanic, Asian and African-American populations in comparison with the white population [2,4,20–24]. The relative rate of 1.89 for African Americans versus whites was also similar to estimates reported in the literature [4,13,14,25–27]. Qureshi *et al.* examined the relation between ethnicity and ICH in NHANES I (First National Health and Nutrition Examination Survey Epidemiological Follow-up Study) and reported that much of the association with ethnicity was mediated through hypertension and education [26].

Hypertension continues to be implicated as the most important risk factor for ICH as more studies are conducted. In a recent Korean study the risk of ICH was 4.9× for stage one hypertension (blood pressure 140–159/90–99 mmHg), 11.6× for stage two hypertension (blood pressure 160–179/100–109 mmHg), and 28.8× for stage three hypertension (blood pressure > 180/> 109 mmHg), as compared with normotensive (blood pressure < 140/< 90 mmHg) subjects [28]. In one study, the odds ratio for ICH was 3.5 with untreated hypertension but only 1.4 for treated hypertension, which suggests that treatment of hypertension can prevent ICH [29]. More direct evidence comes from a study of 4736 patients > 60 years of age with isolated systolic hypertension, wherein treatment resulted in an adjusted relative risk of 0.46 for ICH, and the benefit was observed within one year [30]. Systolic blood pressure > 160 mmHg, also contributes to increased incidence of ICH in patients who are on oral anticoagulation [31].

Pathology of hypertension and intracerebral hemorrhage

Hypertension contributes to decreasing the elasticity of arteries, thereby increasing the likelihood of rupture in response to acute elevations in intravascular pressure [32]. Hypertensive patients suspected of primary intraparenchymal hematoma died and were subsequently autopsied in order to assess the alterations of extraparenchymal and intraparenchymal vascular structures. The spectrum of the lesions due to arterial hypertension, at the level of the intraparenchymal blood vessels, included all steps of vascular wall degeneration, from hypertrophy of smooth muscle layer to complete hyalinization of arterial wall, but with a focal irregular distribution, not related with the proximity of hemorrhagic focus [32]. The capillary walls showed focal or circumferential thickening due to the densification of the type IV collagen material from the basement membrane structure which is attributed to high arterial blood pressure. The CD34 immunostaining showed that endothelial cells kept their structural integrity [32].

Over the course of many years, persistent hypertension leads to cerebral vascular wall damage that can be seen with the hyalinization of excessive fibrillar material from arteriolar wall or from basement membranes, otherwise termed sclerosis (arteriolar and even capillary) with hyalinosis. Hypertensive vasculopathy inhibits the contractile capability of arterioles. The vascular wall resistance to the stress determined by the elevated values of blood pressure in hypertension is weakened by the hyaline material. The presence of hyaline material in the cerebral vascular wall has been correlated with a minimal resistance of the surrounding cerebral parenchyma. It also has been suggested as an explanation as to why the cerebral parenchyma is the only tissue in which blood pressure variations can lead to vascular rupture and cerebral hemorrhage [32,33].

Association of brain microbleeds, hypertension, and intracerebral hemorrhage

Magnetic resonance imaging gradient echo T2 sequences display brain microbleeds as small, homogeneous, round foci of low signal intensity. A systematic review of published literature regarding brain microbleeds revealed the prevalence of brain microbleeds was 5% (95% confidence interval 4–6) in healthy adults, 34% (95% confidence interval 31–36) in people with ischemic stroke, and 60% (95% confidence interval 57–64) in people with non-traumatic ICH [34]. By pooling data that could be extracted from similar studies, it appears that brain microbleeds are associated with hypertension (odds ratio 3.9, 95% confidence interval 2.4–6.4) and diabetes mellitus (odds ratio 2.2, 95% confidence interval 1.2–4.2) in otherwise healthy adults, and they are associated with hypertension (odds ratio 2.3, 95% confidence interval 1.7–3.0) in adults with cerebrovascular diseases [34]. They are also associated with hypertension, left ventricular hypertrophy, advanced small-vessel disease and amyloid angiopathy [35]. Cerebral microbleeds have a topographic distribution similar to that of ICH, suggesting that they are regionally associated [17,36]. Hemorrhages that involve the putamen, globus pallidus, thalamus, internal capsule, periventricular white matter, pons, and cerebellum are often attributed to hypertensive small-vessel disease, particularly in a patient with known hypertension [37]. Further strengthening the association between brain microbleeds and hypertension is a study of hemodialysis patients that did not show an association between hemodialysis and brain microbleeds, instead the authors concluded that the presence of other factors, such as hypertension, strongly contributed [38]. Microbleeds most commonly appear in patients with a history of chronic hypertension [39–42]. Many patients with chronic renal failure have a long history of chronic hypertension.

Acute hypertensive response
Acute systolic blood pressure and mean arterial pressure elevation

Initially, after an acute ICH the blood pressure reaches a maximum and over the course of the next 24 hours declines spontaneously [43,44]. Elevated early-mortality rates have been clearly demonstrated in ICH patients who present with high arterial pressures [45–55]. Stroke patients are frequently chronically hypertensive, and their brain hydraulic autoregulatory curve is shifted to the right [56]. A mean arterial pressure of approximately 50–150 mmHg helps maintain a constant cerebral blood flow in non-stroke patients [57]. Higher mean arterial pressure levels are better tolerated by hypertensive stroke patients. Stroke patients with a history of hypertension are at risk of critical hypoperfusion for mean arterial pressure levels usually well tolerated by normotensive individuals [58]. Mean arterial hypertension should gradually be reduced below 120 mmHg in persons with a history of chronic hypertension, but a reduction of > 20% should be avoided and mean arterial pressure should not be reduced to < 84 mmHg [59,60].

American Heart Association/American Stroke Association guidelines for management of acute hypertensive response

With regards to treating hypertension in patients with ICH hemorrhage the American Heart Association/American Stroke Association distinguishes between those patients with and those without elevated intracranial pressure in their blood pressure management guidelines. The current American Heart Association/American Stroke Association guidelines (see Table 2.1) recommends considering aggressive reduction when systolic blood pressure exceeds 200 mmHg or mean arterial pressure exceeds 150 mmHg. In this case, measurements should be repeated every 5 minutes. In patients in whom systolic blood pressure exceeds 180 mmHg or mean arterial pressure exceeds 130 mmHg, and without evidence or suspicion of elevated intracranial pressure, a modest reduction of blood pressure should be considered, targeting blood pressure at 160/90 mmHg or a mean arterial pressure of 110 mmHg. In this case, measurements should be repeated every 15 minutes. The blood pressure target of 160/90 mmHg is supported by a prospective observational study that showed a trend toward improved outcome in ICH patients in whom

Table 2.1. Recommended American Heart Association/American Stroke Association guidelines for treating elevated blood pressure in spontaneous intracerebral hemorrhage

	SBP	MAP	Suspicion and/or evidence of elevated ICP	CPP	Blood pressure checks/clinical re-examination	Comment
1	> 200 mmHg or if	> 150 mmHg			Every 5 min	Consider aggressive BP reduction with continuous IV infusion
2	> 180 mmHg or if	> 130 mmHg	Yes	> 60–80 mmHg		Consider monitoring ICP and reducing BP using intermittent or continuous IV medications to keep CPP > 60–80 mmHg
3	> 180 mmHg or if	> 130 mmHg	No		Every 15 min	Consider a modest reduction of BP (e.g., MAP of 110 mmHg or target BP of 160/90 mmHg) using intermittent or continuous IV medications to control BP

Notes: BP = blood pressure, CPP = cerebral perfusion pressure, ICP = intracranial pressure, IV = intravenous, SBP = systolic blood pressure, MAP = mean arterial pressure.
Source: Adapted from [62].

Table 2.2. European Stroke Initiative recommendations for treating elevated blood pressure in spontaneous intracerebral hemorrhage [39]

BP lowering is not routinely recommended. Treatment of elevated BP in patients with acute ICH is recommended if BP is elevated above the following levels and confirmed by repeated measurements.

a. 170/100 mmHg (or a MAP of 125 mmHg) is the recommended target BP in patients with a known history of hypertension or have clinical/ECG changes indicative of chronic hypertension who have a SBP > 180 mmHg and/or DBP > 105 mmHg, if treated.

b. 150/90 mmHg (or a MAP of 110 mmHg) is the recommended target BP in patients without a known history of hypertension who have a SBP > 160 mmHg and/or DBP > 95 mmHg, if treated.

c. Avoid reducing the MAP by more than 20%.

d. For patients who are being monitored for elevated ICP the BP limits and targets should be adapted to higher values to guarantee a CPP > 70 mmHg.

Intravenous labetalol or urapidil, intravenous sodium nitroprusside or nitroglycerin and captopril (per os) are the recommended drugs for BP treatment. Oral nifedipine and any drastic blood pressure decreases should be avoided.

Notes: BP = blood pressure, CPP = cerebral perfusion pressure, DBP = diastolic blood pressure, ECG = electrocardiogram, ICH = intracerebral hemorrhage, ICP = intracranial pressure, MAP = mean arterial pressure, SBP = systolic blood pressure.
Source: Adapted from [56].

systolic blood pressure was lowered within six hours of hemorrhage onset; a reduction of systolic blood pressure to a target of less than 160/90 mmHg was associated with neurological deterioration in 7% of patients and with hemorrhagic expansion in 9% [61]. The previous recommendation was to maintain a systolic blood pressure less than or equal to 180 mmHg and/or a mean arterial pressure of less than 130 mmHg.

In patients in whom systolic blood pressure exceeds 180 mmHg or mean arterial pressure exceeds 130 mmHg, and there is evidence or suspicion of elevated intracranial pressure, monitoring of intracranial pressure and cerebral perfusion pressure (cerebral perfusion pressure = mean arterial pressure – intracranial pressure) is recommended and blood pressure lowering should be adapted to maintain cerebral perfusion pressure greater than 60–80 mmHg. In any case, mean arterial pressure should not be lowered by more than 20% of the baseline value. In critically ill patients, blood pressure should preferably be measured continuously, or every 15 minutes if this is not possible [62]. A cerebral perfusion pressure greater than 60 mmHg is supported by studies done with traumatic brain hemorrhage and spontaneous ICH [63–66].

European Stroke Initiative guidelines for management of acute hypertensive response

The European Stroke Initiative recommendation of blood pressure management is based on a history of

hypertension (see Table 2.2). An upper limit of systolic blood pressure of 180 mmHg and a diastolic blood pressure of 105 mmHg is recommended for patients with known prior hypertension or signs of chronic hypertension (left ventricular hypertrophy on electrocardiogram and changes in the retina). If treatment is necessary, the target blood pressure should be 170/100 mmHg (or a mean arterial pressure of 125 mmHg). In patients without known hypertension, the upper recommended limits are 160 mmHg for systolic blood pressure and 95 mmHg for diastolic blood pressure. If treatment is necessary, the target blood pressure should be 150/90 mmHg (or a mean arterial pressure of 110 mmHg) [1,56]. In any case, mean arterial pressure should not be lowered by more than 20% of the baseline value. In critically ill patients, blood pressure should preferably be measured continuously, or every 15 minutes if this is not possible. European Stroke Initiative guidelines also recommend adapting arterial blood pressure thresholds in patients with increased intracranial pressure to maintain a cerebral perfusion pressure of 70 mmHg or greater [1,39].

Pathophysiological consequences of treating acute hypertensive response
Hematoma growth and acute hypertensive response

Blood pressure monitoring and treatment is a critical issue in the treatment of acute ICH because studies

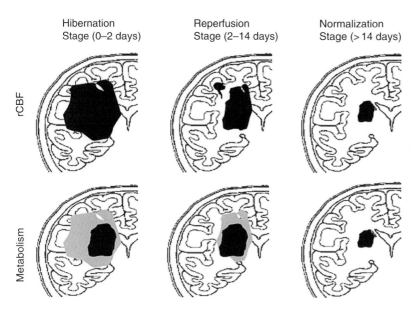

Hibernation Stage (0–2 days) Reperfusion Stage (2–14 days) Normalization Stage (> 14 days)

rCBF

Metabolism

Fig. 2.1 Stages of cerebral blood flow changes associated with ICH. Upper row: light checker pattern demonstrates reduced rCBF (hypoperfusion); dark checker pattern demonstrates increased rCBF (hyperperfusion); lower row: light gray represents regions of hypometabolism. rCBF, regional cerebral blood flow [60].

have shown that reducing the blood pressure in acute ICH may prevent or slow the growth of the hematoma as well as decrease the risk of rebleeding. This is especially true for hemorrhage resulting from a ruptured aneurysm or arteriovenous malformation, in which the risk of continued bleeding or rebleeding is presumed to be highest. Multivariate analyses indicate a strong correlation between elevated systolic blood pressure and subsequent hematoma expansion [67,68]. Retrospective analyses indicate that acute blood pressure reduction has been associated with a decrease in hematoma expansion [69,70]. Several retrospective studies show that elevated systolic blood pressure greater than 160 mmHg on admission has been associated with growth of the hematoma, but this has not been demonstrated in prospective studies of ICH growth [68,71–73].

Hemorrhagic enlargement occurs more frequently in patients with elevated systolic blood pressure, but it is not known whether this is an effect of increased growth of ICH with associated increases in intracerebral pressure or whether increased blood pressure is a contributing cause to the growth of ICH [70]. The risk of hemorrhagic expansion with mild blood pressure elevation may be lower and must be balanced with the theoretical risks of inducing cerebral ischemia in the edematous region that surrounds the hemorrhage in primary ICH, in which a specific large-vessel vasculopathy is not apparent. Baseline blood pressure

was not associated with growth of the ICH in the Recombinant Activated Factor VII ICH trial and in the largest prospective study of intracerebral growth [72–74]. Isolated systolic blood pressure, less than or equal to 210 mmHg, was not clearly related to hemorrhagic expansion or neurological worsening [67].

Hypoperfusion in perihematomal area

There still remains an ongoing debate of whether to aggressively lower blood pressure in the setting of the acute phase of the ICH. An uncertainty exists of whether there is a perihematomal area of critical hypoperfusion that may experience further perilesional ischemia as a result of the lowering of the blood pressure (Fig. 2.1) [75,76]. Decreased cerebral perfusion pressure secondary to the reduced blood pressure could compromise adequate cerebral blood flow due to increased intracranial pressure [61]. While some neuroimaging studies using single-photon emission computerized tomography, functional MRI or perfusion computerized tomography suggest that there may be an area of critical hypoperfusion surrounding the hematoma [77–79], most other studies using positron emission tomography, MRI perfusion imaging or perfusion computerized tomography found reduced cerebral blood flow, but far above ischemic levels, consistent with oligemia [76,80–84].

Contradictive results regarding perilesional hypo-perfusion, hematoma growth, and clinical outcome are observed in clinical studies of blood pressure lowering in ICH [50,61,70–74,85,86].

Decrease in perihematomal edema by reducing blood pressure

The reduction in the volume of the perihematomal edema, which has a direct correlation to hematoma volume, may be associated with the decrease in blood pressure [87,88]. Studies in acute ICH patients using MRI studies provide evidence that edema in acute ICH is plasma derived and oligemia is not an etiological factor [81,82]. A combination of clot retraction, reflecting successful hemostasis and the oncotic force supplied by thrombin and other proteins may lead to fluid formation within the perihematomal region. Edema formation may decrease with the reduction of the blood pressure and subsequently the capillary hydrostatic pressures as a result of altered Starling forces around the hematoma [89].

Pharmacological treatment of acute hypertensive response

Drugs recommended for use in lowering blood pressure in acute stroke include labetalol, hydralazine, nicardipine, and nitroprusside [90,91]. As of yet there is no single agent that is recommended to help reduce blood pressure. Due to the high rates of dysphagia and impaired consciousness, in acute ICH, intravenous therapy is the route of choice for treatment [89]. The advantage of intravenous drugs is that they also have a faster onset of action and the dose can be titrated to achieve a desired blood pressure target (Table 2.3).

Nicardipine

Nicardipine, a dihydropyridine-derivative antagonist of the L-type calcium channel, has an onset of action within minutes. Nicardipine demonstrates greater selectivity for binding of calcium channels in vascular smooth muscle cells than in the cardiac myocytes [92]. This relative tissue selectivity is important in the drug's utility for the treatment of hypertension. In animal studies of cerebral ischemia and myocardial infarction, nicardipine demonstrated a possible membrane-stabilizing action, linked to its lipophilic

Table 2.3. Possible intravenous medications for control of hypertension in patients with intracerebral hemorrhage

Drug	Intravenous bolus dose	Continuous infusion rate
Hydralazine	5–20 mg IVP every 30 min	1.5–5 µg/(kg min)
Enalapril	1.25–5 mg IVP every 6 h*	NA
Esmolol	250 µg/kg IVP loading dose	25–300 µg/(kg min)
Nicardipine	NA	5–15 mg/h
Nipride	NA	0.1–10 µg/(kg min)
Nitroglycerin	NA	20–400 µg/min
Labetalol	5–20 mg every 15 min	2 mg/min (maximum 300 mg/d)
Urapidil	12.5–25 mg bolus	5–40 mg/h

Notes: d = day, h = hour, IVP = intravenous push, NA = not applicable, min = minutes.
*The enalapril first test dose should be 0.625 mg, because of the risk of precipitous blood pressure lowering.
Source: From [56,62].

character [93]. Other dihydropyridine calcium channel blockers do not share this property [94–96]. Nicardipine is photoresistant, water-soluble, and can be administered intravenously, unlike other dihydropyridines. Intravenous nicardipine has a rapid onset of action (1–2 minutes) with an elimination half-life of 40 ± 10 minutes and the major effects last from 10 to 15 minutes. It is also rapidly distributed, extensively metabolized in the liver, and rapidly eliminated [97].

Several studies have been conducted supporting the use of nicardipine in the reduction of blood pressure in the acute ICH patient. Powers et al. evaluated the effect of intravenous nicardipine in seven subjects with ICH (6–22 hours after symptom onset) [85]. Using a positron emission tomography scan with O_{15}-water as the radioactive tracer, regional cerebral blood flow was measured. After baseline measurements of regional cerebral blood flow using the positron emission tomographic scan were made, nicardipine was administered as an initial bolus of 2–8 mg followed by a continuous infusion of 2 to 15 mg/h titrated to reduce mean arterial pressure by 15%. There was no significant difference in the perihematoma regional cerebral blood flow before and after treatment using nicardipine. When used to acutely reduce mean blood pressure below 130 mmHg, nicardipine has also been shown to be safe and effective in acute ICH patients [98]. Qureshi *et al.* used nicardipine to achieve the target blood pressure in 25 of 29 (86%) patients in a single-center prospective study supplemented by retrospective chart review. Prolonged hypotension was observed in one patient and tachycardia in another. Two patients required additional antihypertensive agents. Nicardipine was also used in a separate single-center protocol study for acute blood pressure reduction in ICH patients (n = 188) presenting within 24 hours of symptom onset [99]. All patients were also treated with an antifibrinolytic therapy (tranexamic acid 2 g intravenously over 10 minutes). Nicardipine was administered as a 2–4 mg bolus followed by a continuous intravenous infusion as needed to keep systolic blood pressure less than 150 mmHg. No adverse events associated with nicardipine were reported. Hematoma growth occurred in 4.3% of patients, which is lower than the rate observed in other observational studies [89].

Labetalol

Labetalol is an α- and β-adrenergic antagonist metabolized by the liver that is commonly used in stroke centers throughout the world. Labetalol can be administered either as intermittent boluses or as a continuous infusion. Given intravenously, its hypotensive action begins within 2 minutes, peaks at 5–15 minutes and lasts 2–4 hours [100]. Both European and North American guidelines recommend intravenous labetalol as a first-line agent in ICH patients requiring acute antihypertensive therapy [56,101]. Intravenous boluses of labetalol (10–80 mg bolus every 10 minutes, up to 300 mg) can be used to treat hypertension in the emergency department.

Studies, using intravenous boluses of labetalol, have been conducted in patients with ICH and subarachnoid hemorrhage in hopes of determining the characteristics of blood pressure reduction and its tolerability. Bolus doses (10–25 mg) of intravenous labetalol reduced systolic blood pressure by 6–19% and diastolic blood pressure by 3–26% with no adverse hemodynamic consequences [102]. The time to maximum reduction of blood pressure in the study was 5–35 minutes. There was also a prospective study

evaluating the effectiveness of intravenous labetalol in achieving a blood pressure of less than 160/90 mmHg within 24 hours of symptom onset [61]. Boluses of 10–80 mg of intravenous labetalol were administered provided the heart rate remained greater than 60 beats per minute. The drug was well tolerated, but only 10 patients achieved the target blood pressure with labetalol alone and the other 17 required additional agents (intravenous hydralazine and/or nitroprusside) [61]. Intravenous labetalol treatment has the benefit of minimal side effects with a rapid onset of action and the disadvantage of sustained hypotensive effect with prolonged usage.

Direct acting vasodilators: hydralazine, nitroprusside, and glyceryl trinitrate

Hydralazine, a peripheral vasodilator, acts by relaxing vascular smooth muscle cells leading to the reduction of arterial blood pressure. There is a latency of less than or equal to 15 minutes following an intravenous dose, but thereafter hydralazine reduces blood pressure for less than or equal to 12 hours [100]. Headache, hypotension, and palpitations are the common side effects associated with hydralazine. Hydralazine has been used in conjunction with labetalol to lower systolic blood pressure to less than 160 mmHg [61]. Low rates of neurological deterioration were associated with hydralazine usage and it was well tolerated by the study participants.

Sodium nitroprusside reduces arterial blood pressure because it reduces both preload and afterload. It acts within seconds and lasts for 1–2 minutes with pretreatment blood pressure levels being reached within 1–10 minutes after the infusion is stopped [100].

A prospective feasibility assessment of blood pressure reduction in acute ICH has also used sodium nitroprusside. Infusions of 0.2–5 μg/(kg min) were well tolerated in the ten patients treated with nitroprusside [61]. Nitroprusside is also a spontaneous nitric oxide donor. Nitric oxide is a potent vasodilator and inhibitor of circulating platelets. The spontaneous donation of nitric oxide theoretically makes nitroprusside a non-optimal agent for use in ICH patients, although its effect on platelet function in these patients has not been assessed. One study in ischemic stroke, however, showed impaired platelet aggregation with nitroprusside [103].

Outpatient management of chronic hypertension following intracerebral hemorrhage

Recurrent bleeding rates after hypertensive ICH are as high as 5.4% [104,105]. The European Stroke Initiative and American Heart Association/American Stroke Association guidelines emphasize the control of hypertension as the most important modifiable risk factor for spontaneous ICH in the acute setting. In the non-acute, outpatient setting, treating hypertension is the most important step to reduce the risk of ICH and probably recurrent ICH as well [62]. Modification of the other risk factors, as discussed above, will also contribute to the prevention of ICH. An outpatient regimen of antihypertensive medication begins after the patient is clinically stable, able to swallow medication or take oral medications through a gastrointestinal tube, and near discharge from the acute care hospital. A recent systematic review of blood pressure reduction in the prevention of stroke recurrences, including ICHs, revealed a positive association between the magnitude of blood pressure reduction and the risk of vascular events [106]. These results suggest that continued outpatient blood pressure monitoring and treatment does play a significant role in decreasing ICH recurrence while at the same time suggests there is a need for further studies to determine which if any antihypertensive is superior in its treatment effects [29].

There was no strong evidence until recently that reducing blood pressure after ICH reduces the rate of recurrent ICH. The PROGRESS (Perindopril Protection Against Recurrent Stroke) study has also shown benefits of antihypertensive treatment for high risk, non-hypertensive individuals as well as for those with hypertension, with combination, perindopril (angiotensin converting enzyme inhibitor) and indapamide (diuretic) treatment. PROGRESS, a double-blind randomized trial, comparing perindopril (4 mg daily), with or without indapamide (2–2.5 mg daily), versus placebo for the prevention of recurrent stroke in individuals with a history of non-disabling cerebrovascular disease, irrespective of blood pressure showed that reducing the blood pressure in this patient population also reduced the risk of recurrent strokes [107]. Antihypertensive treatment was initialized at least two weeks after stroke. In the participants being treated with perindopril plus indapamide blood pressure was reduced by a mean of 12 mmHg systolic and 5 mmHg

diastolic and consequently the stroke risk was significantly lower when compared to the double placebo cohort. A reduction of 5 mmHg systolic and 3 mmHg diastolic blood pressure was observed in the group that received perindopril alone, but the stroke risk was not discernibly different from that among participants who received single placebo. In comparison with double placebo, combination therapy was associated with a lower risk of each of the main stroke subtypes: fatal or disabling stroke (60/1770 versus 110/1774; relative risk reduction 46% [95% confidence interval 27–61]), ischemic stroke (126 versus 191; relative risk reduction 36% [95% confidence interval 19–49]), and cerebral hemorrhage (12 versus 49; relative risk reduction 76% [95% confidence interval 55–87]), over the course of four years [107].

Ongoing clinical trials

Until ongoing clinical trials of blood pressure intervention for ICH are completed, physicians must manage blood pressure on the basis of the present incomplete evidence, Class IIb, Level of Evidence C. Blood pressure management represents one of the major controversies in acute ICH treatment. As of 2007, there are five ongoing trials attempting to evaluate the relationship between blood pressure and ICH: Antihypertensive Treatment in Acute Cerebral Hemorrhage (ATACH), Intensive Blood Pressure Reduction in Acute Cerebral Hemorrhage Trial (INTERACT), IntraCerebral Hemorrhage Acutely Decreasing Arterial Pressure Trial (ICH-ADAPT), IntraCerebral Hemorrhage Acutely Decreasing Arterial Pressure Extended Trial (ICH-ADAPT-E) and the Nicardipine for the Treatment of Hypertension in Patients with Ischemic Stroke, Intracerebral Hemorrhage or Subarachnoid Hemorrhage (CARING) trial.

Antihypertensive Treatment in Acute Cerebral Hemorrhage (ATACH)

The Antihypertensive Treatment in Acute Cerebral Hemorrhage (ATACH) trial is a prospective, open-label phase I safety and tolerability study started in 2005 that plans to study 60 patients. The specific goals are to: (1) determine the tolerability of the treatment as assessed by achieving and maintaining three different systolic blood pressure goals with intravenous nicardipine (5–15 mg/h intravenous infusion) for 18–24 hours postictus in subjects with ICH who present within

6 hours of symptom onset; (2) define the safety, assessed by the rate of neurological deterioration during treatment and serious adverse events, of three escalating systolic blood pressure treatment goals using intravenous nicardipine infusion: 170–200 mmHg, 140–170 mmHg and 110–140 mmHg; and (3) obtain preliminary estimates of the treatment effect using the rate of hematoma expansion (within 24 hours) and modified Rankin scale (mRS) and Barthel index at 3 months following symptom onset [108,109].

Intensive Blood Pressure Reduction in Acute Cerebral Hemorrhage Trial (INTERACT)

Started in 2005, the Intensive Blood Pressure Reduction in Acute Cerebral Hemorrhage Trial (INTERACT) is a phase III, randomized, open-label, international, safety/efficacy study. The pilot trial, aiming to study 400 patients, is being done to plan for a major trial that will determine whether lowering high blood pressure levels after the start of a stroke caused by ICH will reduce the chances of a person dying or surviving with a long-term disability. The inclusion criteria for this trial include: (1) patients with acute stroke due to spontaneous ICH confirmed by clinical history and CT scan; (2) at least two systolic blood pressure measurements of greater than or equal to 150 mmHg and less than or equal to 200 mmHg, recorded two or more minutes apart; (3) able to commence randomly assigned blood pressure lowering regimen within six hours of stroke onset; (4) able to be actively treated and admitted to a monitored facility, e.g. intensive care unit/acute stroke unit. Patients randomized to intensive blood pressure lowering are started on locally available, intravenous treatment and changed when feasible to oral agents. The specific treatments that can be used are: labetalol hydrochloride, metoprolol tartrate, hydralazine hydrochloride, glycerol trinitrate, phentolamine mesylate, nicardipine, Urapidil, esmolol, clonidine, enalaprilat and nitroprusside. The primary end point is mortality and dependency according to an mRS score of 3–5 at three months [62,110,111].

Intracerebral Hemorrhage Acutely Decreasing Arterial Pressure Trial (ICH-ADAPT) and ICH-ADAPT-E

Intracerebral Hemorrhage Acutely Decreasing Arterial Pressure Trial (ICH-ADAPT) and the Intracerebral Hemorrhage Acutely Decreasing Arterial Pressure Extended Trial (ICH-ADAPT-E), initiated in 2007, are both multicenter, randomized, open-label, blinded-endpoint trials that are designed to demonstrate whether blood pressure reduction following ICH stroke is safe and does not result in cerebral ischemia. Intracerebral Hemorrhage Acutely Decreasing Arterial Pressure Trial allows for treatment within six hours of the ICH whereas the ICH-ADAPT-E allows treatment within 24 hours of ICH. Both the ICH-ADAPT and the ICH-ADAPT-E plan on studying 82 patients. The trials randomize patients who have acute ICH, confirmed by CT scan. All primary ICH patients, irrespective of location (lobar/subcortical or brainstem), as well as anticoagulant-related hemorrhages will be eligible. Patients must also have two systolic blood pressure measurements greater than or equal to 150 mmHg recorded greater than two minutes apart. Those in the treatment group will receive a 10 mg intravenous bolus of labetalol, administered over one minute, along with a protocol designed to achieve and maintain systolic blood pressure less than or equal to 150 mmHg within one hour of treatment. Patients randomized to the control group will be managed according to current American Stroke Association guidelines.

One hour after initial treatment (two hours after randomization), all patients will undergo a standard non-contrast CT brain scan. Perfusion CT images will be acquired with the administration of intravenous iodinated contrast (40 ml) given over 10 seconds with computed tomography images acquired every 0.5 seconds for 50 seconds. All patients will have a second non-contrast CT brain scan at 24 hours, in order to assess for additional hematoma expansion and perihematomal edema volume. Acute parenteral therapy will be administered only if systolic blood pressure is greater than or equal to 180 mmHg. After 24 hours, the stroke team physician will manage blood pressure in the manner they feel is appropriate. Physicians will be encouraged to start oral antihypertensive therapy, administered via nasogastric feeding tube if necessary, after the initial 24 hours. The primary end point is perihematomal regional cerebral blood flow, as measured with a CT perfusion scan two hours after antihypertensive therapy is initiated [1,112,113].

CARING trial

The CARING trial, Nicardipine for the Treatment of Hypertension in Patients with Ischemic Stroke,

Intracerebral Hemorrhage or Subarachnoid Hemorrhage, is a phase IV, prospective, open-labeled study, that began in 2006. The planned study size is 50 people. It was designed to evaluate the efficacy and safety of double- or triple-concentrated intravenous nicardipine for treatment of hypertension in patients with ischemic stroke, ICH or subarachnoid hemorrhage. Any patients older than 18 years old with ischemic stroke, ICH, or subarachnoid hemorrhage who require blood pressure control will qualify. Twenty-five patients will receive double-concentrated dose; the others (n = 25) the triple-concentrated dose. The treatment period will be determined by the clinician's clinical judgment for the particular patient. An average of 72 hours of infusion may be needed until the blood pressure is ideally controlled by other agents. The primary end point will be the rate of peripheral intravenous phlebitis or irritation in double- or triple-concentrated nicardipine infusion as well as time and dosage adjustment needed to reach the target blood pressure range [114].

References

1. Jüttler E, Steiner T. Treatment and prevention of spontaneous intracerebral hemorrhage: comparison of EUSI and AHA/ASA recommendations. *Expert Rev Neurother* 2007; **7**(10): 1401–16. Review.

2. Ayala C, Croft JB, Greenlund KJ, *et al.* Sex differences in US mortality rates for stroke and stroke subtypes by race/ethnicity and age, 1995–1998. *Stroke* 2002; **33**(5): 1197–1201.

3. Weimar C, Weber C, Wagner M, *et al.* Management patterns and health care use after intracerebral hemorrhage. A cost-of-illness study from a societal perspective in Germany. *Cerebrovasc Dis* 2003; **15**: 29–36.

4. Labovitz DL, Halim A, Boden-Albala B, *et al.* The incidence of deep and lobar intracerebral hemorrhage in whites, blacks, and Hispanics. *Neurology* 2005; **65**(4): 518–522.

5. Jiang B, Wang WZ, Chen H, *et al.* Incidence and trend of stroke and its subtypes in China: results from three large cities. *Stroke* 2006; **37**(1): 63–68.

6. Qureshi AI, Tuhrim S, Broderick JP, *et al.* Spontaneous intracerebral hemorrhage. *N Engl J Med* 2001; **344**(19): 1450–1460.

7. Ariesen MJ, Claus SP, Rinkel GJ, *et al.* Risk factors for intracerebral hemorrhage in the general population: a systematic review. *Stroke* 2003; **34**(8): 2060–2065.

8. Kurth T, Kase CS, Berger K, *et al.* Smoking and the risk of hemorrhagic stroke in men. *Stroke* 2003; **34**: 1151–1155.

9. Kurth T, Kase CS, Berger K, *et al.* Smoking and risk of hemorrhagic stroke in women. *Stroke* 2003; **34**: 2792–2795.

10. Iso H, Baba S, Mannami T, *et al.* Alcohol consumption and risk of stroke among middle-aged men: the JPHC Study Cohort I. *Stroke* 2004; **35**: 1124–1129.

11. Thrift AG, Donnan GA, McNeil JJ. Heavy drinking, but not moderate or intermediate drinking, increases the risk of intracerebral hemorrhage. *Epidemiology* 1999; **10**: 307–312.

12. Feldmann E, Broderick JP, Kernan WN, *et al.* Major risk factors for intracerebral hemorrhage in the young are modifiable. *Stroke* 2005; **36**: 1881–1885.

13. Neaton JD, Wentworth DN, Cutler J, Stamler J, Kuller L. Risk factors for death from different types of stroke. Multiple Risk Factor Intervention Trial Research Group. *Ann Epidemiol* 1993; **3**: 493–499.

14. Iribarren C, Jacobs DR, Sadler M, Claxton AJ, Sidney S. Low total serum cholesterol and intracerebral hemorrhagic stroke: is the association confined to elderly men? The Kaiser Permanente Medical Care Program. *Stroke* 1996; **27**: 1993–1998.

15. Suh I, Jee SH, Kim HC, *et al.* Low serum cholesterol and haemorrhagic stroke in men: Korea Medical Insurance Corporation Study. *Lancet* 2001; **357**: 922–925.

16. Vermeer SE, Algra A, Franke CL, Koudstaal PJ, Rinkel GJ. Long-term prognosis after recovery from primary intracerebral hemorrhage. *Neurology* 2002; **59**: 205–209.

17. Ferro JM. Update on intracerebral haemorrhage. *J Neurol* 2006; **253**(8): 985–999. Epub 2006 May 6. Review.

18. Kase CS, Mohr JP, Caplan LR. Intracerebral hemorrhage. In: Mohr JP, Choi DC, Grotta JC, *et al.*, eds. *Stroke: Pathophysiology, Diagnosis and Management*, 4th edn. Philadelphia, Churchill Livingstone. 2004; 327–376.

19. Caplan LR. Intracerebral hemorrhage. In: Caplan LR, ed. *Caplan's Stroke: A Clinical Approach*, 3rd edn. Boston, Butterworth-Heinemann. 2000; 383–418.

20. Broderick JP, Brott T, Tomsick T, Huster G, Miller R. The risk of subarachnoid and intracerebral hemorrhages in blacks as compared to whites. *N Engl J Med* 1992; **326**(11): 733–736.

21. Sacco RL, Boden-Albala B, Gan R, *et al.* Stroke incidence among white, black and Hispanic residents of an urban community: the Northern Manhattan Stroke Study. *Am J Epidemiol* 1998; **147**: 259–268.

22. Bruno A, Carter S. Possible reason for the higher incidence of spontaneous intracerebral hemorrhage

among Hispanics than non-Hispanic whites in New Mexico. *Neuroepidemiology* 2000; **19**: 51–52.

23. Ayala C, Greenlund KJ, Croft JB, *et al.* Racial/ethnic disparities in mortality by stroke subtype in the United States, 1995–1998. *Am J Epidemiol* 2001; **154**: 1057–1063.

24. Smeeton NC, Heuschmann PU, Rudd AG, *et al.* Incidence of hemorrhagic stroke in black Caribbean, black African, and white populations: the South London stroke register, 1995–2004. *Stroke* 2007; **38**(12): 3133–3138. Epub 2007 Oct 25.

25. Petitti DB, Sidney S, Bernstein A, *et al.* Stroke in users of low-dose oral contraceptives. *N Engl J Med* 1996; **335**: 8–15.

26. Qureshi AI, Giles WH, Croft JB. Racial differences in the incidence of intracerebral hemorrhage: effects of blood pressure and education. *Neurology* 1999; **52**: 1617–1621.

27. Flaherty ML, Woo D, Haverbusch M, *et al.* Racial variations in location and risk of intracerebral hemorrhage. *Stroke* 2005; **36**: 934–937.

28. Song YM, Sung J, Lawlor DA, *et al.* Blood pressure, haemorrhagic stroke, and ischaemic stroke: the Korean national prospective occupational cohort study. *BMJ* 2004; **328**: 324–325.

29. Woo D, Haverbusch M, Sekar P, *et al.* Effect of untreated hypertension on hemorrhagic stroke. *Stroke* 2004; **35**: 1703–1708.

30. Perry HM Jr, Davis BR, Price TR, *et al.* Effect of treating isolated systolic hypertension on the risk of developing various types and subtypes of stroke: the Systolic Hypertension in the Elderly Program (SHEP). *JAMA* 2000; **284**: 465–471.

31. Marietta M, Pedrazzi P, Girardis M, Torelli G. Intracerebral haemorrhage: an often neglected medical emergency. *Intern Emerg Med* 2007; **2**(1): 38–45. Epub 2007 Mar 31. Review.

32. Pleşea IE, Cameniţă A, Georgescu CC, *et al.* Study of cerebral vascular structures in hypertensive intracerebral haemorrhage. *Rom J Morphol Embryol* 2005; **46**(3): 249–256.

33. Sutherland GR, Auer RN. Primary intracerebral hemorrhage *J Clin Neurosci* 2006; **13**(5): 511–517.

34. Cordonnier C, Al-Shahi Salman R, Wardlaw J. Spontaneous brain microbleeds: systematic review, subgroup analyses and standards for study design and reporting. *Brain* 2007; **130**(Pt 8): 1988–2003. Epub 2007 Feb 24.

35. Lee SH, Park JM, Kwon SJ, *et al.* Left ventricular hypertrophy is associated with cerebral microbleeds in hypertensive patients. *Neurology* 2004; **63**: 16–21.

36. Lee SH, Kwon SJ, Kim KS, Yoon BW, Roh JK. Cerebral microbleeds in patients with hypertensive stroke. Topographical distribution in the supratentorial area. *J Neurol* 2004; **251**: 1183–1189.

37. Laissy JP, Normand G, Monroc M, *et al.* Spontaneous intracerebral hematomas from vascular causes. *Neuroradiology* 1991; **33**: 291–295.

38. Watanabe A. Cerebral microbleeds and intracerebral hemorrhages in patients on maintenance hemodialysis. *J Stroke Cerebrovasc Dis* 2007; **16**(1): 30–33.

39. Tanaka A, Ueno Y, Nakayama Y, *et al.* Small chronic hemorrhages and ischemic lesions in association with spontaneous intracerebral hematomas. *Stroke* 1999; **30**: 1637–1642.

40. Roob G, Fazekas F. Magnetic resonance imaging of cerebral microbleeds. *Curr Opin Neurol* 2000; **13**: 69–73.

41. Roob G, Lechner A, Schmidt R, *et al.* Frequency and location of microbleeds in patients with primary intracerebral hemorrhage. *Stroke* 2000; **31**: 2665–2669.

42. Roob G, Schmidt R, Kapeller P, *et al.* MRI evidence of past cerebral microbleeds in a healthy elderly population, *Neurology* 1999; **52**: 991–994.

43. Wallace JD, Levy LL. Blood pressure after stroke. *JAMA* 1981; **246**: 2177–2180.

44. Harper G, Castleden CM, Potter JF. Factors affecting changes in blood pressure after acute stroke. *Stroke* 1994; **25**: 1726–1729.

45. Fogelholm R, Avikainen S, Murros K. Prognostic value and determinants of first-day mean arterial pressure in spontaneous supratentorial intracerebral hemorrhage. *Stroke* 1997; **28**: 1396–1400.

46. Portenoy RK, Lipton RB, Berger AR, Lesser ML, Lantos G. Intracerebral haemorrhage: a model for the prediction of outcome. *J Neurol Neurosurg Psychiatry* 1987; **50**: 976–979.

47. Tuhrim S, Dambrosia JM, Price TR, *et al.* Prediction of intracerebral hemorrhage survival. *Ann Neurol* 1988; **24**: 258–263.

48. Broderick JP, Brott TG, Duldner JE, Tomsick T, Huster G. Volume of intracerebral hemorrhage: a powerful and easy-to-use predictor of 30-day mortality. *Stroke* 1993; **24**: 987–993.

49. Carlberg B, Asplund K, Hagg E. The prognostic value of admission blood pressure in patients with acute stroke. *Stroke* 1993; **24**: 1372–1375.

50. Dandapani BK, Suzuki S, Kelley RE, Reyes-Iglesias Y, Duncan RC. Relation between blood pressure and outcome in intracerebral hemorrhage. *Stroke* 1995; **26**(1): 21–24.

51. Leira R, Dávalos A, Silva Y, *et al.* Early neurologic deterioration in intracerebral hemorrhage: predictors and associated factors. *Neurology* 2004; **63**: 461–467.

52. Qureshi AI, Safdar K, Weil J, *et al.* Predictors of early deterioration and mortality in black Americans with spontaneous intracerebral hemorrhage. *Stroke* 1995; **26**(10): 1764–1767.

53. Terayama Y, Tanahashi N, Fukuuchi Y, Gotoh F. Prognostic value of admission blood pressure in patients with intracerebral hemorrhage: Keio cooperative stroke study. *Stroke* 1997; **28**: 1185–1188.

54. Dunne JW, Chakera T, Kermode S. Cerebellar haemorrhage–diagnosis and treatment: a study of 75 consecutive cases. *QJM* 1987; **64**: 739–754.

55. Meyer JS, Bauer RB. Medical treatment of spontaneous intracranial hemorrhage by the use of hypotensive drugs. *Neurology* 1962; **12**: 36–47.

56. Steiner T, Kaste M, Forsting M, *et al.* Recommendations for the management of intracranial haemorrhage – part I: spontaneous intracerebral haemorrhage. The European Stroke Initiative Writing Committee and the Writing Committee for the EUSI Executive Committee. *Cerebrovasc Dis* 2006; **22**(4): 294–316. Epub 2006 Jul 28. Erratum in: *Cerebrovasc Dis* 2006; **22**(5–6): 461. Katse, Markku [corrected to Kaste, Markku].

57. Tietjen CS, Hurn PD, Ulatowski JA, *et al.* Treatment modalities for hypertensive patients with intracranial pathology: options and risks. *Crit Care Med* 1996; **24**: 311–322.

58. Chillon J-M, Baumbach GI. Autoregulation: arterial and intracranial pressure. In: Edvinsson L, Krause DN, eds. *Cerebral Blood Flow and Metabolism*, 2nd edn. Philadelphia, Lippincott Williams & Wilkins. 2002; 395–412.

59. Morgenstern LB. Medical therapy of intracerebral and intraventricular hemorrhage. In: Mohr JP, Choi DC, Grotta JC, *et al.*, eds. *Stroke: Pathophysiology, Diagnosis and Management*, 4th edn. Philadelphia, Churchill Livingstone. 2004; 1079–1087.

60. Qureshi AI, Bliwise DL, Bliwise NG, *et al.* Rate of 24-h blood pressure decline and mortality after spontaneous intracerebral hemorrhage: a retrospective analysis with a random effects regression model. *Crit Care Med* 1999; **27**: 480–485.

61. Qureshi AI, Mohammad YM, Yahia AM, *et al.* A prospective multicenter study to evaluate the feasibility and safety of aggressive antihypertensive treatment in patients with acute intracerebral hemorrhage. *J Intensive Care Med* 2005; **20**: 34–42.

62. Broderick J, Connolly S, Feldmann E, *et al.* American Heart Association/American Stroke Association Stroke Council; American Heart Association/American Stroke Association High Blood Pressure Research Council; Quality of Care and Outcomes in Research Interdisciplinary Working Group. Guidelines for the management of spontaneous intracerebral hemorrhage in adults: 2007 update: a guideline from the American Heart Association/American Stroke Association Stroke Council, High Blood Pressure Research Council, and the Quality of Care and Outcomes in Research Interdisciplinary Working Group. *Circulation* 2007; **116**(16): e391–413. Republished from: *Stroke* 2007; **38**(6): 2001–2023.

63. Vespa P. What is the optimal threshold for cerebral perfusion pressure following traumatic brain injury? *Neurosurg Focus* 2003; **15**: E4. Review.

64. Robertson CS, Valadka AB, Hannay HJ, *et al.* Prevention of secondary ischemic insults after severe head injury. *Crit Care Med* 1999; **27**: 2086–2095.

65. Chambers IR, Banister K, Mendelow AD. Intracranial pressure within a developing intracerebral haemorrhage. *Br J Neurosurg* 2001; **15**: 140–141.

66. Fernandes HM, Siddique S, Banister K, *et al.* Continuous monitoring of ICP and CPP following ICH and its relationship to clinical, radiological and surgical parameters. *Acta Neurochir Suppl.* 2000; **76**: 463–466.

67. Kazui S, Minematsu K, Yamamoto H, Sawada T, Yamaguchi T. Predisposing factors to enlargement of spontaneous intracerebral hematoma. *Stroke* 1997; **28**: 2370–2375.

68. Fujii Y, Takeuchi S, Sasaki O, Minakawa T, Tanaka R. Multivariate analysis of predictors of hematoma enlargement in spontaneous intracerebral hemorrhage. *Stroke* 1998; **29**: 1160–1166.

69. Qureshi AI, Wilson DA, Hanley DF, Traystman RJ. Pharmacologic reduction of mean arterial pressure does not adversely affect regional cerebral blood flow and intracranial pressure in experimental intracerebral hemorrhage. *Crit Care Med* 1999; **27**: 965–971.

70. Ohwaki K, Yono E, Nagashima H, *et al.* Blood pressure management in acute intracerebral hemorrhage: relationship between elevated blood pressure and hematoma enlargement. *Stroke* 2004; **35**(6): 1364–1367.

71. Kazui S, Naritomi H, Yamamoto H, Sawada T, Yamaguchi T. Enlargement of spontaneous intracerebral hemorrhage: incidence and time course. *Stroke* 1996; **27**: 1783–1787.

72. Brott T, Broderick J, Kothari R, *et al.* Early hemorrhage growth in patients with intracerebral hemorrhage. *Stroke* 1997; **28**(1): 1–5.

73. Broderick JP, Diringer MN, Hill MD, *et al.* Recombinant Activated Factor VII Intracerebral Hemorrhage Trial Investigators. Determinants of

intracerebral hemorrhage growth: an exploratory analysis. *Stroke* 2007; **38**(3): 1072–1075.

74. Jauch EC, Lindsell CJ, Adeoye O, *et al.* Lack of evidence for an association between hemodynamic variables and hematoma growth in spontaneous intracerebral hemorrhage. *Stroke* 2006; **37**: 2061–2065.

75. Adams RE, Powers WJ. Management of hypertension in acute intracerebral hemorrhage. *Crit Care Clin* 1997; **13**(1): 131–161.

76. Herweh C, Juttler E, Schellinger, PD *et al.* Evidence against a perihemorrhagic penumbra provided by perfusion CT. *Stroke* 2007; **38**(11): 2941–2947.

77. Zhao X, Wang Y, Wang C, *et al.* Quantitative evaluation for secondary injury to perihematoma of hypertensive cerebral hemorrhage by functional MR and correlation analysis with ischemic factors. *Neurol Res* 2006; **28**(1): 66–70.

78. Siddique MS, Fernandes HM, Wooldridge TD, *et al.* Reversible ischemia around intracerebral hemorrhage: a single-photon emission computerized tomography study. *J Neurosurg* 2002; **96**(4): 736–741.

79. Rosand J, Eskey C, Yuchiao C, *et al.* Dynamic single-section CT demonstrates reduced cerebral blood flow in acute intracerebral hemorrhage. *Cerebrovasc Dis* 2002; **14**(3–4): 214–220.

80. Fainardi E, Borrelli M, Saletti A, *et al.* Assessment of acute spontaneous intracerebral hematoma by CT perfusion imaging. *J Neuroradiol* 2005; **32**(5): 333–336.

81. Butcher KS, Baird T, MacGregor L, *et al.* Perihematomal edema in primary intracerebral hemorrhage is plasma derived. *Stroke* 2004; **35**(8): 1879–1885.

82. Schellinger PD, Fiebach JB, Hoffmann K, *et al.* Stroke MRI in intracerebral hemorrhage: is there a perihemorrhagic penumbra? *Stroke* 2003; **34**(7): 1674–1679.

83. Kidwell CS, Saver JL, Mattiello J, *et al.* Diffusion–perfusion MR evaluation of perihematomal injury in hyperacute intracerebral hemorrhage. *Neurology* 2001; **57**(11): 1611–1617.

84. Zazulia AR, Diringer MN, Videen TO, *et al.* Hypoperfusion without ischemia surrounding intracerebral hemorrhage. *J Cereb Blood Flow Metab* 2001; **21**(7): 804–810.

85. Powers WJ, Zazulia AR, Videen TO, *et al.* Autoregulation of cerebral blood flow surrounding acute (6–22 h) intracerebral hemorrhage. *Neurology* 2001; **57**(1): 18–24.

86. Becker KJ, Baxter AB, Bybee HM, *et al.* Extravasation of radiographic contrast is an independent predictor of death in primary intracerebral hemorrhage. *Stroke* 1999; **30**(10): 2025–2032.

87. Gebel JM Jr, Jauch EC, Brott TG, *et al.* Natural history of perihematomal edema in patients with hyperacute spontaneous intracerebral hemorrhage. *Stroke* 2002; **33**: 2631–2635.

88. Gebel JM Jr, Jauch EC, Brott TG, *et al.* Relative edema volume is a predictor of outcome in patients with hyperacute spontaneous intracerebral hemorrhage. *Stroke* 2002; **33**: 2636–2641.

89. Asdaghi N, Manawadu D, Butcher K. Therapeutic management of acute intracerebral haemorrhage. *Expert Opin Pharmacother* 2007; **8**(18): 3097–3116. Review.

90. Bereczki D, Liu M, Prado GF, Fekete I. Cochrane report: a systematic review of mannitol therapy for acute ischemic stroke and cerebral parenchymal hemorrhage. *Stroke* 2000; **31**(11): 2719–2722.

91. Interventions for deliberately altering blood pressure in acute stroke. Blood Pressure in Acute Stroke Collaboration (BASC). *Cochrane Database Syst Rev* 2000; (**2**): CD000039.

92. Clarke B, Grant D, Patmore L. Comparative calcium entry blocking properties of nicardipine, nifedipine and PY-108–68 on cardiac and vascular smooth muscle. *Br J Pharmacol* 1983; **79**: 333P.

93. Fischell TA, Maheshwari A. Current applications for nicardipine in invasive and interventional cardiology. *J Invasive Cardiol* 2004; **16**(8): 428–432.

94. Alps BJ, Hass WK. The potential beneficial effect of nicardipine in a rat model of transient forebrain ischemia. *Neurology* 1987; **37**: 809–814.

95. Nakaya H, Kanno M. Effects of nicardipine, a new dihydropyridine vasodilator, on coronary circulation and ischemia-induced conduction delay in dogs. *Arzneimittel-Forschung* 1982; **32**: 626–629.

96. Michel AD, Whiting RL. Cellular action of nicardipine. *Am J Cardiol* 1989; **64**: 3H–7H.

97. Cardene IV [package insert]. Edison, NJ: ESP Pharma, Inc.: 2003.

98. Qureshi AI, Harris-Lane P, Kirmani JF, *et al.* Treatment of acute hypertension in patients with intracerebral hemorrhage using American Heart Association guidelines. *Crit Care Med* 2006; **34**(7): 1975–1980.

99. Sorimachi T, Fujii Y, Morita K, Tanaka R. Predictors of hematoma enlargement in patients with intracerebral hemorrhage treated with rapid administration of antifibrinolytic agents and strict blood pressure control. *J Neurosurg* 2007; **106**(2): 250–254.

100. Varon J, Marik PE. The diagnosis and management of hypertensive crises. *Chest* 2000; **118**(1): 214–227.

101. Broderick JP, Adams HP Jr, Barsan W, *et al.* Guidelines for the management of spontaneous

29

intracerebral hemorrhage: a statement for healthcare professionals from a special writing group of the Stroke Council, American Heart Association. *Stroke* 1999; **30**: 905–915.

102. Patel RV, Kertland HR, Jahns BE, *et al.* Labetalol: response and safety in critically ill hemorrhagic stroke patients. *Ann Pharmacother* 1993; **27**(2): 180–181.

103. Butterworth RJ, Cluckie A, Jackson SH, Buxton-Thomas M, Bath PM. Pathophysiological assessment of nitric oxide (given as sodium nitroprusside) in acute ischaemic stroke. *Cerebrovasc Dis* 1998; **8**(3): 158–165.

104. Bae H, Jeong D, Doh J, *et al.* Recurrence of bleeding in patients with hypertensive intracerebral hemorrhage. *Cerebrovasc Dis* 1999; **9**(2): 102–108.

105. Chen CH, Huang CW, Chen HH, *et al.* Recurrent hypertensive intracerebral hemorrhage among Taiwanese. *Kaohsiung J Med Sci* 2001; **17**(11): 556–563.

106. Rashid P, Leonardi-Bee J, Bath P. Blood pressure reduction and secondary prevention of stroke and other vascular events: a systematic review. *Stroke* 2003; **34**: 2741–2748.

107. PROGRESS Collaborative Group. Randomized trial of a perindopril-based blood-pressure-lowering regimen among 6, 105 individuals with previous stroke or transient ischemic attack. *Lancet* 2001; **358**(9287): 1033–1041.

108. Qureshi AI. Antihypertensive treatment of acute cerebral hemorrhage (ATACH): rationale and design. *Neurocrit Care* 2007; **6**(1): 56–66.

109. Qureshi, A I. *"ATACH: Antihypertensive Treatment in Acute Cerebral Hemorrhage."* www.strokecenter.org.

27 Feb. 2006. UMDNJ, Newark NJ. 3 Jan. 2008 http://www.strokecenter.org/trials/TrialDetail.aspx?tid=602.

110. Anderson C and Neal B. *"Intensive Blood Pressure Reduction in Acute Cerebral Haemorrhage."* ClinicalTrial.Gov. 4 Jan. 2008. The George Institute, National Health and Medical Research Council, Australia. 5 Jan. 2008 http://www.clinicaltrials.gov/ct/show/NCT00226096?order=1.

111. Anderson C. *"INTERACT-Pilot: Intensive Blood Pressure Reduction in Acute Cerebral Hemorrhage – Pilot Study."* Strokecenter.Org. 20 Mar. 2007. Royal Prince Alfred Hospital, Australia. 3 Jan. 2008 http://strokecenter.org/trials/TrialDetail.aspx?tid=569.

112. Butcher K. *"ICH ADAPT: Intracerebral Hemorrhage Acutely Decreasing Arterial Pressure Trial."* Strokecenter.Org. 10 May 2007. Health Sciences Centre, Division of Neurology, Canada. 3 Jan. 2008 http://strokecenter.org/trials/TrialDetail.aspx?tid=748.

113. Butcher K. *"ICH-ADAPT-E: Intracerebral Hemorrhage Acutely Decreasing Arterial Pressure Trial – Extended."* Strokecenter.Org. 10 May 2007. Health Sciences Centre, Division of Neurology, Canada. 3 Jan. 2008 http://strokecenter.org/trials/TrialDetail.aspx?tid=722.

114. Wang DZ. *"CARING: Nicardipine for the Treatment of Hypertension in Patients with Ischemic Stroke, Intracerebral Hemorrhage or Subarachnoid Hemorrhage."* Strokecenter.Org. 25 Apr. 2007. St. Francis Medical Center, IL. 3 Jan. 2008 http://strokecenter.org/trials/TrialDetail.aspx/tid/600.

Chapter 3

Etiology of tumor-related intracranial hemorrhage

Andreas F. Hottinger and Lisa M. DeAngelis

Introduction

Cancer-related intracerebral bleeding is an uncommon cause of hemorrhage and represents only a fraction of all non-traumatic intracranial hemorrhages (ICHs) [1]. In the literature, the incidence of tumoral hemorrhages has been estimated at 0.8–4.4% of all ICHs [2–5]. One study of 144 patients found that tumor-related hemorrhages accounted for 9% of hemorrhages; however, there was an overrepresentation of metastatic brain tumors in this population that explained the majority of their neoplastic ICHs [6].

Intracerebral hemorrhage is relatively common in cancer patients and can be demonstrated in 3–14.6% at autopsy [2,7–11]. The causes of hemorrhage in cancer patients are multiple and include intratumoral bleeding, cerebral metastasis, coagulation disorders, and complications of anticancer treatment (Table 3.1). In addition to metastases, primary brain tumors can also present with or develop an ICH. Recognizing that a neoplasm may be the source of an ICH is of cardinal importance, particularly when it is the presenting manifestation [7].

Tumor-related hemorrhages occur in any part of the central nervous system (CNS) [2]. In most patients, the site of hemorrhage is the brain parenchyma. Subarachnoid (SAH) and subdural hemorrhages are less commonly caused by a neoplasm [12]. Only 0.4% of all SAHs can be attributed to intracranial neoplasms with roughly half linked to primary CNS tumors and half linked to metastatic disease [13]. Subdural hemorrhages secondary to neoplasm occur almost exclusively in patients with metastatic disease and are rarely associated with primary brain tumors [11,12].

Primary brain tumor

In large series of ICH, primary brain neoplasms accounted for only 0.8–0.9% of all non-traumatic hemorrhages [4,14,15], and high-grade gliomas accounted for up to 65% of these [2,16] (Table 3.2). The mechanisms of intratumoral hemorrhage remain unclear, but include tumor necrosis, rupture of tumor blood vessels and invasion of parenchymal blood vessels by tumor [17,18]. The blood supply of intracranial malignant neoplasms depends upon tumor-generated blood vessels that are distinctly different from normal cerebral vessels. Tumor vessels are immature, fenestrated and lack tight junctions, making them more permeable than normal and lacking a blood–brain barrier [19]. These neovessels are associated with high-grade tumors, particularly glioblastoma multiforme (GBM), and are generated in response to tumor secretion of vascular endothelial growth factor (VEGF), which is a significant mediator of angiogenesis [20], and is over–expressed in up to 95% of all glioblastomas [21]. Vascular endothelial growth factor is a 34- to 42-kDa heparin-binding, dimeric, disulfide-bound glycoprotein and exists as five spliced isoforms having 121, 145, 165, 189, and 206 amino acids. It mediates its actions through its receptors Flt-1 and Flk-1 [22]. Experimental evidence demonstrates that certain isoforms of VEGF (121 and 165) are more prone to induce intratumoral hemorrhage than others [23]. Thus, it is not surprising that the grade of malignancy is directly related to the risk of hemorrhage. Up to 8% of all GBMs show ICH, whereas only 1–2% of low-grade gliomas are complicated by hemorrhage [16] (Table 3.2).

Intracerebral Hemorrhage, ed. J. R. Carhuapoma, S. A. Mayer, and D. F. Hanley. Published by Cambridge University Press.
© J. R. Carhuapoma, S. A. Mayer, and D. F. Hanley 2010.

Table 3.1. Etiology and localization of tumor-related intracerebral hemorrhage

Mechanism	Localization	Typical tumor/cause
Tumor related		
Metastatic/primary brain tumor	Hemorrhage in or adjacent to the tumor	Metastatic carcinoma, malignant glioma, oligodendroglioma
Metastatic or primary dural or skull tumor	Subdural or epidural hemorrhage	Carcinoma, leukemia, lymphoma or meningioma
Neoplastic aneurysm	Ruptured aneurysm with parenchymal hemorrhage	Lung carcinoma or choriocarcinoma
Coagulopathy		
DIC	Parenchymal or subdural hemorrhage	Leukemia, especially acute promyelocytic leukemia
Thrombocytopenia	Parenchymal, subdural or subarachnoid hemorrhage	Leukemia, chemotherapy-induced
Microangiopathic hemolytic anemia	Parenchymal hemorrhage	Mucin-producing carcinoma, chemotherapy administration
Treatment related		
Chemotherapy	Parenchymal hemorrhage with or without sagittal sinus occlusion	L-asparaginase, thrombocytopenia, coagulopathy
	Hemolytic uremic syndrome with parenchymal hemorrhage	Following various chemotherapeutic agents: bleomycin, cisplatin, mitomycin C

Note: DIC, disseminated intravascular coagulation.

Liwnicz *et al.* have classified patterns of capillary growth in brain tumors into three groups: axial, retiform, and glomeruloid. Whereas most tumors contain a combination of these capillary types, only the retiform type is associated with significant intratumoral hemorrhage [24]. Retiform capillaries are also present in abundance in all grades of oligodendrogliomas, which may explain the 7–14% incidence of hematomas (greater than that observed in GBM) in this otherwise low-grade tumor [9,11]. However, because this type of tumor is rare, oligodendrogliomas account for only a small fraction of tumor-related hemorrhages.

In other primary CNS tumors, the predisposition to bleed is poorly defined. For instance, meningiomas represent an unusual cause of ICH, which is seen in 0.6–2% of all meningiomas [2,9,11,25] (Table 3.2). Bleeding has not been associated with a particular histological subtype, nor a particular localization [26,27]. It can occur acutely without antecedent symptoms, often masking the tumor [27]. Meningiomas may be complicated by subdural hemorrhages because of their extra-axial location [28].

Pituitary tumors are benign intracranial tumors with a high propensity for bleeding [11,29] (Table 3.2). In approximately 45% of patients the hemorrhage is small, remains asymptomatic, and can be demonstrated only by MRI or CT [30]. However, hemorrhage into a pituitary tumor can cause pituitary apoplexy with acute headache, coma, and pituitary failure. Apoplexy occurs in 2–10% of adenomas and can be a result of hemorrhage or infarction. The diagnosis is established by neuroimaging [31].

Brain metastasis

Metastatic brain tumors can cause intracerebral hemorrhage. The overall incidence has not been as well studied as for primary brain tumors, but in one series, metastases accounted for 21% of tumor-related ICHs [2]. Brain metastases from any primary tumor can cause bleeding, but the different primaries have a wide variability in their tendency to bleed [2,9,32] (Table 3.2). This variability is likely explained by the fact that metastases develop blood vessels similar to those of their primary sites. Malignant melanoma,

Table 3.2. Incidence of intracerebral hemorrhage according to histological type of neoplasm

Type of tumor	Licata and Turazzi [2] (N = 110/7373)	Wakai et al. [11] (N = 94/1861)	Weisberg [32] (CT based study)	Kondziolka et al. [9] N = 49/905	Manganiello [16] N = 7/183	Niiro et al. [25] N = 6/298
All brain tumors	1.5% of all neoplasms, 4.4% of all hematomas	5.0% of all neoplasms		5.4% of all neoplasms		
All gliomas		4.4%			3.8%	
• Astrocytoma	1.4%	4.9% (combination of astrocytoma and AA)		10.9%	2.5%	
• Anaplastic astrocytoma	2.6%			6.1%	6.2%	
• Glioblastoma multiforme	2.5%	7.8%		6.4%	5.5%	
• Oligodendroglioma		7.0%		14.3%		
• Medulloblastoma		1.6%		0%		
• Ependymoma		8.8%		0%	8.0%	
Meningioma	0.6%	1.3%		0.5%		2.0%
Pituitary tumor		15.8%				
Pineoblastoma	20%					
Metastases	3%	2.9%		6.1%		
• Melanoma	25%		40%	35.7%		
• Renal carcinoma			70%			
• Bronchogenic carcinoma			5%			

Notes: Numbers in the table reflect percent of tumors of that category that bled.
AA = anaplastic astrocytoma.

germ-cell tumors, renal cell and thyroid carcinomas can invade and destroy small vessels in the tumor mass and frequently lead to ICH [9,11]. In a CT-based study, Weisberg reported that 40% of brain metastases from melanoma, 70% from renal carcinoma, but only 5% from bronchogenic carcinomas showed evidence of hemorrhage [32]. However, due to the high incidence of bronchogenic carcinoma and its tendency to metastasize to the brain, it represents the most common cause of metastatic intracerebral bleeding [9,11,33,34]. Interestingly, no hemorrhages were associated with metastatic squamous cell carcinoma.

A tumor embolus may cause an aneurysm that can lead to potentially fatal intraparenchymal or subarachnoid hemorrhages [35–37]. Lung carcinoma and choriocarcinoma are the most common primary tumors leading to cerebral neoplastic aneurysms. Embolic aneurysms are typically located in distal arterial branches, usually of the middle cerebral artery.

Other tumor-related ICH

Intracranial hemorrhage can result from coagulopathies associated with cancer or its treatment. These hemorrhages may occur in the cerebral parenchyma, the ventricles, subdural or subarachnoid spaces. Over 90% of patients with systemic cancer will show laboratory evidence of a coagulation abnormality [38–40]. Coagulation protein synthesis may be further compromised when there is liver dysfunction, leading either to deficient fibrinolysis or excessive coagulation [41]. These hemostatic abnormalities can cause cerebral hemorrhage or CNS infarction with secondary hemorrhage from intravascular thrombosis [38,42].

The most frequent form of coagulation dysfunction is thrombocytopenia. Spontaneous hemorrhage may develop if platelet levels drop below $10\,000/mm^3$. In those patients, minor trauma may result in ICH or spinal hemorrhage may complicate a lumbar puncture. Thrombocytopenia may result from invasion of the bone marrow by tumor, damage from chemotherapy or radiotherapy, or when disseminated intravascular coagulation (DIC) develops [38]. Disseminated intravascular coagulation is particularly common in acute promyelocytic leukemia (APL) and has been linked to the release of procoagulants from the degranulation of promyelocytes [43]. It may

be further exacerbated by tumor cell lysis caused by administration of chemotherapy [44]. In APL, DIC typically occurs early in the clinical course and the resulting ICH may lead to death [45]. Recent use of retinoic acid for APL has markedly reduced the risk of ICH early in the course of the disease. Excessive coagulation, due to abnormal platelet aggregation and the procoagulant effect of tumor cells or monocytes, can also lead to CNS infarction with secondary hemorrhage [39,40].

L-asparaginase is used in the induction chemotherapy of acute lymphocytic leukemia and can be complicated in 1–2% of treated patients by cerebral sinus thrombosis or ICH [46–48]. The mechanism of thrombosis is related to drug-induced fibrinolysis or depletion of plasma proteins (especially antithrombin III and fibrinogen) involved in coagulation [49,50]. The most common CNS complication from L-asparaginase is thrombosis of the superior sagittal sinus, which can lead to hemorrhagic venous infarction of the adjacent cortex.

Hemolytic uremic syndrome (HUS) is characterized by microangiopathic hemolytic anemia, fever, thrombocytopenia, and renal failure. It may be complicated by intracerebral hemorrhages [51]. It has been linked to the administration of a number of chemotherapeutic agents, including mitomycin C, bleomycin, and cisplatin. There may be a delay of several months between administration of the drug and the development of HUS.

Irradiation of the brain may induce the formation of vascular abnormalities, including cavernous malformations and aneurysms, which may cause parenchymal or subarachnoid hemorrhage, even after a prolonged interval [52–56]. This has been reported in the brain and spinal cord.

Diagnosis
Clinical

The clinical presentation of intratumoral hemorrhage is often indistinguishable from spontaneous ICH from more typical etiologies such as hypertension. However, the presence of an underlying structural lesion may result in more varied clinical presentations. Therefore, tumor-related ICH can produce a stroke-like episode with rapid onset of focal neurological deficits with or without impairment of consciousness and a rapidly devastating clinical course.

This presentation occurs in 24–67% of patients with tumor-related ICH depending upon the age of the study and means of diagnosis [32,34,57–59]. Typically, older autopsy-based studies are skewed towards large hemorrhages with rapid symptoms and death, whereas CT or MR scan-based studies detect smaller and even asymptomatic hemorrhages. Coma has been reported in 25–54% of the patients in the older autopsy-based studies [14,57], but modern experience suggests that coma is much less frequently associated with ICH. In patients with an ICH, a history of headache or segmental signs preceding the acute ictus should suggest a pre-existing structural lesion. Little *et al.* reported that 8 of 13 patients with brain hemorrhage from intracranial tumor had subtle pre-existing neurological symptoms or signs suggestive of an intracranial mass [14].

The clinical presentation of tumoral intracerebral bleeding can also follow a more protracted course and be manifest as subacute neurological signs that develop over a period of days or even weeks [14,57]. A number of patients will remain asymptomatic, despite radiological evidence of hemorrhage. These asymptomatic hemorrhages have been reported to occur in 20–56% of radiological studies or pathological material obtained at surgery or autopsy [8,11].

Pituitary tumors show a high propensity for intratumoral bleeding [11] (Table 3.2). Because the hemorrhage is usually small in size, only about 65% of radiologically or pathologically proven hemorrhages will cause clinical symptoms [29,30,60]. In approximately 55% of these symptomatic cases, the bleeding will result in pituitary apoplexy characterized by sudden headache, visual impairment, and ophthalmoplegia. Vomiting or meningeal signs may also be present. The differential diagnosis of this syndrome includes rupture of an aneurysm and SAH [61].

Imaging

The rapid onset of lateralizing neurological abnormalities accompanied by decreased level of consciousness suggest ICH, but accurate diagnosis requires imaging of the brain with a CT or MRI scan [62]. As with intracerebral hematoma from any cause, tumor-related hemorrhage appears as a hyperdense lesion on precontrast CT scan [32,33] (Fig. 3.1). Depending upon its age, hemorrhage from any source will have a variable appearance on MRI and may be hypo-, iso- or hyperintense on T1- or T2-weighted

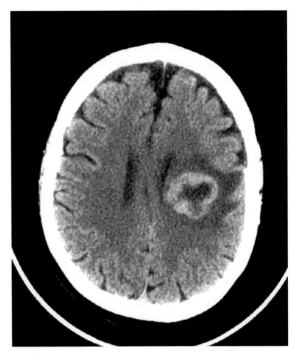

Fig. 3.1 Non-contrast brain CT: acute worsening of right hemiplegia and dysarthria in a patient with glioblastoma multiforme: hyperdense lesion corresponding to intratumoral bleeding. Note the extensive area of peritumoral edema.

images. Hyperacute blood may appear isointense to brain on unenhanced T1 images, but the hematoma becomes hyperintense within several hours. This hyperintensity can persist for weeks. Sometimes hematoma is best appreciated on the gradient echo sequences even when it is not evident on standard T1 or T2 sequences [63].

A number of radiological features may suggest the presence of an underlying tumor (Table 3.3). The location of the hematoma may suggest a mass; unlike the deep basal ganglia or brainstem location of hypertensive hemorrhages, primary tumors tend to occur in the hemispheric white matter and metastases at the junction between the gray and white matter [63]. On neuroimaging obtained within hours of symptom onset, enhancement contiguous to the hemorrhage following contrast administration suggests the bleed occurred within a tumor [64,65]. Hypertensive or traumatic cerebral hemorrhages do not enhance for days to weeks after the ictus. Other lesions that show contrast enhancement in the acute phase of the hemorrhage often have a specific pattern revealing the diagnosis. For instance, arteriovenous malformations typically demonstrate the serpiginous vessels of the lesion itself, whereas neoplastic enhancement is usually nodular, diffuse, or ring-like. The presence of other sites of enhancement in the brain parenchyma suggests brain metastases. Mixed signal intensities within the hemorrhage of either a primary or metastatic brain tumor may be due to subacute low-grade bleeding over time. The presence of significant edema around an acute hemorrhage suggests an underlying mass because it takes several days to develop edema after a traumatic or hypertensive ICH.

Patients often have multiple brain metastases. Simultaneous hemorrhage in multiple brain metastases has been noted especially in melanoma, choriocarcinoma and renal cell carcinoma [32–34] (Fig. 3.2). Therefore, multiple simultaneous parenchymal cerebral hemorrhages of the same age should suggest intracranial metastases.

In every patient presenting with an intracerebral hemorrhage, a platelet count and coagulation studies must be performed. A coagulation abnormality may suggest an underlying hematological malignancy or abnormality. In those patients, the history may reveal easy bruising, mucosal bleeding, or bleeding from the nose or uterus.

Table 3.3. Radiological findings suggesting tumor-related hemorrhage

- Presence of significant edema surrounding an acute hemorrhage
- Contrast enhancement contiguous to an acute hemorrhage
- Areas of enhancement elsewhere in the brain suggest the presence of multiple metastases

If the etiology of the intracerebral hemorrhage remains unclear, but tumor is suspected, evacuation is necessary. Examination of blood clot evacuation specimens can lead to a diagnosis of tumor in a subset of cases, particularly if neural tissue is part of the specimen. A larger quantity of neural tissue submitted for histological evaluation correlates with a higher likelihood of establishing the diagnosis [66].

Etiology-specific treatment algorithm

As with any intracerebral hemorrhage from any cause, the initial treatment of a tumor-related hemorrhage is directed at the mass and the management of increased intracranial pressure or cerebral herniation [67–69]. A patient with a stable neurological deficit following intracerebral hemorrhage may be treated with close monitoring and corticosteroids when peritumoral edema is present. Subdural hematoma due to tumor often requires surgical evacuation. This can often be achieved through a burr hole, so that a craniotomy can be avoided. Occasionally, placing a temporary drain or Ommaya reservoir into the subdural space is required to allow drainage of reaccumulated fluid [70]. The fluid drained should be analyzed cytologically for the presence of tumor cells even though a negative result does not exclude cancer. If the subdural hematoma has resulted from subdural tumor, surgical evacuation of the hematoma should be followed by whole brain radiotherapy.

Corticosteroids have no established role in the acute management of primary supratentorial hemorrhages, but they are effective in treating the vasogenic edema caused by a tumor [71]. Treatment of the edema is important, as it will reduce the total mass

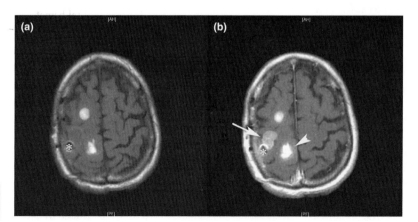

Fig. 3.2 A 77-year-old patient with melanoma and multiple hemorrhagic brain metastases. (a) T1-weighted images: two hyperintense lesions due to hemorrhage into metastases. (There is an artifact due to the presence of a clip: *) (b) T1-weighted images post-contrast: an additional metastasis without hemorrhage is visualized (arrow). Note the enhancement contiguous to one hemorrhage (arrowhead) suggesting the presence of underlying tumoral tissue as well as the appearance of a third lesion, which was not hemorrhagic.

produced by the tumor, hematoma, and edema. The mechanism of action of steroids is not well understood but may be linked to a reduction in the permeability of tumor capillaries [72].

Seizure is a possible presentation of acute hemorrhage and needs to be treated with anticonvulsants [73]. To date, no study has evaluated the indication of prophylactic antiepileptic treatment in patients with hemorrhages from brain tumors. In patients with brain tumors or metastases without hemorrhage, prophylactic administration of antiepileptic drugs does not reduce the incidence of subsequent seizure [74,75]. The Quality Standards Subcommittee of the American Academy of Neurology therefore advises against prophylactic anticonvulsant medications as this does not provide substantial benefit [76]. Even though patients with tumor-associated hemorrhages show an increased risk of seizure, there is no evidence that anticonvulsant prophylaxis is more effective in this subgroup than in the population of patients with brain tumors as a whole. Similarly, there is no evidence that prophylactic antiepileptics reduce the postoperative risk of seizure following craniotomy [77,78]. Therefore, prophylactic anticonvulsants should be avoided.

After the patient has been stabilized acutely, treatment should be directed against the underlying tumor. If the patient appears to have a primary brain tumor, this will likely include neurosurgery. Subsequent treatment with cranial irradiation or chemotherapy will depend upon the pathological diagnosis.

A single brain metastasis should be resected if technically feasible [79]. Patients with multiple brain metastases may benefit from resection if there is a single large hemorrhagic lesion or a hemorrhagic mass is responsible for disabling symptoms. In a patient with a known systemic cancer who suffers an intracerebral hemorrhage, but in whom the CT or MRI does not conclusively establish the presence of a metastasis, careful follow-up with radiological studies repeated a few weeks after the hemorrhage should be performed to exclude an underlying tumor.

Depending upon the tumor type, radiotherapy may either follow resection or be the primary treatment for patients with multiple brain metastases or when the tumor is located in an area that is not surgically accessible. Radiotherapy should be administered according to the appropriate protocol regardless of whether the tumor is associated with hemorrhage. Similarly, radiation should not be delayed because of the presence of a hemorrhage. However, stereotactic radiosurgery is not recommended for a tumor following an acute hemorrhage because of the difficulty defining the target, the potential for increasing cerebral edema and the potential for increased risk of further bleeding [80].

The prognosis of a hemorrhagic neoplasm is primarily determined by the prognosis of the underlying malignancy. If the hemorrhage is asymptomatic or only minimally symptomatic, the overall prognosis will not be different from that of an identical non-hemorrhagic tumor. Therefore, in this situation, the presence of a hemorrhage within an intracranial neoplasm should not alter the therapeutic approach. If the hemorrhage presents with severe neurological deficits or coma, the prognosis will be poor with patients typically surviving only days to weeks [8,14,34,57,58,81].

References

1. Panagos P, Jauch E, Broderick J. Intracerebral hemorrhage. *Emerg Med Clin North Am* 2002; **20**: 631–655.

2. Licata B, Turazzi S. Bleeding cerebral neoplasms with symptomatic hematoma. *J Neurosurg Sci* 2003; **47**: 201–210.

3. Luessenhop A, Shevlin W, Ferrero A, Mccullough D, Barone B. Surgical management of primary intracerebral hemorrhage. *J Neurosurg* 1967; **27**: 419–427.

4. Mutlu N, Berry R, Alpers B. Massive cerebral hemorrhage. Clinical and pathological correlations. *Arch Neurol* 1963; **8**: 644–661.

5. Weisberg L. Computerized tomography in intracranial hemorrhage. *Arch Neurol* 1979; **36**: 422–426.

6. McCormick W, Rosenfield D. Massive brain hemorrhage: a review of 144 cases and an examination of their causes. *Stroke* 1973; **4**: 946–954.

7. Barth H, Fritsch G, Haaks T. [Intracerebral hematoma as an acute manifestation of intracranial tumors]. *Nervenarzt* 1994; **65**: 854–858.

8. Graus F, Rogers L, Posner J. Cerebrovascular complications in patients with cancer. *Medicine (Baltimore)* 1985; **64**: 16–35.

9. Kondziolka D, Bernstein M, Resch L, *et al.* Significance of hemorrhage into brain tumors: clinicopathological study. *J Neurosurg* 1987; **67**: 852–857.

10. Rogers L. Cerebrovascular complications in cancer patients. *Oncology (Huntingt)* 1994; **8**: 23–30.

11. Wakai S, Yamakawa K, Manaka S, Takakura K. Spontaneous intracranial hemorrhage caused by brain

tumor: its incidence and clinical significance. *Neurosurgery* 1982; **10**: 437–444.

12. Minette S, Kimmel D. Subdural hematoma in patients with systemic cancer. *Mayo Clin Proc* 1989; **64**: 637–642.

13. Locksley H, Sahs A, Sandler R. Report on the cooperative study of intracranial aneurysms and subarachnoid hemorrhage. 3. Subarachnoid hemorrhage unrelated to intracranial aneurysm and A–V malformation. A study of associated diseases and prognosis. *J Neurosurg* 1966; **24**: 1034–1056.

14. Little J, Dial B, Belanger G, Carpenter S. Brain hemorrhage from intracranial tumor. *Stroke* 1979; **10**: 283–288.

15. Wakai S, Kumakura N, Nagai M. Lobar intracerebral hemorrhage. A clinical, radiographic, and pathological study of 29 consecutive operated cases with negative angiography. *J Neurosurg* 1992; **76**: 231–238.

16. Manganiello L. Massive spontaneous hemorrhage in gliomas: a report of seven verified cases. *J Nerv Ment Dis* 1949; **110**: 277–298.

17. Lieu A, Hwang S, Howng S, Chai C. Brain tumors with hemorrhage. *J Formos Med Assoc* 1999; **98**: 365–367.

18. Lopes M. Angiogenesis in brain tumors. *Microsc Res Tech* 2003; **60**: 225–230.

19. Nathoo N, Chahlavi A, Barnett G, Toms S. Pathobiology of brain metastases. *J Clin Pathol* 2005; **58**: 237–242.

20. Plate K, Risau W. Angiogenesis in malignant gliomas. *Glia* 1995; **15**: 339–347.

21. Pietsch T, Valter M, Wolf H, *et al.* Expression and distribution of vascular endothelial growth factor protein in human brain tumors. *Acta Neuropathol* 1997; **93**: 109–117.

22. Ferrara N, Houck K, Jakeman L, Leung D. Molecular and biological properties of the vascular endothelial growth factor family of proteins. *Endocr Rev* 1992; **13**: 18–32.

23. Cheng S, Nagane M, Huang H, Cavenee W. Intracerebral tumor-associated hemorrhage caused by overexpression of the vascular endothelial growth factor isoforms VEGF121 and VEGF165 but not VEGF189. *Proc Natl Acad Sci U S A* 1997; **94**: 12081–12087.

24. Liwnicz B, Wu S, Tew J J. The relationship between the capillary structure and hemorrhage in gliomas. *J Neurosurg* 1987; **66**: 536–541.

25. Niiro M, Ishimaru K, Hirano H, Yunoue S, Kuratsu J. Clinico-pathological study of meningiomas with hemorrhagic onset. *Acta Neurochir (Wien)* 2003; **145**: 767–772.

26. Jones N, Blumbergs P. Intracranial hemorrhage from meningiomas: a report of five cases. *Br J Neurosurg* 1989; **3**: 691–698.

27. Lazaro R, Messer H, Brinker R. Intracranial hemorrhage associated with meningioma. *Neurosurgery* 1981; **8**: 96–101.

28. Lefranc F, Nagy N, Dewitte O, Baleriaux D, Brotchi J. Intracranial meningiomas revealed by non-traumatic subdural hematomas: a series of four cases. *Acta Neurochir (Wien)* 2001; **143**: 977–982.

29. Cardoso E, Peterson E. Pituitary apoplexy: a review. *Neurosurgery* 1984; **14**: 363–373.

30. Kaplan B, Day A, Quisling R, Ballinger W. Hemorrhage into pituitary adenomas. *Surg Neurol* 1983; **20**: 280–287.

31. Carral San Laureano F, Gavilan Villarejo I, Olveira Fuster G, Ortego Rojo J, Aguilar Diosdado M. Pituitary apoplexy: retrospective study of 9 patients with hypophyseal adenoma. *An Med Interna* 2001; **18**: 582–586.

32. Weisberg L. Hemorrhagic metastatic intracranial neoplasms: clinical-computed tomographic correlations. *Comput Radiol* 1985; **9**: 105–114.

33. Gildersleeve NJ, Koo A, Mcdonald C. Metastic tumor presenting as intracerebral hemorrhage. Report of 6 cases examined by computed tomography. *Radiology* 1977; **124**: 109–112.

34. Mandybur T. Intracranial hemorrhage caused by metastatic tumors. *Neurology* 1977; **27**: 650–655.

35. Gliemroth J, Nowak G, Kehler U, Arnold H, Gaebel C. Neoplastic cerebral aneurysm from metastatic lung adenocarcinoma associated with cerebral thrombosis and recurrent subarachnoid haemorrhage. *J Neurol Neurosurg Psychiatry* 1999; **66**: 246–247.

36. Murata J, Sawamura Y, Takahashi A, Abe H, Saitoh H. Intracerebral hemorrhage caused by a neoplastic aneurysm from small-cell lung carcinoma: case report. *Neurosurgery* 1993; **32**: 124–126.

37. Schnee C, Flamm E. Unusual aneurysms. *Neuroimaging Clin N Am* 1997; **7**: 803–818.

38. Bick R. Coagulation abnormalities in malignancy: a review. *Semin Thromb Hemost* 1992; **18**: 353–372.

39. Thoron L, Arbit E. Hemostatic changes in patients with brain tumors. *J Neurooncol* 1994; **22**: 87–100.

40. Uchiyama T, Matsumoto M, Kobayashi N. Studies on the pathogenesis of coagulopathy in patients with arterial thromboembolism and malignancy. *Thromb Res* 1990; **59**: 955–965.

41. Nand S, Fisher S, Salgia R, Fisher R. Hemostatic abnormalities in untreated cancer: incidence and

correlation with thrombotic and hemorrhagic complications. *J Clin Oncol* 1987; **5**: 1998–2003.

42. Ey F, Goodnight S. Bleeding disorders in cancer. *Semin Oncol* 1990; **17**: 187–197.

43. Warrell RJ. Pathogenesis and management of acute promyelocytic leukemia. *Annu Rev Med* 1996; **47**: 555–565.

44. Rogers L. Cerebrovascular complications in cancer patients. *Neurol Clin* 2003; **21**: 167–192.

45. Cordonnier C, Vernant J, Brun B, *et al.* Acute promyelocytic leukemia in 57 previously untreated patients. *Cancer* 1985; **55**: 18–25.

46. Feinberg W, Swenson M. Cerebrovascular complications of L-asparaginase therapy. *Neurology* 1988; **38**: 127–133.

47. Gugliotta L, Mazzucconi M, Leone G, *et al.* Incidence of thrombotic complications in adult patients with acute lymphoblastic leukaemia receiving L-asparaginase during induction therapy: a retrospective study. The GIMEMA Group. *Eur J Haematol* 1992; **49**: 63–66.

48. Urban C, Sager W. Intracranial bleeding during therapy with L-asparaginase in childhood acute lymphocytic leukemia. *Eur J Pediatr* 1981; **137**: 323–327.

49. Beinart G, Damon L. Thrombosis associated with L-asparaginase therapy and low fibrinogen levels in adult acute lymphoblastic leukemia. *Am J Hematol* 2004; **77**: 331–335.

50. Nadir Y, Hoffman R, Brenner B. Drug-related thrombosis in hematological malignancies. *Rev Clin Exp Hematol* 2004; **8**: E4.

51. Gordon L, Kwaan H. Thrombotic microangiopathy manifesting as thrombotic thrombocytopenic purpura/hemolytic uremic syndrome in the cancer patient. *Semin Thromb Hemost* 1999; **25**: 217–221.

52. Cheng K, Chan C, Fu Y, *et al.* Acute hemorrhage in late radiation necrosis of the temporal lobe: report of five cases and review of the literature. *J Neurooncol* 2001; **51**: 143–150.

53. Hillemanns A, Kortmann R, Herrlinger U, Skalej M, Krapf H. Recurrent delayed brain hemorrhage over years after irradiation and chemotherapy for astrocytoma. *Eur Radiol* 2003; **13**: 1891–1894.

54. Larson J, Ball W, Bove K, Crone K, Tew JJ. Formation of intracerebral cavernous malformations after radiation treatment for central nervous system neoplasia in children. *J Neurosurg* 1998; **88**: 51–56.

55. Lee J, Chelvarajah R, King A, David K. Rare presentations of delayed radiation injury: a lobar hematoma and a cystic space-occupying lesion appearing more than 15 years after cranial radiotherapy: report of two cases. *Neurosurgery* 2004; **54**: 1010–1013; discussion 1013–4.

56. Malheiros S, Nogueira R, Franco C, Carrete HJ, Gabbai A. Delayed brain hemorrhage after radiotherapy. *Cerebrovasc Dis* 2001; **11**: 141–142.

57. Scott M. Spontaneous intracerebral hematoma caused by cerebral neoplasms. Report of eight verified cases. *J Neurosurg* 1975; **42**: 338–342.

58. Wakai S, Inoh S, Ueda Y, Nagai M. Hemangioblastoma presenting with intraparenchymatous hemorrhage. *J Neurosurg* 1984; **61**: 956–960.

59. Weisberg L. Hemorrhagic primary intracranial neoplasms: clinical-computed tomographic correlations. *Comput Radiol* 1986; **10**: 131–136.

60. Poussaint T, Barnes P, Anthony D, *et al.* Hemorrhagic pituitary adenomas of adolescence. *AJNR Am J Neuroradiol* 1996; **17**: 1907–1912.

61. Levy A. Pituitary disease: presentation, diagnosis, and management. *J Neurol Neurosurg Psychiatry* 2004; **75** Suppl 3: iii47–52.

62. Kim J, Lee J, Lee M. Small primary intracerebral hemorrhage. Clinical presentation of 28 cases. *Stroke* 1994; **25**: 1500–1506.

63. Grossman RI, Yousem DM. Vascular diseases of the brain. In: Grossman RI, Yousem DM, eds. *Neuroradiology. The Requisites*, 2nd edn. St. Louis, Mosby. 2003; 173–242.

64. Leclerc X, Khalil C, Silvera S, *et al.* Imaging of non-traumatic intracerebral hematoma. *J Neuroradiol* 2003; **30**: 303–316.

65. Meyer J, Gorey M. Differential diagnosis of non-traumatic intracranial hemorrhage. *Neuroimaging Clin N Am* 1998; **8**: 263–293.

66. Abrahams N, Prayson R. The role of histopathologic examination of intracranial blood clots removed for hemorrhage of unknown etiology: a clinical pathological analysis of 31 cases. *Ann Diagn Pathol* 2000; **4**: 361–366.

67. Juvela S, Heiskanen O, Poranen A, *et al.* The treatment of spontaneous intracerebral hemorrhage. A prospective randomized trial of surgical and conservative treatment. *J Neurosurg* 1989; **70**: 755–758.

68. Qureshi A, Tuhrim S, Broderick J, *et al.* Spontaneous intracerebral hemorrhage. *N Engl J Med* 2001; **344**: 1450–1460.

69. Rincon F, Mayer S. Novel therapies for intracerebral hemorrhage. *Curr Opin Crit Care* 2004; **10**: 94–100.

70. Stieg P, Kase C. Intracranial hemorrhage: diagnosis and emergency management. *Neurol Clin* 1998; **16**: 373–390.

39

71. Poungvarin N, Bhoopat W, Viriyavejakul A, *et al.* Effects of dexamethasone in primary supratentorial intracerebral hemorrhage. *N Engl J Med* 1987; **316**: 1229–1233.

72. Heiss J, Papavassiliou E, Merrill M, *et al.* Mechanism of dexamethasone suppression of brain tumor-associated vascular permeability in rats. Involvement of the glucocorticoid receptor and vascular permeability factor. *J Clin Invest* 1996; **98**: 1400–1408.

73. Holland K. Efficacy, pharmacology, and adverse effects of antiepileptic drugs. *Neurol Clin* 2001; **19**: 313–345.

74. Forsyth P, Weaver S, Fulton D, *et al.* Prophylactic anticonvulsants in patients with brain tumour. *Can J Neurol Sci* **30**: 106–112.

75. Glantz M, Cole B, Friedberg M, *et al.* A randomized, blinded, placebo-controlled trial of divalproex sodium prophylaxis in adults with newly diagnosed brain tumors. *Neurology* 1996; **46**: 985–991.

76. Glantz M, Cole B, Forsyth P, *et al.* Practice parameter: anticonvulsant prophylaxis in patients with newly diagnosed brain tumors. Report of the Quality Standards Subcommittee of the American Academy of Neurology. *Neurology* 2000; **54**: 1886–1893.

77. Foy P, Chadwick D, Rajgopalan N, Johnson A, Shaw M. Do prophylactic anticonvulsant drugs alter the pattern of seizures after craniotomy. *J Neurol Neurosurg Psychiatry* 1992; **55**: 753–757.

78. Kuijlen J, Teernstra O, Kessels A, Herpers M, Beuls E. Effectiveness of antiepileptic prophylaxis used with supratentorial craniotomies: a meta-analysis. *Seizure* 1996; **5**: 291–298.

79. Patchell R. The management of brain metastases. *Cancer Treat Rev* 2003; **29**: 533–540.

80. Boyd T, Mehta M. Radiosurgery for brain metastases. *Neurosurg Clin N Am* 1999; **10**: 337–350.

81. Richardson R, Siqueira E, Cerullo L. Malignant glioma: its initial presentation as intracranial haemorrhage. *Acta Neurochir (Wien)* 1979; **46**: 77–84.

Cerebral amyloid angiopathy

Steven M. Greenberg

Most human diseases have been recognized clinically many years before they are understood pathologically. In the case of cerebral amyloid angiopathy (CAA), this process has occurred precisely in reverse. Amyloid deposits in small- and medium-sized vessels of the cerebral cortex and leptomeninges (subsequently recognized as congophilic [1]) were described in the German neuropathological literature as early as 1909 and 1910 [2,3]. Cerebral amyloid angiopathy was not linked to clinical disease, however, until the second half of the twentieth century when it was reported as a rare cause of hemorrhagic stroke [4–6]. Even today, with CAA established as a major cause of primary intracerebral hemorrhage (ICH) in the elderly, our understanding of the full spectrum of clinical syndromes associated with CAA remains in evolution.

The current chapter will focus on the pathogenesis of CAA (including the rapidly growing area of transgenic mouse models), clinical and genetic risk factors, presentations and diagnosis, and prospects for treatment. Various aspects of CAA have also been discussed in a large number of excellent review articles from leading contemporary authorities on this disorder [7–16].

Pathogenesis and experimental systems

Advanced CAA (Fig. 4.1) consists of vascular deposition of amyloid and secondary breakdown of amyloid-laden vessel walls. Vessels affected by CAA are the capillaries, arterioles, and small and medium-sized arteries of the cerebral cortex, overlying leptomeninges, and cerebellum; vessels of the white and deep gray matter structures are largely spared. Earliest deposition of amyloid occurs at the border of the vessel media and adventitia, a location postulated to reflect the clearance of ß-amyloid from the brain via interstitial fluid drainage pathways along the periarterial space (Fig. 4.2) [17]. The prevalence of detectable CAA in the aged brain is high, approximately 10–40% in the general elderly and 80% or more among those with concomitant Alzheimer's disease (AD) [13]. The secondary pathological changes associated with advanced CAA include loss of vascular smooth muscle cells, microaneurysms, concentric splitting of the vessel wall, chronic perivascular or transmural inflammation, and fibrinoid necrosis [18–23]. These CAA-related vasculopathic changes are often accompanied by leakage of blood products and appear to comprise the substrate for symptomatic CAA-related ICH [18,19,24–26].

The principal constituent of both vascular amyloid in CAA and plaque amyloid in AD (Fig. 4.1) is the ß-amyloid peptide (Aß), a 39 to 43 amino acid proteolytic fragment of the 695 to 770 residue ß-amyloid precursor protein (APP). Deposition of "long" Aß peptides with carboxyl termini extending to position 42 or 43 (termed Aß42) appears to be a necessary early step in initiation of CAA [27–29], whereas the shorter Aß40 (terminating at position 39 or 40) is the predominant species in vessels with substantial CAA involvement [30–37]. Other proteins or protein fragments detected in association with vascular amyloid include Apolipoprotein E, cystatin C, alpha-synuclein, heparan sulfate proteoglycan, amyloid P component, and complement proteins [38–44].

Major insights into the pathogenesis of human CAA have emerged from the rapidly developing field of transgenic mouse modeling (Fig. 4.3). Mouse lines overexpressing mutant forms of APP demonstrate many of the features of advanced human CAA,

Intracerebral Hemorrhage, ed. J. R. Carhuapoma, S. A. Mayer, and D. F. Hanley. Published by Cambridge University Press.
© J. R. Carhuapoma, S. A. Mayer, and D. F. Hanley 2010.

(a) (b)

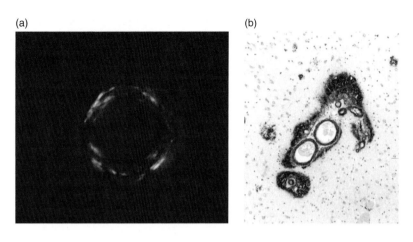

Fig. 4.1 Neuropathological appearance of CAA. Congo red stain (a) shows the characteristic green birefringence under polarized light of a vessel with complete replacement of its wall with amyloid. Another brain with advanced CAA (b) demonstrates extensive ß-amyloid immunostaining in vessels and the immediately surrounding brain parenchyma (sometimes referred to as dyshoric CAA) as well as senile plaques. (Images courtesy of Dr. Matthew P. Frosch, Massachusetts General Hospital and Harvard Medical School, Boston, MA.) See plate section for color version.

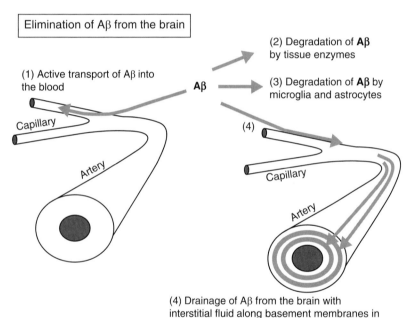

Fig. 4.2 Model for vascular deposition of ß-amyloid. The diagram demonstrates several recognized mechanisms for elimination of Aß from the brain: (1) active transport of Aß into the blood via proteins such as low density lipoprotein receptor-related protein-1 [194,195] and P-glycoprotein [196]; (2) degradation by enzymes in the brain parenchyma [197], (3) microglia [14], and astrocytes [198]; and (4) elimination along the perivascular pathways by which interstitial fluid drains from the brain [17,199]. As mechanisms (1), (2), and (3) fail with age, Aß appears to become increasingly entrapped from the interstitial fluid drainage pathways into the basement membranes of capillaries and small arteries (shown in green) [17,200]. (Figure courtesy of Drs. Roy O. Weller, Roxana Carare-Nnadi, Delphine Boche, and James A. R. Nicoll, University of Southampton School of Medicine, Southampton, UK.) See plate section for color version.

including age-dependent Aß deposition in leptomeningeal and cortical arterioles, loss of vascular smooth muscle cells, aneurysmal dilatation, perivascular microgliosis and astrocytosis, perivascular microhemorrhage, and frank ICH [45–52]. The source of Aß in these mice is largely neuronal, further supporting the model of Aß circulation from brain parenchyma to periarterial space noted above (Fig. 4.2) [17]. Once CAA appears, non-invasive multiphoton imaging of mice at different time points suggests that it progresses primarily by growth of already established deposits [52,53].

Mouse studies have shed particular light on the question of which factors predispose to appearance and growth of CAA in preference to senile plaque formation. One such factor is the structure of the Aß peptide itself: amino acid substitutions associated with hereditary human CAA such as the Dutch [54,55] or Iowa [56] mutations appear to target the peptide for vascular deposition [50,57]. Another

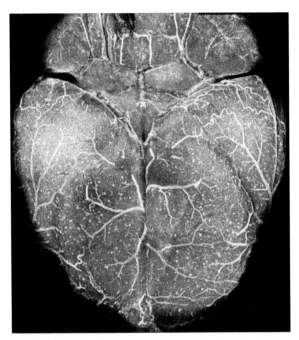

Fig. 4.3 Cerebral amyloid angiopathy in a transgenic mouse. Cerebral amyloid angiopathy in leptomeningeal and superficial cortical vessels and amyloid-containing plaques are demonstrated in the brain of a 22-month old Tg2576 transgenic mouse [201] Amyloid is stained with thioflavin S and imaged by two-photon microscopy [52].

identified factor is Apolipoprotein E. Genetic knock-out of mouse Apolipoprotein E prevented both CAA and CAA-related hemorrhage [49], whereas knockin of the human Apolipoprotein E ϵ4 gene preferentially restored CAA formation [58]. A third factor highlighted by mouse studies is inflammation. Overexpression of transforming growth factor (TGF)-ß1, for example, was found to have inverse effects on plaque and vessel amyloid, decreasing plaque deposits and increasing extent of CAA [59,60].

Another important role for transgenic mouse and other experimental systems has been to investigate physiological and toxic effects of Aß. The peptide has effects on resting vessel diameter [61] and dilatation to pharmacological or physiological stimuli [47, 62,63], possibly reflecting direct physiological or toxic effects of Aß on the contractile/relaxation elements of the vessel wall [64–70]. The β-amyloid peptide also appears to stimulate synthesis and activation of the inflammatory mediator matrix metalloproteinase-9 in cerebrovascular endothelial cells [71], offering another potential cellular mechanism for CAA-related tissue damage [72]. A further in-vitro property of

Aß is to stimulate tissue-type plasminogen activator [73,74], potentially promoting ICH through direct effects on the coagulation/thrombolysis cascade as well as on the integrity of the vessel wall.

Clinical and genetic risk factors

Cerebral amyloid angiopathy-related ICH accounts for a substantial proportion of all spontaneous ICH in the elderly. Typical estimates of 10–20% have been noted in autopsies of elderly ICH patients [13]. Using a different approach of analyzing consecutive clinical ICH patients at the Massachusetts General Hospital (MGH), we have estimated 34% of primary ICH in the elderly as due to CAA (based on the 46% of primary ICH noted to occur in lobar locations multiplied by the 74% of lobar ICH found to have advanced CAA on neuropathological examination [75]). Aging of the population, increasing use of anticoagulants and thrombolytics, and lack of effective preventative strategies suggest that the absolute incidence and proportion of CAA-related ICH will increase.

Advancing age is the strongest clinical risk factor for CAA-related ICH, as predicted by the age-dependence of the underlying pathology [13,76–79]. All 26 patients identified with CAA-related ICH in three large autopsy series [5,80,81] were over age 60 and 23 of 26 (88%) over age 70. Consecutive patients at MGH [82] analyzed for age of first CAA-related ICH demonstrated similar age-dependence, though with slightly younger age distribution (mean age of 76.1±8.3) as expected in a clinical series. Ninety-seven percent of patients were over age 60 at first hemorrhage, 75% over age 70, 39% over age 80 and 4% (4 of 105 patients) in their 90s. There was no marked predilection for *gender* either in our clinical series (54% male, 46% female) or in pathological cases (49% male, 51% female) [7].

Dementia has generally been considered a major risk factor for CAA-related ICH because of the close molecular relationship between CAA and AD. A pathological study of 117 consecutive brains with AD indeed demonstrated advanced CAA to be common, with moderate to severe CAA pathology in 25.6% and CAA-related hemorrhages in 5.1% [83]. An MRI-based study of 59 subjects (mean age 77) with AD found microhemorrhages to be surprisingly prevalent (32%) [84], though the proportion caused by CAA is unclear. Another recent study of consecutive subjects presenting to a memory disorders unit [85] found corticosubcortical microhemorrhages in 9 of 61 (15%), with 7 of the 9 showing multiple microhemorrhage highly suggestive of CAA [75]. Despite these observations, approximately 60–80% of patients diagnosed with CAA-related ICH were *not* cognitively impaired prior to their initial hemorrhagic stroke [7,18,86,87]. It is thus unclear from a clinical standpoint whether the presence or absence of dementia is useful in making the diagnosis of CAA. The association of CAA and AD appears due in part to the shared genetic risk factor Apolipoprotein E ε4 [88].

Despite *hypertension*'s (HTN) clear importance in promoting necrosis and rupture of the deep penetrating vessels [89], there is little evidence for a major role in CAA-related ICH. The estimated prevalence of HTN in CAA is in the range of 32% (determined from 107 pathological cases of CAA reviewed by Vinters [7]) to 52% (measured in our 105 consecutive clinical cases diagnosed with CAA [82]), figures not much greater than the expected rate of HTN for the general elderly. Hypertension is significantly less frequent in lobar ICH than ICH of the deep hemispheres, cerebellum, or pons in most [86,90–92] (though not all [93,94]) studies of the elderly. Most notably, midpoint analysis of the population-based Greater Cincinnati/Northern Kentucky study found no association between HTN and lobar ICH [95], though a more recent analysis in this study suggested that untreated HTN may increase risk [96]. Among other vascular factors, neither *diabetes mellitus* nor *coronary atherosclerosis* has demonstrated an elevated frequency in our CAA cohort.

Other clinical risk factors have been suggested for lobar ICH without specific evidence linking them to CAA. The Greater Cincinnati/Northern Kentucky study identified *previous ischemic stroke* and *frequent alcohol use* in addition to Apolipoprotein E genotype and family history of ICH (see below) as predictors of lobar ICH in a multivariable model [95]. *Low serum cholesterol* has been found to associate with ICH in several other population-based studies [97–102]. The few studies that have analyzed ICH according to location or presumed etiology have not indicated a specific relationship of cholesterol to CAA-related hemorrhages [103,104].

Genetic mutations are rare causes of CAA-related hemorrhage, though those mutations that have been identified have proven highly instructive [105]. Most

of the mutations associated with CAA-related ICH occur in the Aß-coding region of APP [54–56,106–110], a striking contrast to the AD associated mutations that flank the Aß-coding segment [111]. Another interesting aspect to the CAA-associated mutations of APP is that the same amino acid substitution can result in hemorrhagic strokes in one family and CAA without major ICH in another [112,113], suggesting that there are other genetic or non-genetic cofactors required for expression of a full hemorrhagic phenotype. Other familial CAAs with vascular deposition of amyloids unrelated to Aß include the Icelandic cystatin C mutation with early onset and severe ICH [114,115], the dementia syndromes associated with mutations of the BRI protein [116,117], and mutations of the transthyretin gene affecting the central nervous system primarily by meningeal hemorrhage [118–123].

Apolipoprotein E has emerged as the strongest genetic risk factor for the much more common sporadic form of CAA-related ICH. The Apolipoprotein E ε2 and ε4 alleles appear to promote CAA-related ICH at two distinct steps in the disease's pathogenesis, ε4 predicting increased deposition of Aß in vessels (as it does in plaques) [88,124–128] and ε2 associating with the CAA-related vasculopathic changes such as concentric vessel splitting and fibrinoid necrosis [26,129]. Each of these alleles was more than twofold overrepresented among 182 reviewed pathological cases of CAA-related ICH [130]. The general importance of Apolipoprotein E to lobar ICH was further supported by the Greater Cincinnati/Northern Kentucky analysis, in which presence of Apolipoprotein E ε2 or ε4 associated with an adjusted odds ratio for lobar ICH of 2.3 [95]. The Apolipoprotein E alleles had an attributable risk for lobar ICH of 29% in this study, the largest proportion for any risk factor examined. Both Apolipoprotein E ε2 and ε4 appear to associate not only with increased risk for ICH occurrence, but also with a younger age of first hemorrhage [129] and a shorter time till ICH recurrence (see below) [131].

The Greater Cincinnati/Northern Kentucky study found substantial risk for lobar ICH associated with *family history of ICH* even after controlling for Apolipoprotein E genotype [95] suggesting other as yet unidentified genetic risk factors for sporadic CAA. Among the long list of potential candidate genes are those encoding for presenilin-1, neprilysin and TGF-ß1 [132–134].

Clinical presentation and diagnosis
Spontaneous and iatrogenic ICH

Cerebral amyloid angiopathy-related hemorrhages largely follow the distribution of the vascular amyloid, appearing with highest frequency in the cortico-subcortical or lobar regions, less commonly in cerebellum, and generally sparing the brainstem and deep hemispheric structures [7,81]. Among the cortical lobes, CAA-related hemorrhages occur preferentially in the occipital and temporal lobes relative to their cortical volumes (Fig. 4.4) [135]. This pattern of hemorrhage distribution also appears to reflect the distribution of vascular amyloid deposits, reported in several series to favor posterior brain regions [76,77,136]. Although lobar ICH in CAA often dissects into the subarachnoid space [81,137–139], primary subarachnoid hemorrhage due to CAA is rare [138, 140].

Cerebral amyloid angiopathy-related lobar ICH presents similarly to other types of lobar ICH [141] with acute onset of neurological symptoms and the variable presence of headache, seizures, or decreased consciousness according to hemorrhage size and location. Cerebral amyloid angiopathy-related hemorrhages can also be small and clinically silent [6]. These "microbleeds" are well visualized by gradient echo or T2*-weighted MRI techniques (Fig. 4.5),

which enhance the signal dropout associated with deposited hemosiderin [142–145]. By detecting even old hemorrhagic lesions, gradient echo MRI provides a clinical method for demonstrating an individual's lifetime history of hemorrhage and thus for identifying the pattern of multiple lobar lesions characteristic of CAA.

The Boston criteria for CAA codify the typical features of CAA-related ICH into diagnostic categories of "definite," "probable," and "possible" disease as listed in Table 4.1 [75,86]. While diagnosis of *definite CAA* requires demonstration of advanced disease through full postmortem examination, a clinical diagnosis of *probable CAA* can be reached during life by radiographic evidence of two or more strictly lobar or corticosubcortical hemorrhagic lesions without other definite hemorrhagic processes. In a clinical-pathological validation study, 13 of 13 subjects diagnosed clinically with probable CAA also showed CAA pathologically [75], suggesting that the criteria may be sufficiently specific to be useful in practice. In the same study, gradient echo MRI detected the diagnostic pattern in 8 of 11 patients (73%) with pathologically documented CAA, providing an estimate for the sensitivity of the diagnosis. The Boston criteria propose a separate category of *probable CAA with supporting pathology* for patients with lobar ICH and a brain sample (biopsy or resected hematoma

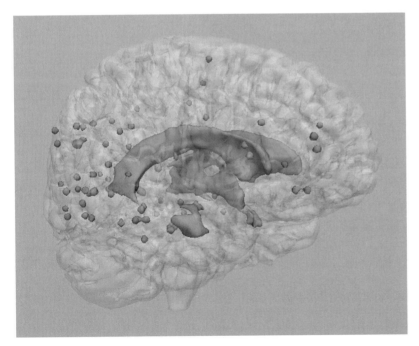

Fig. 4.4 Three-dimensional representation of the distribution of CAA-related hemorrhages. Each dot represents the center of a hemorrhage in a set of 20 patients with probable CAA mapped onto a composite three-dimensional template [135]. See plate section for color version.

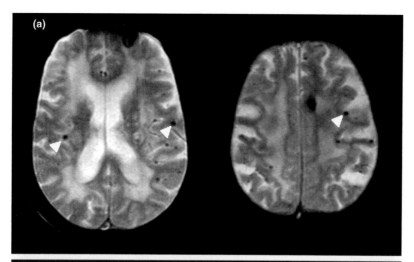

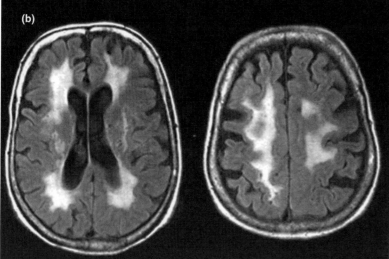

Fig. 4.5 Magnetic resonance imaging appearance of CAA. Axial MRI images are shown for a 76-year-old woman with progressive deficits of cognition and gait and no known vascular risk factors. Gradient echo images (a) demonstrate multiple strictly lobar microbleeds (arrowheads) as well as a larger left frontal hemorrhage, meeting Boston criteria for probable CAA. Fluid attenuated inversion recovery sequences (b) highlight confluent areas of white matter hyperintensity.

Table 4.1. Boston criteria for diagnosis of CAA-related ICH

Definite CAA

Full postmortem examination of brain showing lobar ICH, severe CAA [19], and no other diagnostic lesion

Probable CAA with supporting pathology

Clinical data and pathological tissue (evacuated hematoma or cortical biopsy) showing lobar ICH, some degree of CAA in pathological specimen, and no other diagnostic lesion

Probable CAA

Clinical data and MRI or CT scan showing two or more hemorrhagic lesions restricted to lobar regions (cerebellar hemorrhage allowed), age ≥ 55, and no other cause of hemorrhage*

Possible CAA

Clinical data and MRI or CT scan showing single lobar ICH, age ≥ 55, and no other cause of hemorrhage*

Notes: *Other causes of ICH defined as excessive anticoagulation (International Normalized Ratio > 3.0), antecedent head trauma or ischemic stroke, central nervous system tumor, vascular malformation, or vasculitis, blood dyscrasia or coagulopathy. INR > 3.0 or other non-specific laboratory abnormalities permitted for diagnosis of *possible CAA*.

specimen) with CAA. A validation study for this diagnosis suggested that CAA of at least moderate severity in a random tissue sample was a reasonably specific marker for severe CAA in the brain as a whole [79].

Iatrogenic ICH related to anticoagulation or coronary thrombolysis comprises an important and highly lethal manifestation of CAA. Anticoagulation is hypothesized to promote ICH by allowing small leakages of blood to expand into large symptomatic hemorrhages [146] and might thus be particularly risky in the setting of advanced CAA. This possibility is supported by demonstration of advanced CAA in individual cases of ICH following either coronary thrombolysis [147–149] or anticoagulation [150]. The largest series of consecutive pathological cases found CAA in 3 of 5 lobar ICHs following thrombolysis for acute myocardial infarction [151] and 7 of 11 lobar ICHs occurring on warfarin [152]. The association of CAA with anticoagulation-related ICH was further supported by an increased frequency of the Apolipoprotein E ε2 allele among patients with lobar ICH on warfarin relative to control patients on warfarin without ICH [152]. The apparent link between CAA and iatrogenic ICH might partially explain the noted age-dependence of these complications [153–156].

Presentations without major hemorrhage

A notable finding in very severe cases of CAA is *cognitive impairment* independent of major hemorrhagic stroke. Cognitive impairment has been observed in both familial [56,157,158] and sporadic [159,160] instances of severe CAA, generally in the absence of extensive AD pathology [56,161]. These observations suggest that CAA can cause clinically important cognitive dysfunction in the broader population of elderly with lesser extents of vascular amyloid [162,163]. This possibility has received further support from two population-based studies correlating cognitive testing or dementia status of subjects during life with neuropathological findings at autopsy. Among subjects in the population-based Medical Research Council (MRC) study [164], severe CAA was associated with an impressively elevated odds ratio for dementia of 7.7 (95% confidence intervals [CI] 3.3–20.4). The relationship between CAA and dementia could easily be confounded by potential covariates such as age or the accompanying presence

of AD pathology; the magnitude of the odds for dementia (9.3, 95% CI 2.7–41.0) was no lower, however, in multivariable analysis controlling for age, brain weight, neuritic and diffuse plaques, neocortical and hippocampal neurofibrillary tangles, Lewy bodies, and cerebrovascular disease. In the population-based Honolulu-Asia Aging study (HAAS) [165], AD plus CAA was associated with significantly worse cognitive performance on testing during life than AD without CAA. Like the findings in the MRC study, this effect of CAA remained independent in analysis controlling for potential confounders such as age, tangle and plaque counts, infarctions, and Apolipoprotein E genotype.

Analysis of white matter damage in patients diagnosed with CAA points to the possibility that CAA-related vascular dysfunction may lead to cognitive impairment. White matter damage in advanced CAA (Fig. 4.5) is ascribed to decreased perfusion via amyloid-laden overlying cortical vessels [166], as the white matter itself is largely spared from CAA. Studies of consecutive patients with probable CAA have found white matter lesions to be both common and severe. In one analysis, white matter hypodensity (measured in the hemisphere contralateral to the ICH) was detectable by CT scan in 69 of 88 subjects (78%) and of severe extent (3 or 4 on a 0 to 4 point scale) in 34 of 88 (39%) [87]. An overlapping study using volumetric MRI techniques found nearly double the volume of normalized white matter hyperintensity in 42 subjects with probable CAA compared to 54 similar aged subjects with AD or mild cognitive impairment (19.8 versus 10.8 cm^3, $p = 0.01$) [167]. These studies, together with neuropathological data [168], support an association between CAA and damage of the deep white matter. Further analysis of subjects with probable CAA found that severe white matter hypodensity on CT was independently associated with the presence of pre-ICH cognitive impairment with an odds ratio greater than 3 [87], suggesting that extent of white matter damage might be an important mechanism for the cognitive effects of advanced CAA.

One further group of patients with CAA, white matter lesions, and cognitive impairment is the subgroup with *vascular inflammation*. Although some increase in inflammatory cells may be a common feature of advanced CAA [18,20], this subgroup demonstrates more robust reactions including perivascular mononuclear and multinucleated giant cells

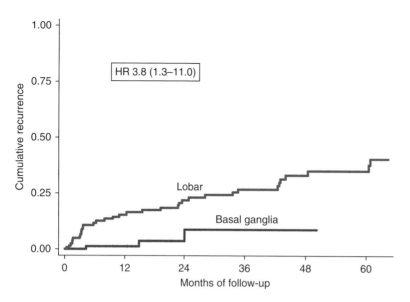

Fig. 4.6 Recurrence risk for lobar and deep hemispheric ICH. A Kaplan-Meier plot demonstrates significantly elevated risk for ICH recurrence among consecutive subjects with lobar (n = 127) relative to basal ganglionic (n = 80) ICH [181]. HR = hazard ratio.

[169] or frank vasculitis [170–174]. In the MGH series, perivascular inflammation was identified in 7 of 42 (17%) consecutive tissue samples from patients pathologically diagnosed with CAA [169], a possible overestimate of the disorder's frequency because of the tendency to perform biopsy in patients with atypical clinical presentations. Patients with CAA-related inflammation generally present with subacute cognitive decline, seizures, or focal or diffuse ischemic injury rather than symptomatic ICH. Many patients show both clinical improvement and partial resolution of their white matter lesions upon treatment with immunosuppression [169,171,175], suggesting that CAA-related inflammation may be a treatable form of CAA.

Cerebral amyloid angiopathy can also present with *transient neurological symptoms* [159,176,177], another syndrome where diagnosis during life is of particular practical importance. The neurological symptoms can include focal weakness, numbness, paresthesias, or language abnormalities, often occurring in a recurrent and stereotyped pattern. Spells typically last for minutes and may spread smoothly from one contiguous body part to another during a single spell. Transient neurological symptoms in CAA appear to be related to the hemorrhagic rather than the ischemic component of the disease, as gradient echo MRI frequently demonstrates otherwise asymptomatic hemorrhage in the cortical region corresponding to the spell [159]. Spells often cease with anticonvulsant treatment. The major practical issue

is to differentiate these episodes by clinical or radiographic means from true transient ischemic attacks, as anticoagulation of patients with advanced CAA may substantially raise the risk for future hemorrhagic stroke.

Clinical course and treatment
Initial outcome and risk of recurrence
Despite improvements in the critical care of stroke, CAA-related lobar ICH remains a highly lethal clinical event: three-month mortality of 28.6% and independent functional outcome of only 30.7% were noted in the MGH study of 184 consecutive non-anticoagulated primary lobar ICH patients age ≥ 55 [178]. Although lobar hemorrhages may be less likely to affect critical brainstem or thalamic structures than deep hemispheric ICH, they also carry several negative prognostic features such as higher age [86] and larger volume [179] that likely account for the comparably poor outcomes of ICH in the two locations [178].

Recurrent hemorrhagic stroke represents a major neurological risk for survivors of an initial CAA-related ICH. A pooled analysis of patients followed after lobar ICH reported a recurrence rate of 4.4% per year [180], with even higher rates noted among consecutive lobar ICH patients seen at MGH [131]. Lobar ICH is associated with substantially higher risk of recurrence compared to deep hemispheric ICH (Fig. 4.6) [181]. The recurrences, like the initial hemorrhages, are typically lobar. Although the site of recurrence is typically distinct from the initial hemorrhage, there is a significant tendency for new hemorrhages to occur in the same lobe as the initial hemorrhage [135].

Identified risk factors for ICH recurrence are the number of previous hemorrhages and Apolipo-protein E genotype [131, 182]. In a study of 94 consecutive lobar ICH patients, the three-year cumulative recurrence risk increased from 14% to 17%, 38%, and 51% for subjects with 1, 2, 3–5, or > 5 hemorrhagic lesions detected at baseline [182]. Possession of either Apolipoprotein E ϵ2 or ϵ4 was also associated with increased risk of recurrence, with highest risk among the subgroup with the rare Apolipoprotein E ϵ2/ϵ4 genotype [131]. Another potential risk for recurrence is the presence of white matter disease [87], though the mechanism for this effect remains unknown. Patient age, sex, and other vascular risk factors such as hypertension or diabetes mellitus were not found to affect risk of ICH recurrence in these studies.

The effect of anticoagulation on risk of ICH recurrence in CAA is unknown, but based on the underlying role played by CAA in some anticoagulant-related hemorrhages (see above), it is presumed to be substantial. Intracerebral hemorrhage during anticoagulation is associated with very poor outcomes [178], raising the question of whether a history of previous lobar ICH should be considered a near absolute contraindication to future anticoagulation. A decision analysis addressing this question for a hypothetical survivor of lobar ICH who also had non-valvular atrial fibrillation found that the risks of anticoagulation outweighed its benefits under a wide range of realistic assumptions [183]. It is therefore reasonable practice to avoid anticoagulation following lobar ICH possibly related to CAA. Antiplatelet medications, conversely, appear not to have large effects on the risk or severity of recurrent ICH [178,181] and may therefore be a safer alternative in lobar ICH patients with strong need for antithrombotic treatment.

Treatment

No evidence has emerged that CAA-related ICH behaves differently from other ICH subtypes in the first hours or days of onset, though this remains an active area of investigation. Lobar location does not appear to affect the likelihood of hematoma expansion [179, 184], and despite theoretical concerns about the fragility of amyloid-laden vessels, CAA does not appear to associate with adverse response to hematoma evacuation [8, 185–189]. It is therefore reasonable to follow the guidelines for acute medical and surgical management of ICH outlined by the American Heart Association Stroke Council [190] without specific modification for CAA. Surgical specimens from hematoma resection (including leptomeningeal tissue if available) should be examined by histochemical and immunochemical methods for the presence and severity of CAA [79].

Future treatments for CAA are likely to focus on preventive or protective therapy aimed at decreasing the deposition or toxicity of vascular amyloid. An example of such an approach is a glycosaminoglycan mimetic designed to interfere with amyloid aggregation and deposition [191] recently evaluated for CAA in a safety, tolerability, and pharmacokinetic study [192]. Our rapidly increasing understanding of the pathogenesis of CAA and AD are likely to supply many new targets for treatment [193], suggesting good prospects for developing effective therapies for this challenging disorder.

References

1. Divry P. Etude histochimique des plaques seniles. *J Belge Neurol Psychiatr* 1927; **27**: 643–657.

2. Fischer O. Die presbyophrene Demenz deren anatomische Grundlage und klinische Abgrenzung. Z. *Gesamte Neurol Psychiatr* 1909; **3**: 371–471.

3. Oppenheim G. Uber drusige Nekrosen in der Grosshirnrinde. *Neurol Centralbl* 1909; **28**: 410–413.

4. Surbek B. L'angiopathie dyshorique (Morel) de l'ecorce cerebrale. *Acta Neuropathol* 1961; **1**: 168–197.

5. Jellinger K. Cerebrovascular amyloidosis with cerebral hemorrhage. *J Neurol* 1977; **214**: 195–206.

6. Okazaki H, Reagan TJ, Campbell RJ. Clinicopathologic studies of primary cerebral amyloid angiopathy. *Mayo Clin Proc* 1979; **54**: 22–31.

7. Vinters HV. Cerebral amyloid angiopathy. A critical review. *Stroke* 1987; **18**: 311–324.

8. Kase CS. Cerebral amyloid angiopathy. In: Kase CS, Caplan LR, eds. *Intracerebral Hemorrhage*. Boston, Butterworth-Heinemann. 1994; 179–200.

9. Yamada M. Cerebral amyloid angiopathy: an overview. *Neuropathology* 2000; **20**: 8–22.

10. Herzig MC, Winkler DT, Walker LC, Jucker M. Transgenic mouse models of cerebral amyloid angiopathy. *Adv Exp Med Biol* 2001; **487**: 123–128.

11. Van Nostrand WE, Melchor JP, Romanov G, Zeigler K, Davis J. Pathogenic effects of cerebral amyloid

angiopathy mutations in the amyloid beta-protein precursor. *Ann N Y Acad Sci* 2002; **977**: 258–265.

12. Kalaria RN. Small vessel disease and Alzheimer's dementia: pathological considerations. *Cerebrovasc Dis* 2002; **13**: 48–52.

13. Jellinger KA. Alzheimer disease and cerebrovascular pathology: an update. *J Neural Transm* 2002; **109**: 813–836.

14. Nicoll JA, Wilkinson D, Holmes C, *et al.* Neuropathology of human Alzheimer disease after immunization with amyloid-beta peptide: a case report. *Nat Med* 2003; **9**: 448–452.

15. Rensink AA, de Waal RM, Kremer B, Verbeek MM. Pathogenesis of cerebral amyloid angiopathy. *Brain Res Brain Res Rev* 2003; **43**: 207–223.

16. Love S. Contribution of cerebral amyloid angiopathy to Alzheimer's disease. *J Neurol Neurosurg Psychiatry* 2004; **75**: 1–4.

17. Weller RO, Massey A, Newman TA, *et al.* Cerebral amyloid angiopathy: amyloid beta accumulates in putative interstitial fluid drainage pathways in Alzheimer's disease. *Am J Pathol* 1998; **153**: 725–733.

18. Mandybur TI. Cerebral amyloid angiopathy: the vascular pathology and complications. *J Neuropathol Exp Neurol* 1986; **45**: 79–90.

19. Vonsattel JP, Myers RH, Hedley-Whyte ET, *et al.* Cerebral amyloid angiopathy without and with cerebral hemorrhages: a comparative histological study. *Ann Neurol* 1991; **30**: 637–649.

20. Yamada M, Itoh Y, Shintaku M, *et al.* Immune reactions associated with cerebral amyloid angiopathy. *Stroke* 1996; **27**: 1155–1162.

21. Maat-Schieman ML, van Duinen SG, Rozemuller AJ, Haan J, Roos RA. Association of vascular amyloid beta and cells of the mononuclear phagocyte system in hereditary cerebral hemorrhage with amyloidosis (Dutch) and Alzheimer disease. *J Neuropathol Exp Neurol* 1997; **56**: 273–284.

22. Uchihara T, Akiyama H, Kondo H, Ikeda K. Activated microglial cells are colocalized with perivascular deposits of amyloid-beta protein in Alzheimer's disease brain. *Stroke* 1997; **28**: 1948–1950.

23. Vinters HV, Natte R, Maat-Schieman ML, *et al.* Secondary microvascular degeneration in amyloid angiopathy of patients with hereditary cerebral hemorrhage with amyloidosis, Dutch type (HCHWA-D). *Acta Neuropathol* 1998; **95**: 235–244.

24. Maeda A, Yamada M, Itoh Y, *et al.* Computer-assisted three-dimensional image analysis of cerebral amyloid angiopathy. *Stroke* 1993; **24**: 1857–1864.

25. Natte R, Vinters HV, Maat-Schieman ML, *et al.* Microvasculopathy is associated with the number of cerebrovascular lesions in hereditary cerebral hemorrhage with amyloidosis, Dutch type. *Stroke.* 1998; **29**: 1588–1594.

26. McCarron MO, Nicoll JA, Stewart J, *et al.* The apolipoprotein E epsilon2 allele and the pathological features in cerebral amyloid angiopathy-related hemorrhage. *J Neuropathol Exp Neurol* 1999; **58**: 711–718.

27. Shinkai Y, Yoshimura M, Ito Y, *et al.* Amyloid ß-proteins 1–40 and 1–42(43) in the soluble fraction of extra- and intracranial blood vessels. *Ann Neurol* 1995; **38**: 421–428.

28. Natte R, Yamaguchi H, Maat-Schieman ML, *et al.* Ultrastructural evidence of early non-fibrillar Abeta42 in the capillary basement membrane of patients with hereditary cerebral hemorrhage with amyloidosis, Dutch type. *Acta Neuropathol* 1999; **98**: 577–582.

29. McGowan E, Pickford F, Kim J, *et al.* Abeta42 is essential for parenchymal and vascular amyloid deposition in mice. *Neuron* 2005; **47**: 191–199.

30. Iwatsubo T, Odaka A, Suzuki N, *et al.* Visualization of A beta 42(43) and A beta 40 in senile plaques with end-specific A beta monoclonals: evidence that an initially deposited species is A beta 42(43). *Neuron* 1994; **13**: 45–53.

31. Mak K, Yang F, Vinters HV, Frautschy SA, Cole GM. Polyclonals to beta-amyloid(1–42) identify most plaque and vascular deposits in Alzheimer cortex, but not striatum. *Brain Res* 1994; **667**: 138–142.

32. Gravina SA, Ho LB, Eckman CB, *et al.* Amyloid beta protein (A-beta) in Alzheimers disease brain – biochemical and immunocytochemical analysis with antibodies specific for forms ending at A beta 40 or A beta 42(43). *J Biol Chem* 1995; **270**: 7013–7016.

33. Iwatsubo T, Mann DM, Odaka A, Suzuki N, Ihara Y. Amyloid beta protein (A beta) deposition: A beta 42 (43) precedes A beta 40 in Down syndrome. *Ann Neurol* 1995; **37**: 294–299.

34. Lemere CA, Blusztajn JK, Yamaguchi H, *et al.* Sequence of deposition of heterogeneous amyloid ß-peptides and Apolipoprotein E in Down syndrome. Implications for initial events in amyloid plaque formation. *Neurobiol Dis* 1996; **3**: 16–32.

35. Castano EM, Prelli F, Soto C, *et al.* The length of amyloid-beta in hereditary cerebral hemorrhage with amyloidosis, Dutch type. Implications for the role of amyloid-beta 1–42 in Alzheimer's disease. *J Biol Chem* 1996; **271**: 32185–32191.

36. Mann DM, Iwatsubo T, Ihara Y, *et al.* Predominant deposition of amyloid-beta 42(43) in plaques in cases of Alzheimer's disease and hereditary cerebral hemorrhage associated with mutations in the amyloid

precursor protein gene. *Am J Pathol* 1996; **148**: 1257–1266.

37. Alonzo NC, Hyman BT, Rebeck GW, Greenberg SM. Progression of cerebral amyloid angiopathy. Accumulation of amyloid-ß40 in already affected vessels. *J Neuropathol Exp Neurol* 1998; **57**: 353–359.

38. Snow AD, Mar H, Nochlin D, *et al.* Early accumulation of heparan sulfate in neurons and in the beta-amyloid protein-containing lesions of Alzheimer's disease and Down's syndrome. *Am J Pathol* 1990; **137**: 1253–1270.

39. Vinters HV, Nishimura GS, Secor DL, Pardridge WM. Immunoreactive A4 and gamma-trace peptide colocalization in amyloidotic arteriolar lesions in brains of patients with Alzheimer's disease. *Am J Pathol* 1990; **137**: 233–240.

40. Namba Y, Tomonaga M, Kawasaki H, Otomo E, Ikeda K. Apolipoprotein E immunoreactivity in cerebral amyloid deposits and neurofibrillary tangles in Alzheimer's disease and kuru plaque amyloid in Creutzfeldt-Jakob disease. *Brain Res* 1991; **541**: 163–166.

41. Kalaria RN, Kroon SN. Complement inhibitor C4-binding protein in amyloid deposits containing serum amyloid P in Alzheimer's disease. *Biochem Biophys Res Commun* 1992; **186**: 461–466.

42. Ueda K, Fukushima H, Masliah E, *et al.* Molecular cloning of cDNA encoding an unrecognized component of amyloid in Alzheimer disease. *Proc Natl Acad Sci U S A* 1993; **90**: 11282–11286.

43. Verbeek MM, Eikelenboom P, de Waal RM. Differences between the pathogenesis of senile plaques and congophilic angiopathy in Alzheimer disease. *J Neuropathol Exp Neurol* 1997; **56**: 751–761.

44. Cho HS, Hyman BT, Greenberg SM, Rebeck GW. Quantitation of apoE domains in Alzheimer disease brain suggests a role for apoE in Abeta aggregation. *J Neuropathol Exp Neurol* 2001; **60**: 342–349.

45. Calhoun ME, Burgermeister P, Phinney AL, *et al.* Neuronal overexpression of mutant amyloid precursor protein results in prominent deposition of cerebrovascular amyloid. *Proc Natl Acad Sci U S A* 1999; **96**: 14088–14093.

46. Van Dorpe J, Smeijers L, Dewachter I, *et al.* Prominent cerebral amyloid angiopathy in transgenic mice overexpressing the London mutant of human APP in neurons. *Am J Pathol* 2000; **157**: 1283–1298.

47. Christie R, Yamada M, Moskowitz M, Hyman B. Structural and functional disruption of vascular smooth muscle cells in a transgenic mouse model of amyloid angiopathy. *Am J Pathol* 2001; **158**: 1065–1071.

48. Winkler DT, Bondolfi L, Herzig MC, *et al.* Spontaneous hemorrhagic stroke in a mouse model of cerebral amyloid angiopathy. *J Neurosci* 2001; **21**: 1619–1627.

49. Fryer JD, Taylor JW, DeMattos RB, *et al.* Apolipoprotein E markedly facilitates age-dependent cerebral amyloid angiopathy and spontaneous hemorrhage in amyloid precursor protein transgenic mice. *J Neurosci* 2003; **23**: 7889–7896.

50. Herzig MC, Winkler DT, Burgermeister P, *et al.* Abeta is targeted to the vasculature in a mouse model of hereditary cerebral hemorrhage with amyloidosis. *Nat Neurosci* 2004; **7**: 954–960.

51. Miao J, Xu F, Davis J, *et al.* Cerebral microvascular amyloid beta protein deposition induces vascular degeneration and neuroinflammation in transgenic mice expressing human vasculotropic mutant amyloid beta precursor protein. *Am J Pathol* 2005; **167**: 505–515.

52. Domnitz SB, Robbins EM, Hoang AW, *et al.* Progression of cerebral amyloid angiopathy in transgenic mouse models of Alzheimer disease. *J Neuropathol Exp Neurol* 2005; **64**: 588–594.

53. Robbins EM, Betensky RA, Domnitz SB, *et al.* Kinetics of cerebral amyloid angiopathy progression in a transgenic mouse model of Alzheimer disease. *J Neurosci* 2006; **26**(2): 365–371.

54. Van Broeckhoven C, Haan J, Bakker E, *et al.* Amyloid beta protein precursor gene and hereditary cerebral hemorrhage with amyloidosis (Dutch). *Science* 1990; **248**: 1120–1122.

55. Levy E, Carman MD, Fernandez Madrid IJ, *et al.* Mutation of the Alzheimer's disease amyloid gene in hereditary cerebral hemorrhage, Dutch type. *Science* 1990; **248**: 1124–1126.

56. Grabowski TJ, Cho HS, Vonsattel JPG, Rebeck GW, Greenberg SM. Novel amyloid precursor protein mutation in an Iowa family with dementia and severe cerebral amyloid angiopathy. *Ann Neurol* 2001; **49**: 697–705.

57. Davis J, Xu F, Deane R, *et al.* Early-onset and robust cerebral microvascular accumulation of amyloid beta-protein in transgenic mice expressing low levels of a vasculotropic Dutch/Iowa mutant form of amyloid beta-protein precursor. *J Biol Chem* 2004; **279**: 20296–20306.

58. Fryer JD, Simmons K, Parsadanian M, *et al.* Human apolipoprotein E4 alters the amyloid-beta 40:42 ratio and promotes the formation of cerebral amyloid angiopathy in an amyloid precursor protein transgenic model. *J Neurosci* 2005; **25**: 2803–2810.

59. Wyss-Coray T, Lin C, Yan F, *et al.* TGF-beta1 promotes microglial amyloid-beta clearance and

reduces plaque burden in transgenic mice. *Nat Med* 2001; **7**: 612–618.

60. Wyss-Coray T, Masliah E, Mallory M, *et al.* Amyloidogenic role of cytokine TGF-ß1 in transgenic mice and in Alzheimer's disease. *Nature* 1997; **389**: 603–606.

61. Kimchi EY, Kajdasz S, Bacskai BJ, Hyman BT. Analysis of cerebral amyloid angiopathy in a transgenic mouse model of Alzheimer disease using in vivo multiphoton microscopy. *J Neuropathol Exp Neurol* 2001; **60**: 274–279.

62. Niwa K, Carlson GA, Iadecola C. Exogenous A beta1–40 reproduces cerebrovascular alterations resulting from amyloid precursor protein overexpression in mice. *J Cereb Blood Flow Metab* 2000; **20**: 1659–1668.

63. Niwa K, Younkin L, Ebeling C, *et al.* Abeta 1–40-related reduction in functional hyperemia in mouse neocortex during somatosensory activation. *Proc Natl Acad Sci U S A* 2000; **97**: 9735–9740.

64. Thomas T, Thomas G, McLendon C, Sutton T, Mullan M. beta-Amyloid-mediated vasoactivity and vascular endothelial damage. *Nature* 1996; **380**: 168–171.

65. Wang Z, Natte R, Berliner JA, van Duinen SG, Vinters HV. Toxicity of dutch (E22Q) and flemish (A21G) mutant amyloid beta proteins to human cerebral microvessel and aortic smooth muscle cells. *Stroke* 2000; **31**: 534–538.

66. Van Nostrand WE, Melchor JP, Ruffini L. Pathologic amyloid beta-protein cell surface fibril assembly on cultured human cerebrovascular smooth muscle cells. *J Neurochem* 1998; **70**: 216–223.

67. Van Nostrand WE, Melchor JP, Cho HS, Greenberg SM, Rebeck GW. Pathogenic effects of D23N Iowa mutant amyloid beta-protein. *J Biol Chem* 2001; **276**: 32860–32866.

68. Eisenhauer PB, Johnson RJ, Wells JM, Davies TA, Fine RE. Toxicity of various amyloid beta peptide species in cultured human blood-brain barrier endothelial cells: increased toxicity of Dutch-type mutant. *J Neurosci Res* 2000; **60**: 804–810.

69. Beckmann N, Schuler A, Mueggler T, *et al.* Age-dependent cerebrovascular abnormalities and blood flow disturbances in APP23 mice modeling Alzheimer's disease. *J Neurosci* 2003; **23**: 8453–8459.

70. Park L, Anrather J, Forster C, *et al.* Abeta-induced vascular oxidative stress and attenuation of functional hyperemia in mouse somatosensory cortex. *J Cereb Blood Flow Metab* 2004; **24**: 334–342.

71. Lee JM, Yin KJ, Hsin I, *et al.* Matrix metalloproteinase-9 and spontaneous hemorrhage in an animal model of cerebral amyloid angiopathy. *Ann Neurol* 2003; **54**: 379–382.

72. Rosenberg GA, Sullivan N, Esiri MM. White matter damage is associated with matrix metalloproteinases in vascular dementia. *Stroke* 2001; **32**: 1162–1168.

73. Kingston IB, Castro MJ, Anderson S. In vitro stimulation of tissue-type plasminogen activator by Alzheimer amyloid beta-peptide analogues. *Nat Med* 1995; **1**: 138–142.

74. Van Nostrand WE, Porter M. Plasmin cleavage of the amyloid beta-protein: alteration of secondary structure and stimulation of tissue plasminogen activator activity. *Biochemistry* 1999; **38**: 11570–11576.

75. Knudsen KA, Rosand J, Karluk D, Greenberg SM. Clinical diagnosis of cerebral amyloid angiopathy: validation of the Boston Criteria. *Neurology* 2001; **56**: 537–539.

76. Tomonaga M. Cerebral amyloid angiopathy in the elderly. *J Am Geriatr Soc* 1981; **29**: 151–157.

77. Vinters HV, Gilbert JJ. Cerebral amyloid angiopathy: incidence and complications in the aging brain. II. The distribution of amyloid vascular changes. *Stroke* 1983; **14**: 924–928.

78. Masuda J, Tanaka K, Ueda K, Omae T. Autopsy study of incidence and distribution of cerebral amyloid angiopathy in Hisayama, Japan. *Stroke* 1988; **19**: 205–210.

79. Greenberg SM, Vonsattel J-PG. Diagnosis of cerebral amyloid angiopathy. Sensitivity and specificity of cortical biopsy. *Stroke* 1997; **28**: 1418–1422.

80. Lee SS, Stemmermann GN. Congophilic angiopathy and cerebral hemorrhage. *Arch Pathol Lab Med* 1978; **102**: 317–321.

81. Itoh Y, Yamada M, Hayakawa M, Otomo E, Miyatake T. Cerebral amyloid angiopathy: a significant cause of cerebellar as well as lobar cerebral hemorrhage in the elderly. *J Neurol Sci* 1993; **116**: 135–141.

82. Greenberg SM. Cerebral amyloid angiopathy. In: Mohr JP, Choi D, Grotta JC, *et al.*, eds. *Stroke: Pathophysiology, Diagnosis and Management*, 4th edn. New York, Harcourt, Inc. 2004; 693–705.

83. Ellis RJ, Olichney JM, Thal LJ, *et al.* Cerebral amyloid angiopathy in the brains of patients with Alzheimer's disease: the CERAD experience, Part XV. *Neurology* 1996; **46**: 1592–1596.

84. Hanyu H, Tanaka Y, Shimizu S, Takasaki M, Abe K. Cerebral microbleeds in Alzheimer's disease. *J Neurol* 2003; **250**: 1496–1497.

85. Atri A, Locascio JJ, Lin JM, *et al.* Prevalence and effects of lobar microhemorrhages in early-stage dementia. *Neuro degenerative Dis* 2005; **2**: 305–312.

86. Greenberg SM, Briggs ME, Hyman BT, *et al.* Apolipoprotein E e4 is associated with the presence

and earlier onset of hemorrhage in cerebral amyloid angiopathy. *Stroke* 1996; **27**: 1333–1337.

87. Smith EE, Gurol ME, Eng JA, *et al.* White matter lesions, cognition, and recurrent hemorrhage in lobar intracerebral hemorrhage. *Neurology* 2004; **63**: 1606–1612.

88. Schmechel DE, Saunders AM, Strittmatter WJ, *et al.* Increased amyloid beta-peptide deposition in cerebral cortex as a consequence of apolipoprotein E genotype in late-onset Alzheimer disease. *Proc Natl Acad Sci U S A* 1993; **90**: 9649–9653.

89. Fisher CM. Pathological observations in hypertensive cerebral hemorrhage. *J Neuropathol Exp Neurol* 1971; **30**: 536–550.

90. Bahemuka M. Primary intracerebral hemorrhage and heart weight: a clinicopathologic case-control review of 218 patients. *Stroke* 1987; **18**: 531–536.

91. Massaro AR, Sacco RL, Mohr JP, *et al.* Clinical discriminators of lobar and deep hemorrhages: the Stroke Data Bank. *Neurology* 1991; **41**: 1881–1885.

92. Schutz H, Bodeker RH, Damian M, Krack P, Dorndorf W. Age-related spontaneous intracerebral hematoma in a German community. *Stroke* 1990; **21**: 1412–1418.

93. Broderick J, Brott T, Tomsick T, Leach A. Lobar hemorrhage in the elderly. The undiminishing importance of hypertension. *Stroke* 1993; **24**: 49–51.

94. Thrift AG, McNeil JJ, Forbes A, Donnan GA. Three important subgroups of hypertensive persons at greater risk of intracerebral hemorrhage. Melbourne Risk Factor Study Group. *Hypertension* 1998; **31**: 1223–1229.

95. Woo D, Sauerbeck LR, Kissela BM, *et al.* Genetic and environmental risk factors for intracerebral hemorrhage: preliminary results of a population-based study. *Stroke* 2002; **33**: 1190–1196.

96. Woo D, Kaushal R, Chakraborty R, *et al.* Association of apolipoprotein E4 and haplotypes of the apolipoprotein e gene with lobar intracerebral hemorrhage. *Stroke* 2005; **36**: 1874–1879.

97. Tanaka H, Ueda Y, Hayashi M, *et al.* Risk factors for cerebral hemorrhage and cerebral infarction in a Japanese rural community. *Stroke* 1982; **13**: 62–73.

98. Iso H, Jacobs DJ, Wentworth D, Neaton JD, Cohen JD. Serum cholesterol levels and six-year mortality from stroke in 350,977 men screened for the multiple risk factor intervention trial [see comments]. *N Engl J Med* 1989; **320**: 904–910.

99. Yano K, Reed DM, MacLean CJ. Serum cholesterol and hemorrhagic stroke in the Honolulu Heart Program. *Stroke* 1989; **20**: 1460–1465.

100. Gatchev O, Rastam L, Lindberg G, *et al.* Subarachnoid hemorrhage, cerebral hemorrhage, and serum cholesterol concentration in men and women. *Ann Epidemiol* 1993; **3**: 403–409.

101. Lindenstrom E, Boysen G, Nyboe J. Influence of total cholesterol, high density lipoprotein cholesterol, and triglycerides on risk of cerebrovascular disease: the Copenhagen City Heart Study. *BMJ* 1994; **309**: 11–15. Erratum in: *BMJ* 1994; **309**(6969): 1619.

102. Iribarren C, Jacobs DR, Sadler M, Claxton AJ, Sidney S. Low total serum cholesterol and intracerebral hemorrhagic stroke: is the association confined to elderly men? *Stroke* 1996; **27**: 1993–1998.

103. Giroud M, Creisson E, Fayolle H, *et al.* Risk factors for primary cerebral hemorrhage: a population-based study–the Stroke Registry of Dijon. *Neuroepidemiology* 1995; **14**: 20–26.

104. Segal AZ, Chiu RI, Eggleston-Sexton PM, Beiser A, Greenberg SM. Low cholesterol as a risk factor for primary intracerebral hemorrhage: a case-control study. *Neuroepidemiology* 1999; **18**: 185–193.

105. Revesz T, Holton JL, Lashley T, *et al.* Sporadic and familial cerebral amyloid angiopathies. *Brain Pathol.* 2002; **12**: 343–357.

106. Hendriks L, van Duijn CM, Cras P, *et al.* Presenile dementia and cerebral haemorrhage linked to a mutation at codon 692 of the beta-amyloid precursor protein gene. *Nat Genet* 1992; **1**: 218–221.

107. Cras P, van Harskamp F, Hendriks L, *et al.* Presenile Alzheimer dementia characterized by amyloid angiopathy and large amyloid core type senile plaques in the APP 692Ala->Gly mutation. *Acta Neuropathol* 1998; **96**: 253–260.

108. Tagliavini F, Rossi G, Padovani A, *et al.* A new ßPP mutation related to hereditary cerebral haemorrhage. *Alzheimers Rep* 1999; **2**: S28.

109. Miravalle L, Tokuda T, Chiarle R, *et al.* Substitutions at codon 22 of Alzheimer's abeta peptide induce diverse conformational changes and apoptotic effects in human cerebral endothelial cells. *J Biol Chem* 2000; **275**: 27110–27116.

110. Obici L, Demarchi A, de Rosa G, *et al.* A novel AbetaPP mutation exclusively associated with cerebral amyloid angiopathy. *Ann Neurol* 2005; **58**: 639–644.

111. Selkoe DJ. The origins of Alzheimer disease. A is for amyloid. *JAMA* 2000; **283**: 1615–1617.

112. Greenberg SM, Shin Y, Grabowski TJ, *et al.* Hemorrhagic stroke associated with the Iowa amyloid precursor protein mutation. *Neurology* 2003; **60**: 1020–1022.

113. Brooks WS, Kwok JB, Halliday GM, *et al.* Hemorrhage is uncommon in new Alzheimer family with Flemish

53

amyloid precursor protein mutation. *Neurology* 2004; **63**: 1613–1617.

114. Palsdottir A, Abrahamson M, Thorsteinsson L, *et al.* Mutation in cystatin C gene causes hereditary brain haemorrhage. *Lancet* 1988; **2**: 603–604.

115. Levy E, Lobez-Otin C, Ghiso J, Geltner D, Frangione B. Stroke in Icelandic patients with hereditary amyloid angiopathy is related to a mutation in the cystatin C gene, an inhibitor of cysteine proteases. *J Exp Med* 1989; **169**: 1771–1778.

116. Vidal R, Frangione B, Rostagno A, *et al.* A stop-codon mutation in the BRI gene associated with familial British dementia. *Nature* 1999; **399**: 776–781.

117. Vidal R, Revesz T, Rostagno A, *et al.* A decamer duplication in the 3′ region of the BRI gene originates an amyloid peptide that is associated with dementia in a danish kindred. *Proc Natl Acad Sci U S A* 2000; **97**: 4920–4925.

118. Vidal R, Garzuly F, Budka H, *et al.* Meningocerebrovascular amyloidosis associated with a novel transthyretin mis-sense mutation at codon 18 (TTRD 18G). *Am J Pathol* 1996; **148**: 361–366.

119. Herrick MK, DeBruyne K, Horoupian DS, *et al.* Massive leptomeningeal amyloidosis associated with a Val30Met transthyretin gene. *Neurology* 1996; **47**: 988–992.

120. Petersen RB, Goren H, Cohen M, *et al.* Transthyretin amyloidosis: a new mutation associated with dementia. *Ann Neurol* 1997; **41**: 307–313.

121. Mascalchi M, Salvi F, Pirini MG, *et al.* Transthyretin amyloidosis and superficial siderosis of the CNS. *Neurology* 1999; **53**: 1498–1503.

122. Brett M, Persey MR, Reilly MM, *et al.* Transthyretin Leu12Pro is associated with systemic, neuropathic and leptomeningeal amyloidosis. *Brain* 1999; **122**: 183–190.

123. Jin K, Sato S, Takahashi T, *et al.* Familial leptomeningeal amyloidosis with a transthyretin variant Asp18Gly representing repeated subarachnoid haemorrhages with superficial siderosis. *J Neurol Neurosurg Psychiatry* 2004; **75**: 1463–1466.

124. Greenberg SM, Rebeck GW, Vonsattel JPV, Gomez-Isla T, Hyman BT. Apolipoprotein E e4 and cerebral hemorrhage associated with amyloid angiopathy. *Ann Neurol* 1995; **38**: 254–259.

125. Premkumar DR, Cohen DL, Hedera P, Friedland RP, Kalaria RN. Apolipoprotein E-epsilon4 alleles in cerebral amyloid angiopathy and cerebrovascular pathology associated with Alzheimer's disease. *Am J Pathol* 1996; **148**: 2083–2095.

126. Olichney JM, Hansen LA, Galasko D, *et al.* The apolipoprotein E epsilon 4 allele is associated with increased neuritic plaques and cerebral amyloid angiopathy in Alzheimer's disease and Lewy body variant. *Neurology* 1996; **47**: 190–196.

127. Zarow C, Zaias B, Lyness SA, Chui H. Cerebral amyloid angiopathy in Alzheimer disease is associated with apolipoprotein E4 and cortical neuron loss. *Alzheimer Dis Assoc Disord* 1999; **13**: 1–8.

128. Walker LC, Pahnke J, Madauss M, *et al.* Apolipoprotein E4 promotes the early deposition of Abeta42 and then Abeta40 in the elderly *Acta Neuropathol* 2000; **100**: 36–42.

129. Greenberg SM, Vonsattel JP, Segal AZ, *et al.* Association of apolipoprotein E epsilon2 and vasculopathy in cerebral amyloid angiopathy. *Neurology* 1998; **50**: 961–965.

130. McCarron MO, Nicoll JAR. Apolipoprotein E genotype in relation to sporadic and Alzheimer-related CAA. In: Verbeek MM, de Waal MW, Vinters HV, eds. *Cerebral Amyloid Angiopathy in Alzheimer's Disease and Related Disorders.* Dordrecht, Kluwer Academic Publishers. 2000; 81–102.

131. O'Donnell HC, Rosand J, Knudsen KA, *et al.* Apolipoprotein E genotype and the risk of recurrent lobar intracerebral hemorrhage. *N Engl J Med* 2000; **342**: 240–245.

132. Yamada M, Sodeyama N, Itoh Y, *et al.* Association of presenilin-1 polymorphism with cerebral amyloid angiopathy in the elderly. *Stroke* 1997; **28**: 2219–2221.

133. Mann DM, Pickering-Brown SM, Takeuchi A, Iwatsubo T. Amyloid angiopathy and variability in amyloid beta deposition is determined by mutation position in presenilin-1-linked Alzheimer's disease. *Am J Pathol* 2001; **158**: 2165–2175.

134. Yamada M. Cerebral amyloid angiopathy and gene polymorphisms. *J Neurol Sci* 2004; **226**: 41–44.

135. Rosand J, Muzikansky A, Kumar A, *et al.* Spatial clustering of hemorrhages in probable cerebral amyloid angiopathy. *Ann Neurol* 2005; **58**: 459–462.

136. Tian J, Shi J, Bailey K, Mann DM. Relationships between arteriosclerosis, cerebral amyloid angiopathy and myelin loss from cerebral cortical white matter in Alzheimer's disease. *Neuropathol Appl Neurobiol* 2004; **30**: 46–56.

137. Gilbert JJ, Vinters HV. Cerebral amyloid angiopathy: incidence and complications in the aging brain. I. Cerebral hemorrhage. *Stroke* 1983; **14**: 915–923.

138. Yamada M, Itoh Y, Otomo E, Hayakawa M, Miyatake T. Subarachnoid haemorrhage in the elderly: a necropsy study of the association with cerebral amyloid angiopathy. *J Neurol Neurosurg Psychiatry* 1993; **56**: 543–547.

139. Miller JH, Wardlaw JM, Lammie GA. Intracerebral haemorrhage and cerebral amyloid angiopathy:

CT features with pathological correlation. *Clin Radiol* 1999; **54**: 422–429.

140. Ohshima T, Endo T, Nukui H, *et al*. Cerebral amyloid angiopathy as a cause of subarachnoid hemorrhage. *Stroke* 1990; **21**: 480–483.

141. Kase CS. Lobar hemorrhage. In: Kase CS, Caplan LR, eds. *Intracerebral Hemorrhage*. Boston, Butterworth-Heinemann. 1994; 363–382.

142. Atlas SW, Mark AS, Grossman RI, Gomori JM. Intracranial hemorrhage: gradient-echo MR imaging at 1.5 T. Comparison with spin-echo imaging and clinical applications. *Radiology* 1988; **168**: 803–807.

143. Greenberg SM, Finklestein SP, Schaefer PW. Petechial hemorrhages accompanying lobar hemorrhage: detection by gradient-echo MRI. *Neurology* 1996; **46**: 1751–1754.

144. Fazekas F, Kleinert R, Roob G, *et al*. Histopathologic analysis of foci of signal loss on gradient-echo T2*- weighted MR images in patients with spontaneous intracerebral hemorrhage: evidence of microangiopathy-related microbleeds. *AJNR Am J Neuroradiol* 1999; **20**: 637–642.

145. Tsushima Y, Tamura T, Unno Y, Kusano S, Endo K. Multifocal low-signal brain lesions on T2*-weighted gradient-echo imaging. *Neuroradiology* 2000; **42**: 499–504.

146. Hart RG, Boop BS, Anderson DC. Oral anticoagulants and intracranial hemorrhage. Facts and hypotheses. *Stroke* 1995; **26**: 1471–1477.

147. Ramsay DA, Penswick JL, Robertson DM. Fatal streptokinase-induced intracerebral haemorrhage in cerebral amyloid angiopathy. *Can J Neurol Sci* 1990; **17**: 336–341.

148. Leblanc R, Haddad G, Robitaille Y. Cerebral hemorrhage from amyloid angiopathy and coronary thrombolysis. *Neurosurgery* 1992; **31**: 586–590.

149. Wijdicks EF, Jack CRJ. Intracerebral hemorrhage after fibrinolytic therapy for acute myocardial infarction. *Stroke* 1993; **24**: 554–557.

150. Melo TP, Bogousslavsky J, Regli F, Janzer R. Fatal hemorrhage during anticoagulation of cardioembolic infarction: role of cerebral amyloid angiopathy. *Eur Neurol* 1993; **33**: 9–12.

151. Sloan MA, Price TR, Petito CK, *et al*. Clinical features and pathogenesis of intracerebral hemorrhage after rt-PA and heparin therapy for acute myocardial infarction: the Thrombolysis in Myocardial Infarction (TIMI) II Pilot and Randomized Clinical Trial combined experience. *Neurology* 1995; **45**: 649–658.

152. Rosand J, Hylek EM, O'Donnell HC, Greenberg SM. Warfarin-associated hemorrhage and cerebral amyloid angiopathy: a genetic and pathologic study. *Neurology* 2000; **55**: 947–951.

153. Anderson JL, Karagounis L, Allen A, *et al*. Older age and elevated blood pressure are risk factors for intracerebral hemorrhage after thrombolysis. *Am J Cardiol* 1991; **68**: 166–170.

154. De Jaegere PP, Arnold AA, Balk AH, Simoons ML. Intracranial hemorrhage in association with thrombolytic therapy: incidence and clinical predictive factors. *J Am Coll Cardiol* 1992; **19**: 289–294.

155. Hylek EM, Singer DE. Risk factors for intracranial hemorrhage in outpatients taking warfarin. *Ann Intern Med* 1994; **120**: 897–902.

156. Bleeding during antithrombotic therapy in patients with atrial fibrillation. The Stroke Prevention in Atrial Fibrillation Investigators. *Arch Intern Med* 1996; **156**: 409–416.

157. Bornebroek M, Haan J, van Buchem MA, *et al*. White matter lesions and cognitive deterioration in presymptomatic carriers of the amyloid precursor protein gene codon 693 mutation. *Arch Neurol* 1996; **53**: 43–48.

158. Mead S, James-Galton M, Revesz T, *et al*. Familial British dementia with amyloid angiopathy: early clinical, neuropsychological and imaging findings. *Brain* 2000; **123**: 975–986.

159. Greenberg SM, Vonsattel JP, Stakes JW, Gruber M, Finklestein SP. The clinical spectrum of cerebral amyloid angiopathy: presentations without lobar hemorrhage. *Neurology* 1993; **43**: 2073–2079.

160. Silbert PL, Bartleson JD, Miller GM, *et al*. Cortical petechial hemorrhage, leukoencephalopathy, and subacute dementia associated with seizures due to cerebral amyloid angiopathy. *Mayo Clin Proc* 1995; **70**: 477–480.

161. Natte R, Maat-Schieman ML, Haan J, *et al*. Dementia in hereditary cerebral hemorrhage with amyloidosis-Dutch type is associated with cerebral amyloid angiopathy but is independent of plaques and neurofibrillary tangles. *Ann Neurol* 2001; **50**: 765–772.

162. Greenberg SM, Gurol ME, Rosand J, Smith EE. Amyloid angiopathy-related vascular cognitive impairment. *Stroke* 2004; **35**: 2616–2619.

163. Greenberg SM. Cerebral amyloid angiopathy and vessel dysfunction. *Cerebrovasc Dis* 2002; **13**: 42–47.

164. Pathological correlates of late-onset dementia in a multicentre, community-based population in England and Wales. Neuropathology Group of the Medical Research Council Cognitive Function and Ageing Study (MRC CFAS). *Lancet* 2001; **357**: 169–175.

165. Pfeifer LA, White LR, Ross GW, Petrovitch H, Launer LJ. Cerebral amyloid angiopathy and cognitive

function: the HAAS autopsy study. *Neurology* 2002; **58**: 1629–1634.

166. Gray F, Dubas F, Roullet E, Escourolle R. Leukoencephalopathy in diffuse hemorrhagic cerebral amyloid angiopathy. *Ann Neurol* 1985; **18**: 54–59.

167. Gurol ME, Irizarry MC, Smith EE, *et al.* Plasma β-amyloid and white matter lesions in AD, MCI, and cerebral amyloid angiopathy. *Neurology* 2006; **66**(1): 23–29.

168. Haglund M, Englund E. Cerebral amyloid angiopathy, white matter lesions and Alzheimer encephalopathy – a histopathological assessment. *Dement Geriatr Cogn Disord* 2002; **14**: 161–166.

169. Eng JA, Frosch MP, Choi K, Rebeck GW, Greenberg SM. Clinical Manifestations of cerebral amyloid angiopathy-related inflammation. *Ann Neurol* 2004; **55**: 246–252.

170. Gray F, Vinters HV, Le Noan H, *et al.* Cerebral amyloid angiopathy and granulomatous angiitis: immunohistochemical study using antibodies to the Alzheimer A4 peptide. *Hum Pathol* 1990; **21**: 1290–1293.

171. Mandybur TI, Balko G. Cerebral amyloid angiopathy with granulomatous angiitis ameliorated by steroid-cytoxan treatment. *Clin Neuropharmacol* 1992; **15**: 241–247.

172. Fountain NB, Eberhard DA. Primary angiitis of the central nervous system associated with cerebral amyloid angiopathy: report of two cases and review of the literature. *Neurology* 1996; **46**: 190–197.

173. Caplan LR, Louis DN. Case records of the Massachusetts General Hospital. Weekly clinicopathological exercises. Case 10–2000. A 63-year-old man with changes in behavior and ataxia. *N Engl J Med* 2000; **342**: 957–965.

174. Scolding NJ, Joseph F, Kirby PA, *et al.* Abeta-related angiitis: primary angiitis of the central nervous system associated with cerebral amyloid angiopathy. *Brain* 2005; **128**: 500–515.

175. Fountain NB, Lopes MB. Control of primary angiitis of the CNS associated with cerebral amyloid angiopathy by cyclophosphamide alone. *Neurology* 1999; **52**: 660–662.

176. Smith DB, Hitchcock M, Philpott PJ. Cerebral amyloid angiopathy presenting as transient ischemic attacks. Case report. *J Neurosurg* 1985; **63**: 963–964.

177. Yong WH, Robert ME, Secor DL, Kleikamp TJ, Vinters HV. Cerebral hemorrhage with biopsy-proved amyloid angiopathy. *Arch Neurol* 1992; **49**: 51–58.

178. Rosand J, Eckman MH, Knudsen KA, Singer DE, Greenberg SM. The effect of warfarin and intensity of anticoagulation on outcome of intracerebral hemorrhage. *Arch Intern Med* 2004; **164**: 880–884.

179. Flibotte JJ, Hagan N, O'Donnell J, Greenberg SM, Rosand J. Warfarin, hematoma expansion, and outcome of intracerebral hemorrhage. *Neurology* 2004; **63**: 1059–1064.

180. Bailey RD, Hart RG, Benavente O, Pearce LA. Recurrent brain hemorrhage is more frequent than ischemic stroke after intracranial hemorrhage. *Neurology* 2001; **56**: 773–777.

181. Viswanathan A, Rakich SM, Engel C, *et al.* Antiplatelet use after intracerebral hemorrhage. *Neurology* 2006; **66**(2): 206–209.

182. Greenberg SM, Eng JA, Ning M, Smith EE, Rosand J. Hemorrhage burden predicts recurrent intracerebral hemorrhage after lobar hemorrhage. *Stroke* 2004; **35**: 1415–1420.

183. Eckman MH, Rosand J, Knudsen KA, Singer DE, Greenberg SM. Can patients be anticoagulated after intracerebral hemorrhage? A decision analysis. *Stroke* 2003; **34**: 1710–1716.

184. Brott T, Broderick J, Kothari R, *et al.* Early hemorrhage growth in patients with intracerebral hemorrhage. *Stroke* 1997; **28**: 1–5.

185. Greene GM, Godersky JC, Biller J, Hart MN, Adams HPJ. Surgical experience with cerebral amyloid angiopathy. *Stroke* 1990; **21**: 1545–1549.

186. Leblanc R, Preul M, Robitaille Y, Villemure JG, Pokrupa R. Surgical considerations in cerebral amyloid angiopathy. *Neurosurgery* 1991; **29**: 712–718.

187. Matkovic Z, Davis S, Gonzales M, Kalnins R, Masters CL. Surgical risk of hemorrhage in cerebral amyloid angiopathy. *Stroke* 1991; **22**: 456–461.

188. Minakawa T, Takeuchi S, Sasaki O, *et al.* Surgical experience with massive lobar haemorrhage caused by cerebral amyloid angiopathy. *Acta Neurochir (Wien)* 1995; **132**: 48–52.

189. Izumihara A, Ishihara T, Iwamoto N, Yamashita K, Ito H. Postoperative outcome of 37 patients with lobar intracerebral hemorrhage related to cerebral amyloid angiopathy. *Stroke* 1999; **30**: 29–33.

190. Broderick JP, Adams HP Jr, Barsan W, *et al.* Guidelines for the management of spontaneous intracerebral hemorrhage: a statement for healthcare professionals from a special writing group of the Stroke Council, American Heart Association. *Stroke* 1999; **30**: 905–915.

191. Kisilevsky R, Lemieux LJ, Fraser PE, *et al.* Arresting amyloidosis in vivo using small-molecule anionic sulphonates or sulphates: implications for Alzheimer's disease. *Nat Med* 1995; **1**: 143–148.

192. Greenberg SM, Rosand J, Schneider AT, *et al.* A phase II study of tramiprosate for cerebral amyloid angiopathy. *Alzheimer Dis Assoc Disord* 2006; **20**: 269–274.

193. Selkoe DJ. Translating cell biology into therapeutic advances in Alzheimer's disease. *Nature* 1999; **399**: A23–31.

194. Shibata M, Yamada S, Kumar SR, *et al.* Clearance of Alzheimer's amyloid-ß(1–40) peptide from brain by LDL receptor-related protein-1 at the blood-brain barrier. *J Clin Invest* 2000; **106**: 1489–1499.

195. Deane R, Wu Z, Sagare A, *et al.* LRP/amyloid beta-peptide interaction mediates differential brain efflux of Abeta isoforms. *Neuron* 2004; **43**: 333–344.

196. Cirrito JR, Deane R, Fagan AM, *et al.* P-glycoprotein deficiency at the blood-brain barrier increases amyloid-beta deposition in an Alzheimer disease mouse model. *J Clin Invest* 2005; **115**: 3285–3290.

197. Iwata N, Takaki Y, Fukami S, Tsubuki S, Saido TC. Region-specific reduction of A beta-degrading endopeptidase, neprilysin, in mouse hippocampus upon aging. *J Neurosci Res* 2002; **70**: 493–500.

198. Wyss-Coray T, Loike JD, Brionne TC, *et al.* Adult mouse astrocytes degrade amyloid-beta in vitro and in situ. *Nat Med* 2003; **9**: 453–457.

199. Weller RO. Drainage pathways of CSF and interstitial fluid. In: Kalimo H, ed. *Pathology and Genetics. Cerebrovascular Diseases.* Basel, ISN Neuropath Press. 2005; 50–55.

200. Preston SD, Steart PV, Wilkinson A, Nicoll JA, Weller RO. Capillary and arterial cerebral amyloid angiopathy in Alzheimer's disease: defining the perivascular route for the elimination of amyloid beta from the human brain. *Neuropathol Appl Neurobiol* 2003; **29**: 106–117.

201. Hsiao K, Chapman P, Nilsen S, *et al.* Correlative memory deficits, Abeta elevation, and amyloid plaques in transgenic mice. *Science* 1996; **274**: 99–102.

57

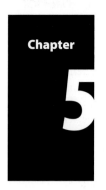

Coagulopathy-related intracerebral hemorrhage

Hagen B. Huttner and Thorsten Steiner

INTRACEREBRAL HEMORRHAGE RELATED TO ORAL ANTICOAGULANT THERAPY

Introduction

Over the recent years, there has been significant progress on the understanding of spontaneous intracerebral hemorrhage (ICH) concerning its pathophysiology, hematoma expansion, treatment, and the critical time window for controlling the bleeding. On the contrary, the current understanding of ICH related to oral anticoagulant therapy (OAT) is rather limited. The pathophysiology, incidence, and time course of hematoma expansion, as well as critical time window for treatment of OAT-related ICH (OAT-ICH) are not well defined. Furthermore, despite the fact that ICH is the most serious and fatal complication of OAT, currently there are no universally accepted guidelines on treatment. Treatment modalities vary and supportive evidence from randomized controlled trials does not exist. With respect to the established benefit of OAT in the prevention of stroke in patients with atrial fibrillation [1] and taking the increasing number of aging population into account, application of OAT is expected to increase and thus the number of patients who suffer from OAT-ICH.

This chapter provides information about the epidemiology of OAT-associated ICH, its pathophysiology, and treatment options based on the currently available data. The open questions regarding the optimal treatments and time window for controlling the bleeding will also be discussed and future research fields depicted in which randomized controlled clinical trials are urgently needed. This chapter considers the scientifically relevant findings and represents a clinically orientated foundation of how to manage OAT-ICH.

Epidemiology

Worldwide, the incidence of spontaneous intracranial hemorrhage ranges from 10 to 20 per 100 000 population per year [2]. The incidence is higher in the Afro-Caribbean and Japanese, around 55 per 100 000 population [3]. The reported incidence of OAT-ICH ranges from 0.25 to 1.1 per 100 patient-years [4–8] and is seven- to tenfold higher than in patients who are not on OAT [9–12]. Approximately 70% of OAT-associated intracranial bleedings are ICH, the majority of the remainder are subdural hematomas [10].

One of the most common indications for OAT is to prevent stroke in patients with atrial fibrillation. Unfortunately, while OAT effectively decreases the risk for thromboembolic stroke in this group of patients, OAT also increases the risk for ICH (placebo [0.1%] *versus* warfarin [0.3%–3.7%]) [1,10,13]. Furthermore, the use of warfarin is associated with worse outcome in patients with ICH. Flibotte *et al.* found that the use of warfarin significantly increases the likelihood of death when controlling for baseline ICH and intraventricular hemorrhage volumes [14]. In addition, the use of warfarin and increased intensity of anticoagulation are independent predictors of three-month mortality [12]. These described risks strongly affect the decision to use OAT in atrial fibrillation, resulting in an underuse in patients who will benefit from the treatment particularly among the elderly [15]. With the growing number of elderly individuals, the prevalence of atrial fibrillation is expected to rise dramatically [16]; hence the increased number of patients on OAT and patients with

Intracerebral Hemorrhage, ed. J. R. Carhuapoma, S. A. Mayer, and D. F. Hanley. Published by Cambridge University Press.
© J. R. Carhuapoma, S. A. Mayer, and D. F. Hanley 2010.

OAT-ICH [17,18]. Identifying effective treatments for OAT-ICH might decrease mortality and improve the outcome in this group of patients. As a result, it might also help optimize the use of OAT in patients with atrial fibrillation.

Outcome

Intracerebral hemorrhage is the deadliest form of stroke, with a mortality rate between 30% and 55% [11,19,20]. The mortality rate is increased to as high as 67% in patients who are on oral anticoagulants [11,12]. An overall poor outcome after three months in patients with primary ICH and OAT-ICH has been described [14,20–25] and the majority of surviving patients with OAT-ICH remains severely disabled [12,14]. The use of warfarin and an increased intensity of anticoagulation were shown to be independent predictors of three-months mortality [12,26]. Hematoma volume is the most powerful predictor of neurological deterioration, functional outcome, and mortality in both spontaneous ICH and OAT-ICH [21,27]. However, earlier data did not find a strong correlation between hematoma volume and outcome in OAT-ICH patients [28], whereas more recent data suggested a strong correlation [27]. This correlation may be dominated by the effect of hematoma volume on mortality [27]. Moreover, there is a relationship between ICH volume and mortality at 30 days and 6 months [29]. Treatments that stop the bleeding quickly will limit the hematoma expansion and decrease the hematoma volume which would likely be associated with decreased mortality and better outcome [14,30].

Pathophysiology

Over the recent years, we have gained significant insights into the pathophysiology of spontaneous ICH. On the contrary, the pathophysiology of OAT-ICH remains poorly understood. This section discusses the current concepts of OAT-ICH and highlights the areas where further studies are required.

What causes ICH during OAT: current concepts

Hart and colleagues have hypothesized that the use of OAT merely unmasks pre-existing subclinical intracerebral bleeding especially in patients with underlying hypertension and cerebrovascular disease [31].

This hypothesis is based on the following findings. First, a study by Roob et al. using gradient echo MRI, indicated that microbleeds may be found even in neurologically normal individuals and are strongly associated with higher age and hypertension [32]. Second, cerebral amyloid angiopathy is most commonly found in people over 65 years old and has been identified as a major risk factor for spontaneous ICH in the elderly [33]. Both advancing age and cerebral amyloid angiopathy are also important contributory factors to lobar ICH in patients who are on OAT [34] and the bleeding rate is increasing with age [35], implying that both spontaneous and OAT-ICH have the same underlying cause. Third, data from the Stroke Prevention in Reversible Ischemia Trial (SPIRIT) and the European Atrial Fibrillation Trial (EAFT) revealed that those patients who were on OAT with an average INR > 3 were at a remarkably higher risk of suffering from fatal primary cerebrovascular event (i.e., OAT-ICH) than patients with atrial fibrillation being treated with aspirin [36,37]. Moreover, the studies showed that the presence of white matter lesions, so-called "leukoaraiosis" on CT scans, was an independent predictor of ICH [36]. In summary, all the mentioned findings indicate that the underlying causes of both spontaneous and OAT-ICH might be the same, and OAT might only be a precipitating factor. Nonetheless, so far, supportive evidence is based on a limited number of patients.

It is also possible that OAT directly causes ICH. Oral anticoagulants interfere with the synthesis of vitamin K-dependent clotting factors resulting in dysfunctional factors VII, IX, X, and prothrombin [38–40]. Adequate levels and functional forms of these clotting factors are essential to counteract the burden placed on blood vessels as part of normal daily activities and prevent spontaneous bleeding [39,41]. Patients who are on OAT are at an increased risk for not only intracerebral bleeding but also bleeding in other organ systems [5,10]. The bleeding could be a direct result of the insufficient levels of functional factors VII, IX, X, and prothrombin [40].

Clearly, further studies which include larger numbers of patients are required to understand better the pathogenesis of OAT-ICH. Furthermore, if the underlying causes of spontaneous ICH are indeed the same as those of OAT-ICH, it will be useful to know whether screening for underlying conditions such as leukoaraiosis or microbleeds can identify patients who are at high risk of developing ICH.

59

Genetic aspects

Coumarins inhibit the vitamin K epoxide reductase multiprotein complex (VKOR), which is essential for the formation of several blood coagulation factors [42]. Recently published data indicate that there might be a so called warfarin resistance both in animals and humans [42–44]. The VKOR is thought to be involved in two diseases, the combined deficiency of vitamin K-dependent clotting factors type 2 (VKCFD2) and the warfarin resistance, due to a mutated gene vitamin K epoxide reductase complex subunit 1 (VKORC1) [42]. Further research will hopefully provide a better understanding of the pharmacological action of coumarins and may lead to more rational design of anticoagulants targeting VKOR.

With regard to the cerebral amyloid angiopathy, the presence of specific alleles such as the ϵ2 or ϵ4 alleles of the Apolipoprotein E gene appears to increase the risk of ICH by augmenting the vasculopathic effects of amyloid deposition in cerebral vessels [33,45]. Although these genotypes predict the recurrence of lobar ICH [45], up to now the sensitivity and specificity of genotype screening are not sufficient to be used as an indicator of amyloid angiopathy [34]. At present, there is no accurate diagnostic test for asymptomatic cerebral amyloid angiopathy; hence improvements in testing are needed. Subsequently, clinical trials will be required to determine whether such a test can help stratify the risk of ICH in patients who are under OAT.

Imaging

Hematoma shape

Oral anticoagulant therapy – related intracerebral hemorrhage might occur at the same sites as spontaneous ICH, although a slightly more frequently lobar location has been reported [31,46,47]. Compared to primary spontaneous ICH, OAT-ICHs have been thought to occur in more "irregular" shapes [48,49]. According to a study from Fujii, who focused on hematoma enlargement but also characterized three hematoma shapes [48], our group hypothesized that OAT-ICH significantly more often shows other than the common round-to-ellipsoid shape. We categorized the hematoma shape into (i) round-to-ellipsoid with smooth margins, (ii) irregular with frayed margins, and (iii) multinodular to separated (Fig. 5.1). Interestingly, we found OAT-ICH to occur in over 60% in irregular and separated forms [50].

Hematoma volume can easily be estimated using the so-called ABC/2 formula, a bed side technique, which is derived from an approximation according to the formula for ellipsoids, in which A is the greatest hemorrhage diameter, B is the diameter 90 degrees to A, and C is the approximate number of CT slices with hemorrhage multiplied by the slice thickness [51–53]. In consequence to our findings, the ABC/2 formula, which therefore calculates hematoma volume most precisely in round-to-ellipsoid shapes of hematomas, overestimated ICH volume in OAT-ICH. Alteration of the denominator to 3 revealed a more precise volume estimation in cases of irregularly and separate shaped ICH [50]. As hematoma volume is one of the most important predictors for poor outcome [21,25], a falsely large estimated hematoma volume might influence initial treatment decisions, such as "do not resuscitate" orders, and therefore lead to undesirable self-fulfilling prophecies with regard to outcome [54]. Accurate hematoma measurements are also of importance for clinical trials, where ICH volume change may be a surrogate end point.

Hematoma expansion in OAT-ICH

Intracerebral hemorrhage is a dynamic process. In spontaneous ICH, hematoma expansion occurs in

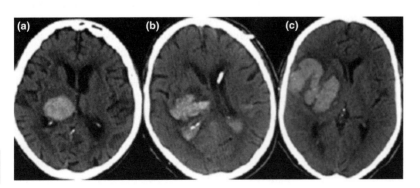

Fig. 5.1 Examples of various shapes of hematoma in OAT-ICH (a) round-to-ellipsoid, (b) irregular, and (c) separated.

nearly 38% of patients in the early hours after onset [19], and extravasation of contrast agents within the hematoma, a possible indicator of ongoing bleeding, has been detected in 46% of spontaneous ICH [55]. In contrast, incidence and time course of hematoma expansion in OAT-ICH remain poorly understood. In a retrospective study based on 47 patients with ICH associated with OAT, hematoma expansion was found in 28% of patients within 24 hours of onset [56]. However, apart from vitamin K, patients also received fresh frozen plasma (FFP) and prothrombin complex concentrates (PCC), and it remained unclear which treatments those patients with hematoma expansion had received. In another study, based on a follow-up CT scan up to seven days, hematoma expansion was found in 16% (9/57) of patients who were not on OAT compared with 54% (7/13) in those who received OAT [14]. Furthermore, expansion was also found later in the clinical course compared with patients with ICH who were not on OAT, suggesting that OAT prolongs the bleeding episode. In addition, the use of warfarin was an independent predictor of hematoma expansion (odds ratio [OR] 6.2, 95% confidence intervals [CI] 1.7–22.9) but interestingly no relationship between an exceeded INR and ICH volume at presentation could be demonstrated [14,56–58]. In spontaneous ICH, it has been proposed that hematoma expansion results from persistent bleeding or rebleeding from a single site of arterial rupture or secondary bleeding in the perilesional tissue [59]. Oral anticoagulants not only impair the formation of a fibrin clot but also cause premature clot lysis. Therefore, the mechanisms underlying hematoma expansion in OAT-ICH are likely to be the same as that in spontaneous ICH, but with a higher degree of severity.

In summary, the incidence and dynamics of hematoma expansion in OAT-ICH remain to be established. Current data suggest that the natural course of hematoma expansion in this group of patients is more prolonged as compared to spontaneous ICH. This may provide a longer time window for treatment of OAT-ICH.

Brain edema in OAT-ICH

Cerebral hematoma leads to the development of edema in the surrounding parenchyma. It has been proposed that factors released from activated platelets at the site of bleeding, for example vascular endothelial growth factor, may interact with thrombin to increase vascular permeability and contribute to the development of edema [60]. Thrombin was found to play a key role in edema formation [60]. Several studies in spontaneous ICH have proposed that the role of perihematomal ischemia is small [61]. In OAT-ICH, however, no similar studies have been undertaken. Results from clinical trials on recombinant coagulation factor VIIa, a drug which enhances thrombin generation, showed that edema was decreased in the treated group as compared to placebo, which may be due to the short time window until applied (< 4 hours) [62]. Whatever the role of thrombin in the development of edema might be, it appears that an early and effective hemostatic treatment ameliorates the process. Nevertheless, further research on the precise mechanism of edema is needed.

Current treatment strategies

Coumarins are vitamin K antagonists that produce their anticoagulant effect by interfering with the cyclic interconversion of vitamin K and its 2,3-epoxide, resulting in the synthesis of non-functional vitamin K-dependent coagulation proteins (i.e., factors II, VII, IX, and X) [39,40]. The decreased levels of functional coagulation factors lead to an increased risk of bleeding complications. The commonly used coumarin derivative (the coumadin warfarin) has a half-life of 36–42 hours and other coumarin derivatives have a half-life up to 7 days [40,63]. Hence, the aims of OAT-ICH management are to control bleeding, limit hematoma expansion, and prevent rebleeding by prompt reversal of the anticoagulant effect. Treatment options include the use of vitamin K, FFP and PCC [64]. In addition, recent data indicate that activated recombinant factor VII (rFVIIa) might be an effective treatment as well [30,65,66].

Despite ICH being the most fatal complication of OAT, currently there are no standardized guidelines for the reversal of anticoagulant effect in this group of patients. The United Kingdom (UK) guidelines recommend intravenous vitamin K (5–10 mg), and the use of factor concentrate, because rapid reversal of over-coagulation is more readily achieved than with FFP [67]. Another UK guideline issued by the Northern Region Hematologists' Group recommends intravenous vitamin K (5 mg) and PCC (30 U/kg) [40]. The United States guidelines state that intravenous vitamin K (10 mg) and PCC should be given but do not state the dose of PCC [63]. The guidelines of the American Heart Association (AHA) and the European Stroke Initiative (EUSI) recommend the use of intravenous vitamin K (10 mg) to reverse the effect of warfarin and to replace clotting factors. Concerning the latter both recommendations mention PCC and FFP, while the AHA is also considering factor IX complex concentrates and rFVIIa [68,69]. Both recommendations make the point that factor concentrates may act faster but may have an increased thromboembolic risk, while FFP is associated with greater volumes and much longer infusion time. This following section discusses the use of vitamin K, FFP, PCC, and rFVIIa based on currently available data.

Vitamin K

The effect of vitamin K on the correction of abnormal hemostasis is not immediate and it takes at least 2–6 hours for an initial effect, and even up to 4 days for an adequate response. Consequently, the use of vitamin K alone is not a treatment of choice for acute management of ICH and concomitant treatment with coagulation factor replacement is required. Nevertheless, the administration of 5–20 mg of vitamin K intravenously is necessary to achieve a sustained reversal of anticoagulant effect [40,63,67]. Side effects of intravenous vitamin K include allergic reactions and therefore it should be injected slowly.

Fresh frozen plasma

Fresh frozen plasma (FFP) contains all coagulation factors in a non-concentrated form. Hence, a large volume is required by each patient to achieve effective hemostasis [9,38,70]. In principle, 1 ml of FFP per kg body weight increases the levels of coagulation factors by 1–2 IU/dl [71]. However, the actual contents of vitamin K-dependent coagulation factors in each unit of FFP vary considerably [38] because of donors' biological and process variabilities. Consequently, the efficacy of FFP in controlling bleeding is unpredictable and it may not fully reverse an increased INR [38,67]. Moreover, FFP will not raise the level of factor IX more than 20% and this effect is not reflected by an INR [67].

Fresh frozen plasma units require compatibility testing and have to be thawed before transfusion. From the time a request has been made to the time the FFP units are available, it takes at least 45 minutes.

Furthermore, the large volume required and a rapid transfusion rate might lead to circulatory overload. Therefore, in the case of life-threatening bleeding such as ICH, FFP is not an ideal treatment option. In addition, FFP transfusion is associated with several potential adverse reactions including citrate toxicity, allergic reactions, transfusion-related acute lung injury (TRALI), and blood-borne infections [72,73].

Prothrombin complex concentrates

Prothrombin complex concentrates (PCC) contain coagulation factors VII, IX, X, and prothrombin as well as proteins C, S, and Z in a more concentrated form as compared to FFP. The potency of a PCC is expressed as factor IX content in International Units (IU) and it varies from preparation to preparation [41,74]. Based on data obtained from patients with hemophilia B, a dose of 1 IU of factor IX per kg body weight increases the level of plasma factor IX by 1 IU/dl [41,74].

Studies based on small numbers of patients showed that PCC were superior to FFP for the reversal of anticoagulant effect of OAT in terms of complete INR-reversal [38,64]. The effect of PCC was also significantly more pronounced and faster compared with FFP [75]. Moreover, neurological deterioration was significantly less in patients treated with PCC than those with FFP [75]. Therefore, in the case of OAT-ICH, the use of PCC may result in an improved neurological status [9]. Nonetheless, a retrospective study by Sjöblom and coworkers comparing vitamin K, FFP, PCC, and no treatment in 151 patients with OAT-ICH treated at ten Swedish hospitals did not find any evidence that any treatment was superior to the others, based on mortality rate at three months [29].

Prothrombin complex concentrates are manufactured from pooled plasma. Similarly to any plasma-derived products, there is a risk of transfusion-transmitted infection. Because the manufacturing process of a PCC incorporates a viral inactivation step, the risk of transmission of transfusion-transmitted known pathogens is small but cannot totally be excluded [76]. Furthermore, the risk of emerging pathogens of which the pathogenesis and clinical relevance are not fully understood is increasing [76]. Other potential adverse effects of PCC are allergic and anaphylactic reactions. In addition, some preparations of PCC are associated with high degrees of thrombogenicity increasing the risk of thromboembolic events such as deep vein thrombosis, pulmonary embolism, myocardial infarction, and disseminated intravascular coagulation (DIC) [41,74].

Recombinant coagulation factor VIIa

Among all the vitamin K-dependent coagulation factors, factor VII has the shortest half-life and has been reported to be the most affected coagulation factor protein during treatment with OAT [65]. Activated recombinant factor VII (rFVIIa) is the physiological initiator of coagulation, and it is therefore plausible that factor VIIa could be an alternative treatment to FFP and PCC in OAT-ICH (Fig. 5.2).

A recent publication by Mayer *et al.* based on a double-blind, randomized, placebo-controlled trial involving 399 patients with primary ICH, has shown that a single dose of rFVIIa given within four hours after the onset of ICH effectively limits hematoma expansion, reduces mortality, and improves functional outcomes at three months [62].

Regarding the use of rFVIIa in OAT-ICH, there are limited data. In healthy individuals receiving OAT, rFVIIa successfully normalized the INR, and the effect lasted longer when higher doses were used [65,77]. However, only a few patients have been treated with rFVIIa so far [30,66,77–79]. Boffard and colleagues found a significant reduction in the need of red blood cell transfusions when using rFVIIa in patients with blunt trauma [79]. Freeman *et al.* showed that rFVIIa rapidly lowered elevated INR levels and moreover seemed to be safe in ICH patients [30]. Furthermore, when administered in addition to FFP, a significant decrease in FFP requirement was shown resulting in a facilitating faster correction of increased INR levels [78]. Nonetheless, several features of rFVIIa are desirable for acute treatment of OAT-ICH patients. These include rapid and local action at the site of vascular injury, low volume, and the promising efficacy and safety profiles based on a recent study in primary ICH [62,80]. Furthermore the meaning of the INR as a measurement for the effect of rFVIIa in OAT-ICH is unclear (see below).

Guidelines for reversal of anticoagulant effect

Standardized guidelines for treatment of intracerebral bleeding in patients who are under OAT are still lacking. Although it is generally agreed that vitamin K

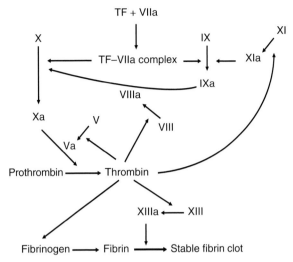

Fig. 5.2 Coagulation is initiated by the binding of FVIIa to the exposed tissue factor (TF) on subendothelium at the site of vascular injury. TF–FVIIa complex activates FIX and FX. Factor IXa also activates FX. FXa, in turn, rapidly converts prothrombin to thrombin, generating small amounts of thrombin. Thrombin activates FV and FVIII accelerating the activation of prothrombin and FX, respectively. Thrombin also activates FXI to FXa which, in turn, activates FIX. The generation of large amounts of FXa by FIXa and FVIIIa ensures that sufficient amounts of thrombin are continuously generated to convert fibrinogen to fibrin. Thrombin activates FXIII to FXIIIa which then cross-links the soluble fibrin monomers to form a stable fibrin clot.

administration is essential, the recommended dose varies considerably. Currently, PCC appears to be the preferred treatment of choice for an immediate reversal of the anticoagulant effect. However, there is no supportive evidence which is based on a large-scale randomized controlled trial. Data are mainly derived from retrospective studies or prospective studies that included only limited numbers of patients. Similarly to vitamin K, there is considerable variability in the recommended dose of PCC. Large-scale, randomized controlled trials are needed to prove whether one treatment is superior to the others. Furthermore, the potential role of rFVIIa requires further investigation.

The guidelines from the American Thoracic Society state that 10 mg of intravenous vitamin K and PCC should be given but do not specify the dose of PCC [63]. The guidelines issued by the Australasian Society of Thrombosis and Hemostasis recommend 5–10 mg of intravenous vitamin K, 25–50 IU/kg of PCC, and 150–300 ml FFP [81]. The recommendation for the concomitant use of PCC and FFP is because the PCC preparation licensed in Australia and New Zealand at the time the guidelines were published in

2004 did not contain FVII. The AHA and EUSI guidelines also recommend intravenous vitamin K (10 mg) and the application of factor concentrates [68,69].

We recommend administering 10 mg vitamin K with every treatment to support the supply of pro-thrombin-dependent clotting factors. Currently, PCC appears to be a logical treatment for an immediate reversal of the anticoagulant effect, keeping in mind, however, that concerns about thromboembolic side effects persist. While FFP is widely available, its efficacy is difficult to predict due to the variable contents of coagulation factors in each unit. Furthermore, the large volumes required limit its use in patients with impaired cardiac function. Treatment should be repeated as long as the INR is not normalized. The alternative use of rFVIIa in OAT-ICH may be considered but requires further investigation as other treatments do.

Considerations central to the decision of whether and when to resume therapeutic anticoagulation in patients who have suffered OAT-ICH include whether intracranial bleeding has been fully arrested, the estimated ongoing risk of thromboembolism, and the presumed pathophysiology of the ICH, which will determine the risk of hemorrhage recurrence [82–85]. Costs of these treatments are difficult to predict for medical (interindividual variability of effect, variability of product), economic, and political reasons (in a patient of 70 kg with an INR of 3 on admission the costs to decrease the INR to 1.4 or lower may be €330–€550 for FFP (2000–3500 ml), €400–€900 for PCC ($\approx$ 2000 units), and €3500–€5500 for rFVIIa (single dose). However, it is of utmost importance to realize that the clinical effect of a treatment should finally determine the clinical decision of treatment and still neither treatment has prospectively shown to be effective.

Unresolved issues on treatment
Time window for treatment

In spontaneous ICH, evidence suggests that significant hematoma expansion occurs during the first three hours of onset, and this is the critical time window for a hemostatic treatment [59,80]. In OAT-ICH, it is likely that the natural course of hematoma expansion is more prolonged, perhaps up to 24 or 48 hours [14,86]. This, on the one hand, might be beneficial as it will provide a longer time window for treatment. On the other hand, it could make the designing of a trial protocol more complicated in terms of the timing of treatment and number of doses needed.

Dose regimen

In spontaneous ICH, the administration of an effective hemostatic agent at an early stage accelerates the formation of a fibrin clot which stops the bleeding [62,80]. In this case, it seems that only one single dose is sufficient, provided that other supportive cares such as control of blood pressure are optimized. However, in OAT-ICH the underlying coagulopathy prolongs the time course of bleeding or rebleeding, and repeated dosing or a higher dose might be essential. In this respect, the interval and duration of treatment required for reversal of INR may differ. Due to a different half-life, this may be different for warfarin and coumarin as well.

Restarting oral anticoagulants

During the acute phase of OAT-ICH, the oral anticoagulants are usually suspended. However, there is no consensus on how long OAT should be suspended and whether the use of an alternative anticoagulant is essential during this period. In addition, there are no data on the risk of rebleeding after OAT is re-initiated.

Data from a retrospective study in 39 patients with OAT-ICH revealed that warfarin could be withdrawn for two days to three months without causing thromboembolism [82]. Furthermore, a second bleeding was not observed after anticoagulants or antiplatelet agents were reinstated [82]. In another retrospective study based on 141 patients, warfarin was withheld for a median of 10 days [83,87]; only 3 patients had an ischemic stroke within 30 days.

In contrast to the above studies, we used heparin in 15 patients with OAT-ICH during the period in which OAT was withheld [85]. During the acute phase, the INR was completely normalized and subsequently OAT was substituted by either full- or low-dose heparin. In 4 (out of 15) patients receiving full-dose heparin (partial thromboplastin time 1.5- to 2.0-fold of normal), there were no complications. However, three of seven patients given low-dose heparin developed severe cerebral embolism. Furthermore, three of four patients in whom the INR was partially corrected developed rebleeding. Due to the limited number of patients, we were unable to draw a definitive conclusion.

Recently, ximelagatran and warfarin have been compared with regard to stroke prevention in the SPORTIF V trial in patients with non-valvular atrial fibrillation, and for the treatment of deep vein thrombosis in the THRIVE trial [88,89]. After a mean follow-up of 20 months in SPORTIF V, the primary end point of stroke or systemic embolic events occurred in 37 patients in the warfarin group (out of 1962) and 51 in the ximelagatran group (out of 1960 patients). There was no significant difference between the groups with respect to a major bleeding. In THRIVE, the primary efficacy end point of recurrent venous thromboembolism occurred in 26 out of 1240 patients in the ximelagatran group and 24 out of 1249 patients in the warfarin group. In conclusion, the trials comparing ximelagatran with warfarin as prophylaxis for stroke in atrial fibrillation and in the treatment of venous thromboembolism showed a non-inferiority of ximelagatran. However, severe side effects on the hepatic function in the ximelagatran group were observed and until now no US Food and Drug Administration (FDA) approval for ximelagatran has been applied.

In summary, current data suggest that OAT can be withheld for at least 2–3 weeks without increasing the risk of thromboembolism [82–84]. Moreover, the risk of thromboembolism in patients who have developed ICH remains high and restarting OAT does not seem to increase the risk of recurrent ICH [9]. Nevertheless, so far, all data are based on retrospective studies.

Monitoring the hemostasis status during the reversal of anticoagulant effect

Because of the narrow therapeutic range of OAT, patients who are on OAT require close monitoring. The INR has been widely employed for this purpose. However, results from the Stroke Prevention in Atrial Fibrillation Study showed that warfarin increases the risk of ICH even when an INR is maintained within the therapeutic range of 2 to 4.5 (placebo vs. warfarin, 0.1% vs. 0.3–3.7%) [1,13]. Furthermore, around 70% of OAT-ICH occur at an INR of ≥ 3.0 [12]. When an INR is greater than 4.0, the reported risk of ICH is 2% per year [26].

The INR is designed specifically for patients receiving OAT who are in a stable state, consequently the use of an INR alone provides an adequate assessment of the hemostatic status of patients with OAT-ICH during replacement therapy with FFP or PCC [38]. This is due to the test system being more sensitive to decreased levels of factors VII and X, and prothrombin, but not to decreased levels of factor IX. Makris *et al.* demonstrated that during a stable state, factor IX levels in patients who are on OAT are correlated with INR. By contrast, following FFP transfusion, the correction of INR does not concomitantly correct the factor IX levels [38]. Therefore, the use of INR as an indicator of anticoagulant reversal might not reflect the actual status of all vitamin K-dependent coagulation factors. The measurement of individual coagulation factors provides a better indicator of the patient's hemostatic status but is not practical particularly in case of emergency. An alternative practical monitoring test is currently not available.

Thromboelastography is a system which records a profile of clot formation in whole blood [90]. The system provides an overall picture of the coagulation and fibrinolytic status. Based on seven patients with central nervous system bleeding during OAT who were treated with rFVIIa, Sorensen and colleagues showed that it may be feasible to use thromboelastography to monitor the hemostatic status of these patients [77]. Nevertheless, more data on the application of thromboelastography in monitoring the reversal of the anticoagulant effect is needed to prove the usefulness of the system.

Summary

The current knowledge on ICH associated with OAT is still limited and far behind spontaneous ICH. Despite the fact that ICH is the most serious complication of OAT, there are no standardized guidelines for treatment of bleeding. Current treatments are aiming at the normalization of the iatrogenic coagulation disorder, and are not based on evidence from randomized controlled trials. Moreover, many patients with OAT-ICH are at high risk of thromboembolism. The risk of thromboembolism that is associated with current hemostatic treatment strategies which aim to normalize coagulation is unknown.

Further studies are needed to establish the incidence, pathophysiology, and time course of hematoma expansion in patients with OAT-ICH. Moreover, as the bleeding period in ICH patients who are on OAT is likely to be more prolonged and extensive than that in spontaneous ICH, effective treatment regimens might also differ in terms of the time window, dose, repeated dose, and duration of treatment. In addition, an optimal treatment for patients who are on warfarin and coumarin might not be the same. These are important issues which require further investigation.

As the aging population is increasing, the number of patients with atrial fibrillation who require prophylactic OAT will increase. Consequently, the frequency of OAT-ICH is expected to rise as well. Hence, identifying an effective treatment for controlling the bleeding will lead to decreased mortality and improve outcome.

INTRACEREBRAL HEMORRHAGE RELATED TO OTHER ANTICOAGULANT TREATMENT

Heparin

Heparin, the cofactor of antithrombin III in low dose antagonizes factor Xa, in high dose directly antagonizes thrombin [91–93]. The half-life is dose-dependent between 1.5 and 5 hours [92]. Administration must be parenteral, the degradation is carried out by heparinases and the elimination via the kidneys [91]. Side effects include thrombocytopenia, loss of hair, anaphylaxy, and in chronic use osteoporosis [94]. Intracerebral hemorrhage associated with the heparin therapy has been reported about previously (IST/CAST studies) [85,95–97]. However, low-dose heparin seems to be safe in patients with ICH to prevent thromboembolic complications [97].

Thrombolysis-associated ICH

With the increasing appropriateness of thrombolysis using recombinant tissue plasminogen activator (rt-PA) in cerebral ischemia, over the last few years the risk of thrombolysis-associated ICH has grown. Thrombolysis-related ICH can occur either after systemic intravenous or after intra-arterial thrombolysis (ECASS I–II/ATLANTIS/PROACT) [96,98–100]. Risk factors for hemorrhagic transformation after thrombolysis are severity of the neurological deficit, age, increased serum glucose levels on admission, and elevated systolic blood pressure [99]. Thrombolysis must be stopped and CT scan performed immediately in cases of neurological deterioration.

The half-life of t-PA is about 8 minutes; however, decomposition products may be effective for several hours. Treatment includes FFP or PCC, but neither option has been reliably evaluated. Furthermore, in animal studies matrix-metalloproteinases are currently being tested [101].

References

1. Risk factors for stroke and efficacy of antithrombotic therapy in atrial fibrillations. Analysis of pooled data from five randomized controlled trials. *Arch Intern Med* 1994; **154**: 1449–1457.

2. Broderick JP, Brott T, Tomsick T, Huster G, Miller R. The risk of subarachnoid and intracerebral hemorrhages in blacks as compared with whites. *N Engl J Med* 1992; **326**: 733–736.

3. Qureshi AI, Saad M, Zaidat OO, *et al.* Intracerebral hemorrhages associated with neurointerventional procedures using a combination of antithrombotic agents including abciximab. *Stroke* 2002; **33**: 1916–1919.

4. Cannegieter SC, Rosendaal FR, Wintzen AR, *et al.* Optimal oral anticoagulant therapy in patients with mechanical heart valves. *N Engl J Med* 1995; **333**: 11–17.

5. Fihn SD, McDonell M, Martin D, *et al.* Risk factors for complications of chronic anticoagulation. A multicenter study. Warfarin Optimized Outpatient Follow-up Study Group. *Ann Intern Med* 1993; **118**: 511–520.

6. Palareti G, Leali N, Coccheri S, *et al.* Bleeding complications of oral anticoagulant treatment: an inception-cohort, prospective collaborative study (ISCOAT). Italian Study on Complications of Oral Anticoagulant Therapy. *Lancet* 1996; **348**: 423–428.

7. Turpie AG, Gent M, Laupacis A, *et al.* A comparison of aspirin with placebo in patients treated with warfarin after heart-valve replacement. *N Engl J Med* 1993; **329**: 524–529.

8. van der Meer FJ, Rosendaal FR, Vandenbroucke JP, Briet E. Bleeding complications in oral anticoagulant therapy. An analysis of risk factors. *Arch Intern Med* 1993; **153**: 1557–1562.

9. Butler AC, Tait RC. Management of oral anticoagulant-induced intracranial haemorrhage. *Blood Rev* 1998; **12**: 35–44.

10. Hart RG, Boop BS, Anderson DC. Oral anticoagulants and intracranial hemorrhage. Facts and hypotheses. *Stroke* 1995; **26**: 1471–1477.

11. Franke CL, de Jonge J, van Swieten JC, Op de Coul AA, van Gijn J. Intracerebral hematomas during anticoagulant treatment. *Stroke* 1990; **21**: 726–730.

12. Rosand J, Eckman MH, Knudsen KA, Singer DE, Greenberg SM. The effect of warfarin and intensity of anticoagulation on outcome of intracerebral hemorrhage. *Arch Intern Med* 2004; **164**: 880–884.

13. Bleeding during antithrombotic therapy in patients with atrial fibrillation. The Stroke Prevention in Atrial Fibrillation Investigators. *Arch Intern Med* 1996; **156**: 409–416.

14. Flibotte JJ, Hagan N, O'Donnell J, Greenberg SM, Rosand J. Warfarin, hematoma expansion, and outcome of intracerebral hemorrhage. *Neurology* 2004; **63**: 1059–1064.

15. Vasishta S, Toor F, Johansen A, Hasan M. Stroke prevention in atrial fibrillation: physicians' attitudes to anticoagulation in older people. *Arch Gerontol Geriatr* 2001; **33**: 219–226.

16. Go AS, Hylek EM, Phillips KA, *et al.* Prevalence of diagnosed atrial fibrillation in adults: national implications for rhythm management and stroke prevention: the AnTicoagulation and Risk Factors in Atrial Fibrillation (ATRIA) Study. *JAMA* 2001; **285**: 2370–2375.

17. Flaherty ML, Haverbusch M, Sekar P, *et al.* Location and outcome of anticoagulant-associated intracerebral hemorrhage. *Neurocrit Care* 2006; **5**: 197–201.

18. Flaherty ML, Kissela B, Woo D, *et al.* The increasing incidence of anticoagulant-associated intracerebral hemorrhage. *Neurology* 2007; **68**: 116–121.

19. Brott T, Broderick J, Kothari R, *et al.* Early hemorrhage growth in patients with intracerebral hemorrhage. *Stroke* 1997; **28**: 1–5.

20. Juvela S. Risk factors for impaired outcome after spontaneous intracerebral hemorrhage. *Arch Neurol* 1995; **52**: 1193–1200.

21. Broderick JP, Brott TG, Duldner JE, Tomsick T, Huster G. Volume of intracerebral hemorrhage. A powerful and easy-to-use predictor of 30-day mortality. *Stroke* 1993; **24**: 987–993.

22. Nilsson OG, Lindgren A, Brandt L, Saveland H. Prediction of death in patients with primary intracerebral hemorrhage: a prospective study of a defined population. *J Neurosurg* 2002; **97**: 531–536.

23. Kazui S, Minematsu K, Yamamoto H, Sawada T, Yamaguchi T. Predisposing factors to enlargement of spontaneous intracerebral hematoma. *Stroke* 1997; **28**: 2370–2375.

24. Daverat P, Castel JP, Dartigues JF, Orgogozo JM. Death and functional outcome after spontaneous intracerebral hemorrhage. A prospective study of 166 cases using multivariate analysis. *Stroke* 1991; **22**: 1–6.

25. Tuhrim S, Dambrosia JM, Price TR, *et al.* Prediction of intracerebral hemorrhage survival. *Ann Neurol* 1988; **24**: 258–263.

26. Hylek EM, Singer DE. Risk factors for intracranial hemorrhage in outpatients taking warfarin. *Ann Intern Med* 1994; **120**: 897–902.

27. Berwaerts J, Dijkhuizen RS, Robb OJ, Webster J. Prediction of functional outcome and in-hospital mortality after admission with oral anticoagulant-related intracerebral hemorrhage. *Stroke* 2000; **31**: 2558–2562.

28. Mathiesen T, Benediktsdottir K, Johnsson H, Lindqvist M, von Holst H. Intracranial traumatic and non-traumatic haemorrhagic complications of warfarin treatment. *Acta Neurol Scand* 1995; **91**: 208–214.

29. Sjöblom L, Hardemark HG, Lindgren A, *et al.* Management and prognostic features of intracerebral hemorrhage during anticoagulant therapy: a Swedish multicenter study. *Stroke* 2001; **32**: 2567–2574.

30. Freeman WD, Brott TG, Barrett KM, *et al.* Recombinant factor VIIa for rapid reversal of warfarin anticoagulation in acute intracranial hemorrhage. *Mayo Clin Proc* 2004; **79**: 1495–1500.

31. Hart RG. What causes intracerebral hemorrhage during warfarin therapy? *Neurology* 2000; **55**: 907–908.

32. Roob G, Schmidt R, Kapeller P, *et al.* MRI evidence of past cerebral microbleeds in a healthy elderly population. *Neurology* 1999; **52**: 991–994.

33. Revesz T, Ghiso J, Lashley T, *et al.* Cerebral amyloid angiopathies: a pathologic, biochemical, and genetic view. *J Neuropathol Exp Neurol* 2003; **62**: 885–898.

34. Rosand J, Hylek EM, O'Donnell HC, Greenberg SM. Warfarin-associated hemorrhage and cerebral amyloid angiopathy: a genetic and pathologic study. *Neurology* 2000; **55**: 947–951.

35. Yasaka M, Minematsu K, Yamaguchi T. Optimal intensity of international normalized ratio in warfarin therapy for secondary prevention of stroke in patients with non-valvular atrial fibrillation. *Intern Med* 2001; **40**: 1183–1188.

36. Gorter JW. Major bleeding during anticoagulation after cerebral ischemia: patterns and risk factors. Stroke Prevention In Reversible Ischemia Trial (SPIRIT). European Atrial Fibrillation Trial (EAFT) study groups. *Neurology* 1999; **53**: 1319–1327.

37. A randomized trial of anticoagulants versus aspirin after cerebral ischemia of presumed arterial origin. The Stroke Prevention in Reversible Ischemia Trial (SPIRIT) Study Group. *Ann Neurol* 1997; **42**: 857–865.

38. Makris M, Greaves M, Phillips WS, *et al.* Emergency oral anticoagulant reversal: the relative efficacy of

infusions of fresh frozen plasma and clotting factor concentrate on correction of the coagulopathy. *Thromb Haemost* 1997; **77**: 477–480.

39. Hirsh J, Dalen J, Anderson DR, *et al.* Oral anticoagulants: mechanism of action, clinical effectiveness, and optimal therapeutic range. *Chest* 2001; **119**: 8S–21S.

40. Hanley JP. Warfarin reversal. *J Clin Pathol* 2004; **57**: 1132–1139.

41. Hellstern P. Production and composition of prothrombin complex concentrates: correlation between composition and therapeutic efficiency. *Thromb Res* 1999; **95**: S7–12.

42. Rost S, Fregin A, Ivaskevicius V, *et al.* Mutations in VKORC1 cause warfarin resistance and multiple coagulation factor deficiency type 2. *Nature* 2004; **427**: 537–541.

43. Fregin A, Rost S, Wolz W, *et al.* Homozygosity mapping of a second gene locus for hereditary combined deficiency of vitamin K-dependent clotting factors to the centromeric region of chromosome 16. *Blood* 2002; **100**: 3229–3232.

44. Oldenburg J, von Brederlow B, Fregin A, *et al.* Congenital deficiency of vitamin K dependent coagulation factors in two families presents as a genetic defect of the vitamin K-epoxide-reductase-complex. *Thromb Haemost* 2000; **84**: 937–941.

45. O'Donnell HC, Rosand J, Knudsen KA, *et al.* Apolipoprotein E genotype and the risk of recurrent lobar intracerebral hemorrhage. *N Engl J Med* 2000; **342**: 240–245.

46. Mendelow AD, Gregson BA, Fernandes HM, *et al.*; STICH investigators. Early surgery versus initial conservative treatment in patients with spontaneous supratentorial intracerebral hematomas in the International Surgical Trial in Intracerebral Haemorrhage (STICH): a randomised trial. *Lancet* 2005; **365** (9457): 387–397.

47. Lipton RB, Berger AR, Lesser ML, Lantos G, Portenoy RK. Lobar vs thalamic and basal ganglion hemorrhage: clinical and radiographic features. *J Neurol* 1987; **234**: 86–90.

48. Fujii Y, Tanaka R, Takeuchi S, *et al.* Hematoma enlargement in spontaneous intracerebral hemorrhage. *J Neurosurg* 1994; **80**: 51–57.

49. Gebel JM, Sila CA, Sloan MA, *et al.* Thrombolysis-related intracranial hemorrhage: a radiographic analysis of 244 cases from the GUSTO-1 trial with clinical correlation. Global Utilization of Streptokinase and Tissue Plasminogen Activator for Occluded Coronary Arteries. *Stroke* 1998; **29**: 563–569.

50. Huttner HB, Steiner T, Hartmann M, *et al.* Comparison of ABC/2 estimation technique to computer-assisted planimetric analysis in warfarin related intracerebral parenchymal hemorrhage. *Stroke* 2006; **47**: 404–408.

51. Kothari RU, Brott T, Broderick JP, *et al.* The ABCs of measuring intracerebral hemorrhage volumes. *Stroke* 1996; **27**: 1304–1305.

52. Kwak R, Kadoya S, Suzuki T. Factors affecting the prognosis in thalamic hemorrhage. *Stroke* 1983; **14**: 493–500.

53. Gebel JM, Sila CA, Sloan MA, *et al.* Comparison of the ABC/2 estimation technique to computer-assisted volumetric analysis of intraparenchymal and subdural hematomas complicating the GUSTO-1 trial. *Stroke* 1998; **29**: 1799–1801.

54. Becker KJ, Baxter AB, Cohen WA, *et al.* Withdrawal of support in intracerebral hemorrhage may lead to self-fulfilling prophecies. *Neurology* 2001; **56**: 766–772.

55. Becker KJ, Baxter AB, Bybee HM, *et al.* Extravasation of radiographic contrast is an independent predictor of death in primary intracerebral hemorrhage. *Stroke* 1999; **30**: 2025–2032.

56. Yasaka M, Minematsu K, Naritomi H, Sakata T, Yamaguchi T. Predisposing factors for enlargement of intracerebral hemorrhage in patients treated with warfarin. *Thromb Haemost* 2003; **89**: 278–283.

57. Fogelholm R, Eskola K, Kiminkinen T, Kunnamo I. Anticoagulant treatment as a risk factor for primary intracerebral haemorrhage. *J Neurol Neurosurg Psychiatry* 1992; **55**: 1121–1124.

58. Radberg JA, Olsson JE, Radberg CT. Prognostic parameters in spontaneous intracerebral hematomas with special reference to anticoagulant treatment. *Stroke* 1991; **22**: 571–576.

59. Mayer SA. Ultra-early hemostatic therapy for intracerebral hemorrhage. *Stroke* 2003; **34**: 224–229.

60. Sansing LH, Kaznatcheeva EA, Perkins CJ, *et al.* Edema after intracerebral hemorrhage: correlations with coagulation parameters and treatment. *J Neurosurg* 2003; **98**: 985–992.

61. Schellinger PD, Fiebach JB, Hoffmann K, *et al.* Stroke MRI in intracerebral hemorrhage: is there a perihemorrhagic penumbra? *Stroke* 2003; **34**: 1674–1679.

62. Mayer SA, Brun NC, Begtrup K, *et al.* Recombinant activated factor VII for acute intracerebral hemorrhage. *N Engl J Med* 2005; **352**: 777–785.

63. Ansell J, Hirsh J, Dalen J, *et al.* Managing oral anticoagulant therapy. *Chest* 2001; **119**: 22S–38S.

64. Boulis NM, Bobek MP, Schmaier A, Hoff JT. Use of factor IX complex in warfarin-related intracranial hemorrhage. *Neurosurgery* 1999; **45**: 1113–1118; discussion 1118–1119.

65. Erhardtsen E, Nony P, Dechavanne M, *et al.* The effect of recombinant factor VIIa (NovoSeven) in healthy volunteers receiving acenocoumarol to an International Normalized Ratio above 2.0. *Blood Coagul Fibrinolysis* 1998; **9**: 741–748.

66. Deveras RA, Kessler CM. Reversal of warfarin-induced excessive anticoagulation with recombinant human factor VIIa concentrate. *Ann Intern Med* 2002; **137**: 884–888.

67. Baglin TP, Keeling DM, Watson HG. Guidelines on oral anticoagulation (warfarin): third edition–2005 update. *Br J Haematol* 2006; **132**: 277–285.

68. Broderick JP, Connolly ES, Feldman E, *et al.*; American Heart Association/American Stroke Association Stroke Council; American Heart Association/American Stroke Association High Blood Pressure Research Council; Quality of Care and Outcomes in Research Interdisciplinary Working Group. Guidelines for the management of spontaneous intracerebral hemorrhage in adults: 2007 update: a guideline from the American Heart Association, American Stroke Association Stroke Council, High Blood Pressure Research Council, and the Quality of Care and Outcomes in Research Interdisciplinary Working Group. *Stroke* 2007; **38**(6): 2001–23. Epub 2007 May 3.

69. Steiner T, Kaste M, Forsting M, *et al.* Recommendations for the management of intracranial haemorrhage – part I: spontaneous intracerebral haemorrhage. The European Stroke Initiative Writing Committee and the Writing Committee for the EUSI Executive Committee. *Cerebrovasc Dis* 2006; **22**(4): 294–316. Epub 2006 Jul 28. Erratum in: *Cerebrovasc Dis* 2006; **22** (5–6): 461. Katse Markku [corrected to Kaste, Markku].

70. Pindur G, Morsdorf S, Schenk JF, *et al.* The overdosed patient and bleedings with oral anticoagulation. *Semin Thromb Hemost* 1999; **25**: 85–88.

71. Hellstern P, Muntean W, Schramm W, Seifried E, Solheim BG. Practical guidelines for the clinical use of plasma. *Thromb Res* 2002; **107** Suppl 1: S53–57.

72. Gilstad CW. Anaphylactic transfusion reactions. *Curr Opin Hematol* 2003; **10**: 419–423.

73. Pomper GJ, Wu Y, Snyder EL. Risks of transfusion-transmitted infections: 2003. *Curr Opin Hematol* 2003; **10**: 412–418.

74. Hellstern P, Halbmayer WM, Kohler M, Seitz R, Muller-Berghaus G. Prothrombin complex concentrates: indications, contraindications, and risks: a task force summary. *Thromb Res* 1999; **95**: S3–6.

75. Fredriksson K, Norrving B, Stromblad LG. Emergency reversal of anticoagulation after intracerebral hemorrhage. *Stroke* 1992; **23**: 972–977.

76. Seitz R, Dodt J. Virus safety of prothrombin complex concentrates and factor IX concentrates. *Thromb Res* 1999; **95**: S19–23.

77. Sorensen B, Johansen P, Nielsen GL, Sorensen JC, Ingerslev J. Reversal of the International Normalized Ratio with recombinant activated factor VII in central nervous system bleeding during warfarin thromboprophylaxis: clinical and biochemical aspects. *Blood Coagul Fibrinolysis* 2003; **14**: 469–477.

78. Brody DL, Aiyagari V, Shackleford AM, Diringer MN. Use of recombinant factor VIIa in patients with warfarin-associated intracranial hemorrhage. *Neurocrit Care* 2005; **2**: 263–267.

79. Boffard KD, Riou B, Warren B, *et al.* Recombinant factor VIIa as adjunctive therapy for bleeding control in severely injured trauma patients: two parallel randomized, placebo-controlled, double-blind clinical trials. *J Trauma* 2005; **59**: 8–15; discussion 15–18.

80. Mayer SA, Brun NC, Broderick J, *et al.* Safety and feasibility of recombinant factor VIIa for acute intracerebral hemorrhage. *Stroke* 2005; **36**: 74–79.

81. Baker RI, Coughlin PB, Gallus AS, *et al.* Warfarin reversal: consensus guidelines, on behalf of the Australasian Society of Thrombosis and Hemostasis. *Med J Aust* 2004; **181**: 492–497.

82. Wijdicks EF, Schievink WI, Brown RD, Mullany CJ. The dilemma of discontinuation of anticoagulation therapy for patients with intracranial hemorrhage and mechanical heart valves. *Neurosurgery* 1998; **42**: 769–773.

83. Phan TG, Koh M, Wijdicks EF. Safety of discontinuation of anticoagulation in patients with intracranial hemorrhage at high thromboembolic risk. *Arch Neurol* 2000; **57**: 1710–1713.

84. Ananthasubramaniam K, Beattie JN, Rosman HS, Jayam V, Borzak S. How safely and for how long can warfarin therapy be withheld in prosthetic heart valve patients hospitalized with a major hemorrhage? *Chest* 2001; **119**: 478–484.

85. Bertram M, Bonsanto M, Hacke W, Schwab S. Managing the therapeutic dilemma: patients with spontaneous intracerebral hemorrhage and urgent need for anticoagulation. *J Neurol* 2000; **247**: 209–214.

86. Leira R, Davalos A, Silva Y, *et al.* Early neurologic deterioration in intracerebral hemorrhage: predictors and associated factors. *Neurology* 2004; **63**: 461–467.

87. Phan TG, Koh M, Vierkant RA, Wijdicks EF. Hydrocephalus is a determinant of early mortality in putaminal hemorrhage. *Stroke* 2000; **31**: 2157–2162.

88. Albers GW, Diener HC, Frison L, *et al.* Ximelagatran vs warfarin for stroke prevention in patients with

nonvalvular atrial fibrillation: a randomized trial. *JAMA* 2005; **293**: 690–698.

89. Fiessinger JN, Huisman MV, Davidson BL, *et al.* Ximelagatran vs low-molecular-weight heparin and warfarin for the treatment of deep vein thrombosis: a randomized trial. *JAMA* 2005; **293**: 681–689.

90. Sorensen B, Johansen P, Christiansen K, Woelke M, Ingerslev J. Whole blood coagulation thrombelastographic profiles employing minimal tissue factor activation. *J Thromb Haemost* 2003; **1**: 551–558.

91. Weitz JI, Bates SM. New anticoagulants. *J Thromb Haemost* 2005; **3**: 1843–1853.

92. Bates SM, Weitz JI. New anticoagulants: beyond heparin, low-molecular-weight heparin and warfarin. *Br J Pharmacol* 2005; **144**: 1017–1028.

93. Bates SM, Weitz JI. Coagulation assays. *Circulation* 2005; **112**: e 53–60.

94. Gibaldi M, Wittkowsky AK. Contemporary use of and future roles for heparin in antithrombotic therapy. *J Clin Pharmacol* 1995; **35**: 1031–1045.

95. Sloan MA, Price TR, Petito CK, *et al.* Clinical features and pathogenesis of intracerebral hemorrhage after rt-PA and heparin therapy for acute myocardial infarction: the Thrombolysis in Myocardial Infarction (TIMI) II Pilot and Randomized Clinical Trial combined experience. *Neurology* 1995; **45**: 649–658.

96. Schmulling S, Rudolf J, Strotmann-Tack T, *et al.* Acetylsalicylic acid pretreatment, concomitant heparin therapy and the risk of early intracranial hemorrhage following systemic thrombolysis for acute ischemic stroke. *Cerebrovasc Dis* 2003; **16**: 183–190.

97. Boeer A, Voth E, Henze T, Prange HW. Early heparin therapy in patients with spontaneous intracerebral haemorrhage. *J Neurol Neurosurg Psychiatry* 1991; **54**: 466–467.

98. Kase CS, Furlan AJ, Wechsler LR, *et al.* Cerebral hemorrhage after intra-arterial thrombolysis for ischemic stroke: the PROACT II trial. *Neurology* 2001; **57**: 1603–1610.

99. Tanne D, Kasner SE, Demchuk AM, *et al.* Markers of increased risk of intracerebral hemorrhage after intravenous recombinant tissue plasminogen activator therapy for acute ischemic stroke in clinical practice: the Multicenter rt-PA Stroke Survey. *Circulation* 2002; **105**: 1679–1685.

100. Selim M, Fink JN, Kumar S, *et al.* Predictors of hemorrhagic transformation after intravenous recombinant tissue plasminogen activator: prognostic value of the initial apparent diffusion coefficient and diffusion-weighted lesion volume. *Stroke* 2002; **33**: 2047–2052.

101. Lapchak PA, Chapman DF, Zivin JA. Metalloproteinase inhibition reduces thrombolytic (tissue plasminogen activator)-induced hemorrhage after thromboembolic stroke. *Stroke* 2000; **31**: 3034–3040.

Vascular malformations of the brain

Christian Stapf and J. P. Mohr

Vascular malformations constitute an important cause of intracranial hemorrhage especially in younger patients. However, this group of pathologies is quite heterogeneous and comprises a large spectrum ranging from sporadic congenital lesions (such as brain arteriovenous malformations [AVMs]) to genetically determined familial disorders that may progress over time (e.g., hereditary hemorrhagic telangiectasia, familial cerebral cavernous malformations, etc.).

No defined strategies exist for the diagnostic workup after acute intracerebral hemorrhage (ICH), and no diagnostic criteria have been established or prospectively validated so far. Therefore, the timing and use of currently available diagnostic tools (such as angio-CT, MRI, MRA, MRV, and cerebral angiography) varies depending on individual attitudes, local routine, regional traditions, and national healthcare plans. Data from a recent prospective series suggested that cerebral angiography may have a low yield in identifying an underlying vascular malformation in ICH patients older than 45 years with a history of hypertension and who present with a thalamic, putaminal, or posterior fossa bleed [1]. Current recommendations favor angiography for all cases without a clear cause of hemorrhage, particularly for young, normotensive patients [2,3]. Nonetheless, timing of cerebral angiography after acute ICH depends usually on the patient's clinical state and the neurosurgeon's judgment about the need for surgical intervention. Consequently, the underlying pathology may be missed in those who die or who have severe morbidity at initial presentation. In other cases, an underlying AVM or aneurysm may be compressed by mass effect of the initial hematoma and only be visible on follow-up angiography. Cavernous malformations presenting with hemorrhage beyond the limits of the actual malformations may only be identified on MRI after hematoma resorption, i.e. several months after the index bleed. The outdated concept of so-called "primary intracerebral hemorrhage" adds to the possibility that intracranial vascular malformations may still be under-diagnosed in ICH patients [4].

In principle, vascular malformations may arise from any segment of the different functional units of the brain vasculature, including arteries, arterioles, capillaries, venules, and veins. This may be due to developmental derangement during the time of the vessel formation, or may occur later in time based on external risk factors and genetic predisposition (Fig. 6.1). Many of these anomalies are associated with an increased risk of hemorrhage, as structural changes of the vascular wall lead to often progressive hemodynamic changes and lower resistance to intraluminal volume and pressure. As a general rule, the average risk of spontaneous hemorrhage appears to be rather low if the vascular malformation is diagnosed unruptured. Most types have been associated with higher bleeding rates if hemorrhage occurred at initial presentation.

Anomalies of the arterial wall
Aneurysms

Aneurysms do not constitute vascular malformations sensu stricto, but their formation represents the most frequently observed structural anomaly of intracranial arteries after endoluminal changes due to atherosclerosis. Aneurysm rupture constitutes the principal cause of non-traumatic subarachnoid hemorrhage (SAH) with an overall crude annual incidence between 10 and 15 per 100 000 in the western world and up to 30 per 100 000 in high-risk populations such

Intracerebral Hemorrhage, ed. J. R. Carhuapoma, S. A. Mayer, and D. F. Hanley. Published by Cambridge University Press.
© J. R. Carhuapoma, S. A. Mayer, and D. F. Hanley 2010.

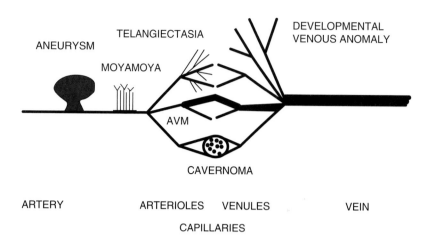

Fig. 6.1 Schematic overview of cerebral vascular malformations and anomalies.

as Asia or Finland [5]. Both aneurysm development and growth depend on familial predisposition and additional risk factors such as increasing age, female sex, smoking, and alcohol consumption. Looking at age alone, most prospective and retrospective studies have independently demonstrated an almost steady increase of annual incidence rates with age, with values ranging from below 5 per 100 000 for those younger than 35 years and rates between 30 and 40 per 100 000 for individuals aged 75 or older [6,7]. Morphological factors favoring hemorrhage from previously unruptured aneurysm include increasing aneurysm size and location in the posterior (i.e. vertebrobasilar) circulation [8].

Recent US population estimates suggest an overall mortality rate of 2.77 per 100 000 person-years attributable to aneurysm rupture [9]. Most of the larger outcome studies indicate that roughly one-third of patients who suffer a first-ever SAH die in the acute state, another third will survive with a disabling deficit, and only one-third will not be disabled from the event. The probability of survival seems to be lower in women [9] and has been shown to depend on the degree of initial neurological impairment [10], commonly graded according to the Glasgow Coma Scale [11] or by the grading system as proposed by Hunt and Hess [12].

In some instances, rupture of an intracranial aneurysm may lead to intraparenchymatous cerebral hemorrhage, particularly if located on middle cerebral artery (MCA) branches, or in distinct etiological subtypes, such as dissecting or mycotic aneurysms (Fig. 6.2). Therefore, whenever an intracerebral hematoma reaches down to the level of the carotid

tip or circle of Willis arteries or if ICH is associated with subarachnoid bleeding into the basal cisterns, an underlying aneurysm should be excluded by MRA, CT angiography (CTA) or conventional angiography in the acute phase as re-rupture rates seem to be similarly high as in cases with isolated SAH. Some arterial aneurysms develop in the context of an AVM and may add to the potential hazard of intracranial hemorrhage associated with such lesions (see below).

No systematic data exist on whether endovascular or surgical techniques should be preferred after intracerebral (i.e., intraparenchymatous) aneurysm bleeding. Recent outcome data on aneurysm treatment after SAH favor endovascular embolization [13,14]. Individual treatment decisions should be based on a multidisciplinary consideration of the patient's age and clinical condition, aneurysm anatomy, and the indication for additional hematoma evacuation or placement of a ventricular drain.

Telangiectasias

At the level of the arterioles, telangiectasias may develop as clusters of pencil-like vessels located mainly in the brainstem or cerebellum. Even though considered true vascular malformations, they have long been considered curiosities for the pathologist and are of only minor clinical significance, as they may not be an actual source of symptomatic bleeding [15]. They may demonstrate small microhemorrhages on histological examination, but the size of the hemorrhage does not appear to be massive enough to create a clinical syndrome. Nowadays, telangiectasias may be detected on MRI with and without contrast injection (Fig. 6.3).

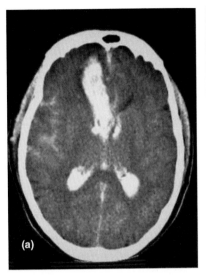
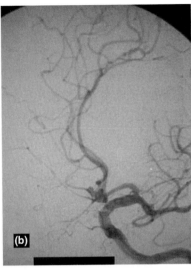

Fig. 6.2 Right frontal hematoma with ventricular extension and subarachnoid hemorrhage. (a) (Non-contrast CT scan) due to rupture of an aneurysm of the anterior communicating artery; (b) diagnostic angiography with left carotid injection.

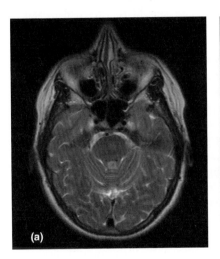
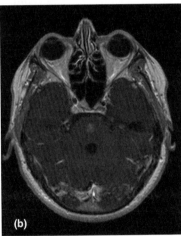

Fig. 6.3 Asymptomatic pontine telangiectasia with hyperintense signal on T2-weighted MR images (a) and on T1-weighted images after contrast injection (b).

So-called familial hemorrhagic telangiectasia or Osler-Weber-Rendu syndrome is an autosomal dominant disorder associated with multiple "telangiectasias" elsewhere in the body, which actually constitute tiny vascular nodules with arteriovenous shunting. Their number may increase during lifetime with the mostly affected organs being the mucosa, skin, and lungs. If located in the brain, these lesions may behave similar to sporadic AVM and may cause spontaneous rupture with intracranial hemorrhage (see below) [16].

Moyamoya

Moyamoya is a rare form of chronic cerebrovascular occlusive disease with angiographic findings of progressive stenosis or occlusion of the circle of Willis arteries together with a network of dilated perforating neovessels in the vicinity of the occlusion [17]. The initial description arose from the angiographic appearance of this pathological vascularization at the base of the brain: the tiny size and large number of vessels imaged made the combination look like a "cloud" or a "puff of smoke" instead of single arteries [18]. The numerous, dilated small neovessels have also been termed "rete mirabile."

In the vascular network of perforating arteries (the so-called moyamoya vessels) various histological changes can be observed: the distal portion of the carotid arteries as well as those constituting the circle of Willis often show fibrocellular intimal thickening,

73

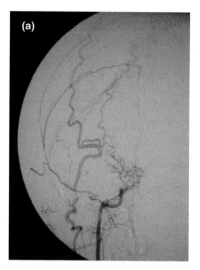 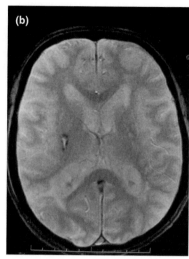 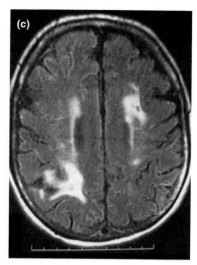

Fig. 6.4 Moyamoya disease with typical angiographic and MR imaging features: After injection of the right common carotid artery (a) visualization of distal internal carotid artery (ICA) occlusion with filling of dilated neovessels (moyamoya vessels). The gradient echo (T2*) MR shows subacute ICH at the level of the right lateral lenticulostriate arteries (b). Old ischemic lesions in the distal right MCA and deep left MCA territory can be seen on FLAIR (c).

waving of the internal elastic lamina, and attenuation of the media. Dilated neovessels are found around the circle of Willis, and reticular conglomerates of small vessels may appear in the pia mater. With hemodynamic stress or aging, the dilated arteries with attenuated walls may predispose to the formation of microaneurysms, and their rupture is considered one of the mechanisms leading to parenchymatous hemorrhages in moyamoya patients.

Annual incidence estimates of symptomatic moyamoya range between 0.06 per 100 000 in whites and 0.54 per 100 000 in Japan, but seem to be almost twice as high in women, and show two age distribution peaks around 10–20 and 40–50 years [19–22]. Clinically, ischemic and hemorrhagic symptoms are encountered. The ischemic type dominates in childhood, and clinically transient ischemic events occur more often than infarctions with persistent neurological deficits. Hemorrhagic complications are more frequent in adult patients. Bleeding occurs often in repetitive intervals, and massive bleeding, although infrequent, is the principal cause of death.

Hereditary factors and ethnic origin may play a role in the occurrence or susceptibility to idiopathic moyamoya disease, as suggested by the occasional familial occurrence (12% in Japanese cases) [22]. A secondary moyamoya syndrome may be seen in association with other congenital diseases such as sickle cell anemia, von Recklinghausen disease (neurofibromatosis type 1),

and Down syndrome (trisomy 21) [23]. However, the clinical manifestation and disease progression is not congenital and may also be seen as secondary complication of early-onset intracranial atherosclerosis, autoimmune disease, vasculitis, meningitis, post-radiation changes, cranial trauma, and brain neoplasm [17,24].

Typical angiographic findings were considered indispensable for the diagnosis of moyamoya, but as the quality of MRI and MRA greatly improved, the diagnosis was also made if they clearly demonstrated all the findings indicative of moyamoya (Fig. 6.4) [17].

In advanced stages of moyamoya, some degree of early venous drainage may be seen on angiograms suggesting arteriovenous shunting at the level of the neovessel network. On the other hand, moyamoya-type vascular changes have been observed on high-flow feeding arteries in brain AVMs. Whether the two entities are linked biologically, or whether the moyamoya type vascular pathology observed in AVM patients merely results from hemodynamic changes associated with the AVM remains as yet unclear.

Anomalies of the capillary junction
Brain arteriovenous malformations

Among vascular malformations causing intracranial hemorrhage, brain AVMs are among the most frequently encountered. Brain AVMs commonly affect

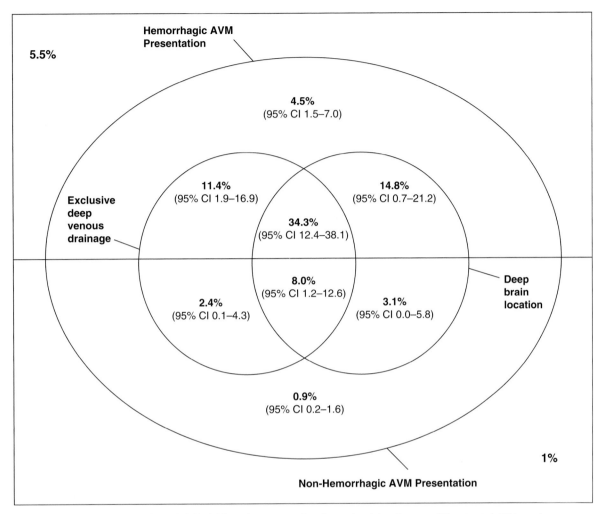

Fig. 6.5 Columbia AVM Hemorrhage Risk Model (based on prospective observational data from n = 622 untreated AVM cases). (Modified from [27]).

distal arterial branches and in roughly half of the cases, the malformation is found in the borderzone region shared by the distal anterior, middle, and/or posterior cerebral arteries [15]. Morphologically they resemble tortuous agglomerations of abnormally dilated arteries with drainage into deep and/or superficial veins. In its core region or "nidus," the AVM lacks a capillary bed, thereby allowing high-flow arteriovenous shunting through one or more fistulae. The lack of capillary resistance turns an AVM into a high-flow and low-pressure lesion that may not directly depend on the systemic blood pressure (explaining why AVMs tend not to rupture in a context of physical exercise).

The annual incidence of AVM hemorrhage in the general population is 0.5 per 100 000, but with the increasing availability of MR brain imaging, even more unruptured AVMs are diagnosed every year in the western world and typical symptoms include seizures or headaches. Some present with progressive or fluctuating neurological deficits without signs of hemorrhage. An increasing number of patients are diagnosed with an incidental finding of an asymptomatic malformation. Overall, women and men are equally affected with a mean age at diagnosis around 40 years [25]. Familial AVMs are extremely rare and have been described in only 25 pedigrees world wide [26].

Risk factors for spontaneous bleeding include mainly a history of prior hemorrhage, but also morphological characteristics such as deep AVM location and exclusive deep venous drainage (Fig. 6.5) [27].

Brain AVMs without these risk factors seem to carry a rather low hemorrhage risk (< 1% per year). Whether or not associated aneurysms on feeding arteries or within the AVM nidus constitute an additional risk is subject to current debates. Overall, Hispanic Americans seem to carry a higher risk of AVM rupture as compared to whites [28]. If rupture occurs, the clinical deficits tend to be less severe and the associated mortality far lower as compared to ICH from other causes [29].

Even though many AVMs can be detected on MR brain imaging, diagnostic four-vessel angiography remains the gold standard for the correct diagnosis on anatomic characterization of these malformations (Fig. 6.6). Cerebral angiography may also help to differentiate brain AVMs from other types of intracranial anomalies with arteriovenous shunting (Table 6.1). In a standard description of a newly diagnosed brain AVM, important morphological baseline variables include the maximal AVM diameter, the topographic nidus location in the brain, the arterial supply (number and type of feeding artery), the presence of associated (i.e., feeding-artery or intranidal) aneurysms, arterial stenosis with or without moyamoya-type changes, deep and/or superficial venous drainage, as well as the presence of any venous outflow stenosis and/or ectasia.

As a complex neurovascular disorder, brain AVMs are ideally managed by a multidisciplinary team of vascular neurologists, neuroradiologists, neurosurgeons, and radiotherapists. Seizures, headaches and chronic disability require symptomatic treatment and follow-up by a neurologist, while people with AVMs that have bled need appropriate monitoring in a dedicated neuroscience or stroke unit [30]. Current interventional treatment options comprise any combination of endovascular embolization (interventional neuroradiology), microsurgical removal (neurosurgery), and/or stereotactic radiotherapy (radiosurgery) [31]. Despite technical advances in these treatments during recent decades, none – either individually or in combination – has been tested in a controlled study.

The reported associated morbidity from any intervention is around 10% in most recent endovascular, neurosurgical, and radiotherapy series. The best possible treatment strategy should be discussed in view of the topographic and morphological characteristics and possible risk factors for natural history and

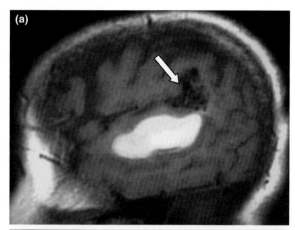

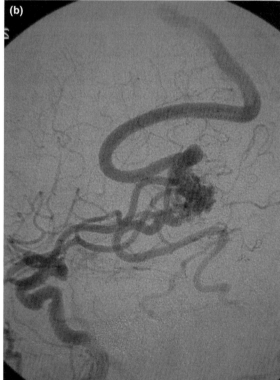

Fig. 6.6 Intracerebral hemorrhage due to an arteriovenous malformation. T1-weighted MRI (a) showing a hyperintense left temporal hematoma with an AVM nidus (arrow) visualized in the vicinity of the hemorrhage. Carotid artery angiography confirms the presence of a brain AVM fed by cortical MCA branches and with superficial venous drainage (b).

treatment risk. Intervention seems justified in many ruptured brain AVMs, mainly to prevent subsequent hemorrhage. No systematic data exist on the best timing for intervention (early versus late after AVM

Table 6.1. Brain AVM differential diagnosis: intracranial arteriovenous fistulae

Entity	Pathogenesis	Clinical characteristics
Vein of Galen aneurysmal malformation [46,47]	Persistent dilated embryonic vein of the prosencephalon, posterior choroidal artery affected	Congestive heart failure in neonates, intracranial hemorrhage in infants
Dural arteriovenous fistula [35]	Different types (traumatic, secondary to venous occlusion, etc.)	Arterial supply through meningeal arterial branches. High recurrence rate
Hereditary hemorrhagic telangiectasia (Osler-Weber-Rendu)	Capillary regression leads to multiple small AV-shunts in various tissues	Vascular abnormalities in nose, skin, lung, brain, and gastrointestinal tract
Encephalo-trigeminal syndrome (Sturge-Weber) [48]	Phakomatosis	Neurocutaneous syndrome affecting the meninges, not the brain
Cerebro-retinal angiomatosis (von Hippel-Lindau) [48]	Phakomatosis	Associated malignancy
Wyburn-Mason (or Bonnet-Dechaume-Blanc) syndrome [49,50]	Phakomatosis	Neurocutaneous syndrome with metameric brainstem AVM in newborns
Neovascular collaterals	Venous thrombosis or arterial occlusion may lead to focal angioneogenesis with early AV shunting	Postthrombotic syndrome, moyamoya syndrome, etc.

rupture), but recent series suggest the risk of re-rupture seems particularly high (18% within the first year after the initial hemorrhage) [32]. The benefit from prophylactic intervention in patients with unruptured brain AVMs is currently unproven and subject to an ongoing international treatment trial [33,34].

Dural arteriovenous fistulae

Dural arteriovenous fistulae (DAVFs) constitute arteriovenous shunts at the level of the meninges that are usually supplied by branches of the external carotid and/or vertebral artery. They are generally considered acquired lesions due to trauma or venous occlusion and have an extracerebral location. Often they present with pulse-synchronic bruits, headaches, and signs of increased intracranial pressure, but they may also cause progressive neurological deficits and intracranial bleeding, including ICH. Those with direct or retrograde venous outflow into cerebral veins have been associated with hemorrhagic presentation or progressive neurological symptoms at initial

diagnosis, but no controlled longitudinal data exist on the actual longitudinal risk of these lesions. Nonetheless, the most widely used classification as proposed by Merland and Cognard is mainly based on the venous outflow pattern as these characteristics may also impact on the endovascular treatment approach: in type I fistulae, meningeal branches shunt directly into a dural sinus without retrograde venous filling. Type II lesions are similar to type I but show venous reflux from the dural sinus into subarachnoid veins. Type III fistulae connect directly to cortical veins. If the latter type shows venous ectasias, it is labeled type IV. The rare infratentorial type V lesions show retrograde venous drainage into the spinal venous system [35].

A common presentation of a dural arteriovenous shunt is the carotid-cavernous fistula. This subtype consists of mainly a single shunt (rarely several transdural feeders) which links the internal carotid artery during its passage through the cavernous sinus with a portion of the cavernous sinus. Although they often arise following trauma, they are also known to occur spontaneously, especially in the elderly. The classic

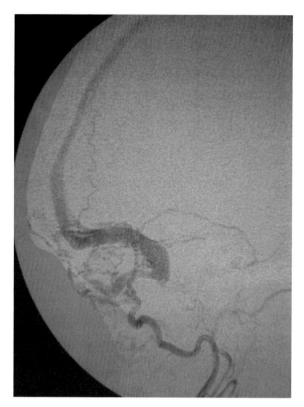

Fig. 6.7 Dural arteriovenous fistula visualized on angiography after injection of the right external carotid artery showing arteriovenous shunting into the right transverse sinus, occlusion of the distal sigmoid sinus, and retrograde venous outflow into the superior sagittal sinus.

symptom complex features an injected sclera of the affected eye, chemosis, ophthalmoplegia, a bruit, and, in severe cases, even loss of vision [36].

Quite commonly, DAVFs are missed on standard CT, MRI, and MRA images, and their definite diagnosis is mainly based on diagnostic cerebral angiography after obligatory injection of the common carotid and vertebral arteries (Fig. 6.7).

Most often, DAVFs are treated using an endovascular approach, either via the feeding artery system, or via retrograde occlusion of the draining veins. Depending on the topographic location, direct embolization via transcranial puncture or neurosurgical occlusion of the venous draining system constitute alternative therapeutic strategies.

Cavernous malformations

Cerebral cavernous malformations (CCMs) or cavernomas constitute abnormally enlarged capillary

cavities without intervening brain parenchyma. The lesions may occur anywhere including the cortical surface, white matter pathways, basal ganglia, or deep in the brainstem. They rarely occupy a clinically significant amount of space in the brain but may be located in clinically important regions and are occasionally multiple. Their cavernous channels often show multiple areas of thrombosis and hemosiderin deposits as remnants of prior intracavernomatous (less often extra-cavernomatous) hemorrhage. Blood flow through these lesions is minimal, and therefore they are generally not seen on diagnostic angiograms.

They may be recognized as round, slightly hyperdense lesions on non-contrast head CT showing some ring enhancement after injection (Fig. 6.8a and b). In most cases, the diagnosis is easily established on brain MRI with a typical popcorn-shaped, mixed hyper- and hypointense appearance and usually a hypointense perilesional signal on FLAIR and T2-weighted images (Fig. 6.8c). Gradient echo (T2*-weighted) imaging carries the highest sensitivity for the detection of CCM revealing intralesional paramagnetic hemosiderin deposits as hypointense signals (Fig. 6.8d). Extracerebral manifestations may affect cranial nerves (rare, but most commonly the trigeminal, optic, or oculomotor nerves), the spinal cord, the retina (in up to 5% of familial CCM cases), and the skin (visible as isolated hyperkeratotic cutaneous capillary venous malformations, so far described in cases with familial CCMs only).

Based on autopsy data, prevalence estimates for CCMs in the general population range between 100 and 500 per 100 000. Women and men appear to be equally affected. The mean age at diagnosis spreads around age 30 in most recent series, with an estimated annual detection rate of 0.56 per 100 000 [37]. The proportion of familial cases ranges between 10% and 40% in most western populations, but the highest frequency (50%) has been reported in Hispanic Americans, suggesting a genetic founder effect [38]. Patients harboring multiple CCMs have a high likelihood of carrying a genetic mutation.

Clinically, it is often difficult to determine a one-to-one relationship between lesion and symptoms. At initial diagnosis the latter include epileptic seizures in 45%, symptomatic hemorrhage in 40%, and headaches or other/unrelated symptoms leading to diagnostic imaging in 15%. Among patients with familial CCMs, 60% will become symptomatic. The

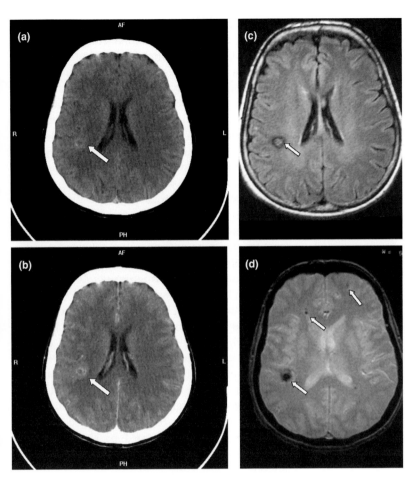

Fig. 6.8 Multiple cerebral cavernomatosis in a patient with proven CCM1/KRIT1 mutation. A subcortical right hemispheric CCM with hyperdense "ring" can be appreciated on non-contrast, (a) (arrow) and post-contrast, (b) (arrow) cranial CT. Brain MRI shows the same malformation with a mixed hyperintense/hypointense "popcorn" signal and a hypointense perilesional rim on FLAIR, (c) (arrow) and presence of multiple hypointense CCMs using the T2*-weighted (gradient echo) sequence, (d) (arrows).

proportion of symptomatic patients among sporadic cases remains as yet unknown. Three different gene loci have been defined so far, all leading to autosomal dominant pattern of inheritance: CCM1 or KRIT1 is located on chromosome 7q and accounts for over 40% of familial cases (up to 70% in Hispanic Americans); CCM2 or MGC4607 is on chromosome 7p and can be found in roughly 30%; finally CCM3 or PDCD10 has been mapped to chromosome 3q and is the underlying defect in 15%. Another 15% of familial cases show no mutation in the three loci, which is why at least one more gene defect can be suspected [38].

In routine clinical practice, the diagnosis of CCMs should be stratified by patient history (symptomatic versus asymptomatic, family history), MR imaging data (anatomic location, single versus multiple CCMs, hemorrhagic versus non-hemorrhagic, with or without associated developmental venous anomaly), and genetic test results (if performed). Ideally, the hemorrhage status is specified based on extra- versus intracavernomatous bleeding, and whether the MRI signal suggests acute blood or chronic hemosiderin deposits (Table 6.2). In the early days of MR imaging in surgical CCM patients, an initial morphological classification has been proposed based on their appearance on T1- and T2-weighted sequences: Type 1 cavernomas are hyperintense lesions indicating recent hemorrhage. Type 2 malformations are those most often seen in daily practice; they harbor mixed hyper- and hypointense signals suggestive of mixed subacute and chronic hemorrhage signs or calcifications. Type 3 lesions are hypointense and mostly asymptomatic. Type 4 CCMs are also assumed to be asymptomatic and can be detected on gradient echo (T2*) imaging alone. The latter group, however, may be difficult to differentiate from other causes

Table 6.2. Neurological classification of cerebral cavernous malformation

Parameter		
Clinical	Symptomatic	Asymptomatic
	• Seizures	
	• Hemorrhage	
	• Headache	
Family history	Positive	Negative
	• Pedigree	
	• Pattern of inheritance	
Imaging	MRI (T1 +/− contrast, T2 or FLAIR, T2*)	
Number	Multiple	Single
	• Anatomic location	• Anatomic location
Size	Maximum cavernoma diameter	
Hemorrhage	Acute bleeding	Chronic hemosiderin
	Extra-cavernomatous	Intra lesional
DVA	Present	Absent
Genetic testing	Positive	Negative
	• CCM1 (KRIT1)	
	• CCM2 (MGC4607)	
	• CCM3 (PDCD10)	

Note: DVA, developmental venous anomaly.
Source: Adjusted after [51].

of cerebral microbleeds, such as amyloid angiopathy, arteriolosclerotic small-vessel disease, cerebral autosomal dominant anteriopathy with subcortical infarcts and leucoencephalopathy (CADASIL), vasculitis, and others [39].

On longitudinal patient follow-up the number of CCMs may increase over time, especially in genetic CCM types. A given cavernoma may remain stable, increase in volume or even regress [40]. The crude average hemorrhage risk of a cavernoma seems to be as low as 0.6% per year [41]. Factors favoring symptomatic hemorrhage include a history of prior cavernoma hemorrhage, strategic locations such as the brainstem and basal ganglia, and anticoagulation therapy [42]. Pregnancy as a risk factor for cavernoma hemorrhage remains controversial. No data exist on whether or not antiplatelet drugs modify the risk of bleeding. Overall, even in genetically determined cases, the long-term prognosis is favorable with 80% preserved long-term autonomy, with less favorable outcome seen in patients with brainstem CCM [38].

If indicated, neurosurgical excision is the treatment of choice as outcome after stereotactic radiotherapy appears to have less favorable results [43,44]. The decision for intervention is ideally based on a multidisciplinary discussion considering the overall profile of the patient (Table 6.2). Surgery is generally limited to symptomatic CCMs associated with therapy-resistant epilepsy, progressive CCM enlargement, or after symptomtic CCM hemorrhage. If extra-lesional CCM bleeding has occurred, surgical excision may not only eliminate the risk of subsequent hemorrhage, but the risk of intervention itself may also be lower as the surgical approach in the post-acute phase is facilitated by the pre-existing bleeding cavity. Due to the progressive multiplication of lesions over time, surgical intervention is not generally recommended in patients with familial CCM. Resection of an associated developmental venous anomaly (see below) is contraindicated as its occlusion may lead to venous stasis, brain edema, and eventual hemorrhage.

Anomalies of cerebral veins
Developmental venous anomaly

A developmental venous anomaly (DVA) is found in up to 30% of CCM patients [45]. In the pre-MRI era, so-called "venous malformations" were considered a possible cause of ICH. The term is now obsolete, as DVAs constitute mainly asymptomatic variants of the physiological white matter or tectal venous drainage system. They are represented by a deep prominent vein which shows late on the venous phase of an arteriogram and is associated with a finger-like projection from the main vein. An associated cavernoma

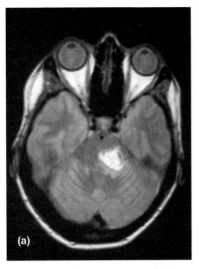 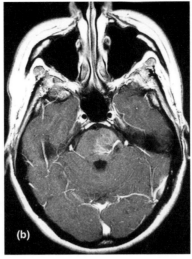 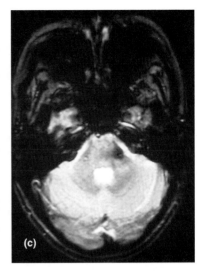

Fig. 6.9 Subacute pontine hemorrhage on non-contrast T1-weighted MRI in a 32-year-old patient without significant prior medical history. (a) Follow-up imaging after hematoma resorption reveals a developmental venous anomaly (b) (T1 after gadolinium injection) with an associated cavernous malformation (c) (hypointense on T2*-weighted image).

constitutes the actual bleeding source, if hemorrhage occurs in the vicinity of a DVA (Fig. 6.9).

References

1. Zhu XL, Chan MS, Poon WS. Spontaneous intracranial hemorrhage: which patients need diagnostic cerebral angiography? A prospective study of 206 cases and a review of literature. *Stroke* 1997; **28**: 1406–1409.

2. Broderick JP, Adams HP, Barsan W, *et al.* Guidelines for the management of spontaneous intracerebral hemorrhage. A statement for healthcare professionals from a special writing group of the Stroke Council, American Heart Association. *Stroke* 1999; **30**: 905–915.

3. Steiner T, Kaste M, Forsting M, *et al.* Recommendations for the management of intracranial hemorrhage-part I: spontaneous intracerebral hemorrhage. The European Stroke Initiative Writing Committee and the Writing Committee for the EUSI Executive Committee. *Cerebrovasc Dis* 2006; **22**(4): 294–316. Epub 2006 Jul 28. Erratum in: *Cerebrovasc Dis* 2006; **22**(5–6): 461. Katse Mankku [corrected to Kaste, Markku].

4. Stapf C, Van der Worp HB, Steiner T, *et al.* Stroke research priorities for the next decade – a supplement statement on intracranial hemorrhage. *Cerebrovasc Dis* 2007; **23**: 318–319.

5. Stapf C, Mohr JP. Aneurysms and subarachnoid hemorrhage – epidemiology. In: Le Roux PD, Winn RH, eds. *Management of Cerebral Aneurysms*. Philadelphia, Saunders. 2004; 183–187.

6. Phillips LH, Whisnant JP, O'Fallon M, *et al.* The unchanging pattern of subarachnoid hemorrhage in a community. *Neurology* 1980; **30**: 1034–1040.

7. The ACROSS Group Epidemiology of aneurysmal subarachnoid hemorrhage in Australia and New Zealand. Incidence and case fatality from the Australasian Cooperative Research on Subarachnoid Hemorrhage Study (ACROSS). *Stroke* 2000; **31**: 1843–1850.

8. Wiebers DO, Whisnant JP, Huston J 3rd, *et al.* International Study of Intracranial Aneurysms Investigators. Unruptured intracranial aneurysms: natural history, clinical outcome, and risks of surgical and endovascular treatment. *Lancet* 2003; **362**: 103–110.

9. Johnston SC, Selvin S, Gress DR. The burden, trends, and demographics of mortality from subarachnoid hemorrhage. *Neurology* 1998; **50**: 1413–1418.

10. Longstrength WT Jr, Nelson LM, Koepsell TD, *et al.* Subarachnoid hemorrhage and hormonal factors in women. A population-based case-control study. *Ann Int Med* 1994; **121**: 168–173.

11. Jennett B, Teasdale G. *Management of Head Injuries.* Philadelphia, FA Davis, 1981.

12. Hunt WE, Hess RM. Surgical risk as related to time of intervention in the repair of intracranial aneurysms. *J Neurosurg* 1968; **28**: 14–20.

13. Johnston SC, Wilson CB, Halbach VV, *et al.* Endovascular and surgical treatment of unruptured

cerebral aneurysms: comparison of risks. *Ann Neurol* 2000; **48**: 11–19.

14. International Subarachnoid Aneurysm Trial (ISAT) Collaborative Group. International Subarachnoid Aneurysm Trial (ISAT) of neurosurgical clipping versus endovascular coiling in 2143 patients with ruptured intracranial aneurysms: a randomised trial. *Lancet* 2002; **360**: 1267–1274.

15. Farrell DF, Forno LS. Symptomatic capillary telangiectasis of the brainstem without hemorrhage. Report of an unusual case. *Neurology* 1970; **20**(4): 341–346.

16. Jessurun GA, Kamphuis DJ, van der Zande FH, Nossent JC. Cerebral arteriovenous malformations in The Netherlands Antilles. High prevalence of hereditary hemorrhagic telangiectasia-related single and multiple cerebral arteriovenous malformations. *Clin Neurol Neurosurg* 1993; **95**(3): 193–198.

17. Fukui M. Guidelines for the diagnosis and treatment of spontaneous occlusion of the circle of Willis ("moyamoya" disease). Research Committee on Spontaneous Occlusion of the Circle of Willis (Moyamoya Disease) of the Ministry of Health and Welfare, Japan. *Clin Neurol Neurosurg* 1997; **99** Suppl 2: S238–240.

18. Suzuki J. *Moyamoya Disease*. Berlin, Springer-Verlag, 1986.

19. Goto Y, Yonekawa Y. Worldwide distribution of moyamoya disease. *Neurol Med Chir (Tokyo)* 1992; **32**: 883–886.

20. Kuroda S, Ishikawa T, Houkin K, *et al.* Incidence and clinical features of disease progression in adult moyamoya disease. *Stroke* 2005; **36**: 2148–2153.

21. Uchino K, Johnston CS, Becker KJ, Tirschwell DL. Moyamoya disease in Washington State and California. *Neurology* 2005; **65**: 956–958.

22. Kuriyama S, Kusaka Y, Fujimura M, *et al.* Prevalence and clinicoepidemiological features of moyamoya disease in Japan. Findings from a nationwide epidemiological survey. *Stroke* 2008; **39**: 42–47.

23. Merkel KH, Ginsberg PL, Parker JC Jr, Post MJ. Cerebrovascular disease in sickle cell anemia: a clinical, pathological and radiological correlation. *Stroke* 1978; **9**: 45–52.

24. Ullrich NJ, Robertson R, Kinnamon DD, *et al.* Moyamoya following cranial irradiation for primary brain tumors in children. *Neurology* 2007; **68**: 932–938.

25. Stapf C, Mast H, Sciacca RR, *et al.* The New York Islands AVM Study: design, study progress and initial results. *Stroke* 2003; **34**: e29–33.

26. Van Beijnum J, van der Worp HB, Schippers HM, *et al.* Familial occurrence of brain arteriovenous malformations: a systematic review. *J Neurol Neurosurg Psychiatry* 2007; **78**: 1213–1217.

27. Stapf C, Mast H, Sciacca RR, *et al.* Predictors of hemorrhage in patients with untreated brain arteriovenous malformation. *Neurology* 2006; **66**: 1350–1355.

28. Kim H, Sidney S, McCulloch CE, *et al.* for the UCSF BAVM Study Project. Racial/ethnic differences in longitudinal risk of intracranial hemorrhage in brain arteriovenous malformation patients. *Stroke* 2007; **38**: 2430–2437.

29. Choi JH, Mast H, Sciacca RR, *et al.* Clinical outcome after first and recurrent hemorrhage in patients with untreated brain arteriovenous malformation. *Stroke* 2006; **37**: 1243–1247.

30. Al-Shahi R, Stapf C. The prognosis and treatment of arteriovenous malformations of the brain. *Pract Neurol* 2005; **5**: 194–205.

31. Ogilvy CS, Stieg PE, Awad I, *et al.* AMA Scientific Statement. Recommendations for the management of intracranial arteriovenous malformations: a statement for healthcare professionals from a special writing group of the Stroke Council, American Stroke Association. *Stroke* 2001; **32**: 1458–1471.

32. Mast H, Young WL, Koennecke HC, *et al.* Risk of spontaneous hemorrhage after diagnosis of cerebral arteriovenous malformations. *Lancet* 1997; **350**: 1065–1068.

33. Stapf C, Mohr JP, Choi JH, Mast H. Invasive treatment of unruptured brain arteriovenous malformations is experimental therapy. *Curr Opin Neurol* 2006; **19**: 63–68.

34. Wedderburn CJ, van Beijnum J, Bhattacharya JJ, *et al.* on behalf of the SIVMS Collaborators. Outcome after interventional or conservative management of unruptured brain arteriovenous malformations: a prospective, population-based cohort study. *Lancet Neurol* 2008; **7**(3): 223–230. Epub 2008 Feb 1.

35. Cognard C, Gobin YP, Pierot L, *et al.* Cerebral dural arteriovenous fistulae: clinical and angiographic correlation with a revised classification of venous drainage. *Radiology* 1995; **194**: 671–680.

36. Theaudin M, Saint-Maurice JP, Chapot R, *et al.* Diagnosis and treatment of dural carotid-cavernous fistulae: a consecutive series of 27 patients. *J Neurol Neurosurg Psychiatry* 2007; **78**: 174–179.

37. Al-Shahi R, Bhattacharya JJ, Currie DG, *et al.* and Scottish Intracranial Vascular Malformation Study Collaborators. Prospective, population-based detection of intracranial vascular malformations in adults: The Scottish Intracranial Vascular Malformation Study (SIVMS). *Stroke* 2003; **34**: 1163–1169.

38. Labauge P, Denier C, Bergametti F, Tournier-Lasserve E. Genetics of cavernous angiomas. *Lancet Neurol* 2007; **6**: 237–244.

39. Viswanathan A, Chabriat H. Cerebral microhemorrhage. *Stroke* 2006; **37**: 550–555.

40. Clatterbuck RE, Moriarity JL, Elmaci I, *et al.* Dynamic nature of cavernous malformations: a prospective magnetic resonance imaging study with volumetric analysis. *J Neurosurg* 2000; **93**: 981–986.

41. Labauge P, Brunerau L, Laberge S, Houtteville JP. Prospective follow-up of 33 asymptomatic patients with familial cerebral cavernous malformations. *Neurology* 2001; **57**: 1825–1828.

42. Lehnhardt FG, von Smekal U, Rückriem B, *et al.* Value of gradient echo magnetic resonance imaging in the diagnosis of familial cerebral cavernous malformation. *Arch Neurol* 2005; **62**: 653–658.

43. Mathiesen T, Edner G, Kihlström L. Deep and brainstem cavernomas: a consecutive 8-year series. *J Neurosurg* 2003; **99**: 31–37.

44. Pollock BE, Garces YI, Stafford SL, *et al.* Stereotactic radiosurgery for cavernous malformations. *J Neurosurg* 2000; **93**: 987–991.

45. Rabinov JD. Diagnostic imaging of angiographically occult vascular malformations. *Neurosurg Clin N Am* 1999; **10**: 419–432.

46. Raybaud CA, Strother CM, Hald JK. Aneurysms of the vein of Galen: embryonic considerations and anatomical features relating to the pathogenesis of the malformation. *Neuroradiology* 1989; **31**: 109–128.

47. Lasjaunias P. *Vascular Diseases in Neonates, Infants and Children. Interventional Neuroradiology Management*, 1st edn. Berlin, Springer-Verlag, 1997.

48. Alberts MJ. Intracerebral hemorrhage and vascular malformations. In: Alberts MJ, ed. *Genetics of Cerebrovascular Disease*. Armonk, NY, Futura Publishing Company. 1999; 209–236.

49. Patel U, Gupta SC. Wyburn-Mason syndrome. A case report and review of the literature. *Neuroradiology* 1990; **31**: 544–546.

50. Ponce FA, Han PP, Spetzler RF, Canady A, Feiz-Erfan I. Associated arteriovenous malformation of the orbit and brain: a case of Wyburn-Mason syndrome without retinal involvement. Case report. *J Neurosurg* 2001; **95**: 346–349.

51. Al-Shahi Salman R, Berg MJ, Morrison L, Awad IA. Hemorrhage from cavernous malformations of the brain: definition and reporting standards. *Stroke* 2008; **40**: 3222–3230.

Cerebral venous thrombosis and intracerebral hemorrhage

Isabelle Crassard and Marie-Germaine Bousser

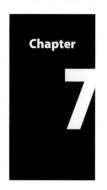

Introduction

Cerebral venous thrombosis (CVT), a rare variety of cerebrovascular disease, is a well-established cause of intracerebral hemorrhage (ICH). Indeed, recognized since the beginning of the nineteenth century [1], this disease was mostly diagnosed at autopsy which usually showed hemorrhagic lesions which were long thought to contraindicate the use of heparin [2,3]. In the last 25 years, the widespread use of neuroimaging has allowed early diagnosis of CVT and has thus completely modified our knowledge of this condition. More common than previously thought, CVT is characterized by a wide spectrum of clinical presentations and of neuroimaging changes, with hemorrhagic lesions in about one-third of cases. The overall outcome is frequently favorable with a mortality rate well below 10% but hemorrhagic varieties of CVT (H-CVT) are usually associated with a more severe clinical presentation and a worse outcome than non-hemorrhagic varieties. Cerebral venous thrombosis as a cause of ICH is crucial to recognize because it is the only variety of ICH that should be treated with heparin.

Anatomy of the cerebral venous system

Blood from the brain is drained by cerebral veins that empty into dural sinuses, themselves mostly drained by the internal jugular veins [4,5,6] (Fig. 7.1).

Cerebral veins

Three groups of veins drain the venous blood of the brain.

Superficial cerebral veins

Some of the cortical veins (frontal, parietal, and occipital superior cortical veins) drain the venous blood of the cortex into the superior sagittal sinus (SSS) whereas others, mainly the middle cerebral vein drain into the cavernous sinuses. They are linked by numerous anastomoses allowing, in case of thrombosis, the development of collateral circulation. The main collateral veins are the vein of Labbé connecting the middle cerebral veins to the lateral sinus (LS) and the great anastomotic vein of Trolard connecting the SSS to the middle cerebral veins. These cortical veins are characterized by the presence of thin walls, the absence of muscle fibers and valves, permitting both dilatation and reversal of flow when the sinus into which they drain is occluded. Because of their thin walls and their ability to dilate, cortical veins, by contrast to arteries, may rupture if the venous pressure increases. The number and location of cortical veins are variable, which explains both the difficulty in their angiographic diagnosis and the absence of well-delineated cortical venous territories, and hence the absence of well-identified "venous" clinical syndromes similar to the arterial clinical syndromes.

Deep cerebral veins

Internal cerebral and basal veins drain the blood from the deep white matter of the cerebral hemispheres and from basal ganglia. They join to form the great vein of Galen followed by the straight sinus (SS). By contrast to the superficial veins, the deep venous system is constant and well visualized on imaging, so that its occlusion or absence is easily recognized.

Intracerebral Hemorrhage, ed. J. R. Carhuapoma, S. A. Mayer, and D. F. Hanley. Published by Cambridge University Press.
© J. R. Carhuapoma, S. A. Mayer, and D. F. Hanley 2010.

(a)

(b)

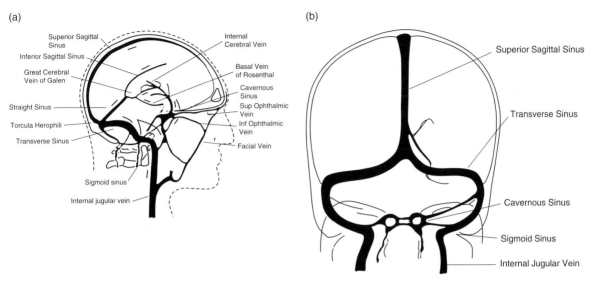

Fig. 7.1 Anatomy of dural sinuses and cerebral veins. Anatomic drawings of lateral view (a) and anteroposterior view (b).

Veins of the posterior fossa

These are divided into three groups: the superior veins drain into the galenic system; the anterior ones into the petrosal sinus; and the posterior ones into the torcula, the SSS, and the lateral sinuses. They are also variable so that the diagnosis of their rare thrombosis is very difficult.

Dural sinuses

Superior sagittal sinus (SSS)

The SSS lies in the attached border of the falx cerebri and extends from the foramen cecum to the occipital protuberance where it joins the SS and the LSs to form the torcular Herophili. Its anterior part can be narrow or even missing, mimicking an occlusion. It is then replaced by two superior cerebral veins that join behind the coronal suture. The SSS drains the major part of the cortex but it also receives diploic veins that are connected to scalp veins by emissary veins (explaining some CVT after minor head trauma by local spreading of a thrombosed scalp vein).

Lateral sinuses (LSs)

The LSs start at the torcular Herophili to reach the jugular bulbs. They consist of two portions: the transverse sinus lying in the attached border of the tentorium and the sigmoid sinus directly applied to the inner aspect of the mastoid process. The LSs drain the blood flow of the cerebellum, the brainstem, and

the posterior part of the cerebral hemispheres. They also receive some diploic veins and some small veins from the middle ear. There are numerous LS anatomical variations: the two most frequent are the absence of transverse sinus replaced by a large cortical vein draining directly into the sigmoid sinus and hypoplasia of the left LS [2].

The dural sinuses contain most of the arachnoid villi and granulations in which cerebrospinal fluid (CSF) absorption takes place. In this way dural sinuses play a major role in CSF circulation and pressure, which explains the high frequency of raised intracranial pressure in CVT involving the dural sinuses.

Cavernous sinuses

These consist of trabeculated cavities formed by the separation of the layers of the dura. They are located on both sides of the sella turcica, just above and outside the sphenoid air sinuses. They drain the blood flow from the orbits by the ophthalmic veins and from the anterior part of the base of the brain through the sphenoparietal sinus and the middle cerebral veins. They themselves drain into the superior petrosal and inferior petrosal sinuses then into the internal jugular veins.

Topography

All studies show that the frequency of sinus thrombosis far outweighs that of cerebral veins thrombosis

85

Table 7.1. The sites of thrombosis in large series of CVT

	ISCVT N = 624	Authors' series N = 234		
			Hemorrhagic forms N = 58	Non-Hemorrhagic forms N = 176
Superior sagittal sinus	313 62%	124 53%	34 58%	90 51%
Lateral sinus		184 79%	40 69%	144 81%
– Right	257 41%	44 19%	16 28%	28 16%
– Left	279 45%	97 41%	25 43%	72 41%
Straight sinus/deep venous system	180 29%	39 17%	6 10%	33 19%
Cortical veins	107 17%	44 19%	21 36%	23 13%

Note: 49 patients of the authors' series have been included in ISCVT.

but it should be emphasized again that the diagnosis of cortical vein thrombosis on angiography or even on MRI T2* is extremely difficult so that cortical vein thrombosis is likely to be vastly overlooked [7–13]. The most commonly affected vessels are LS and SSS followed by cortical veins, deep venous system, and cavernous sinus (Table 7.1).

In a majority of cases thrombosis involves several sinuses and veins, the most frequent association being SSS + LS, SSS + cortical veins, LS + temporal veins, deep veins with SS. This frequent multiple sinus and vein involvement also accounts for the lack of well-defined topographical clinical syndromes in CVT. The pattern of distribution of sinus and veins involvement differs in hemorrhagic and non-hemorrhagic varieties of CVT with an at least four times more frequent involvement of cortical veins in hemorrhagic varieties (Table 7.1).

Pathology and pathophysiology

Thrombosis within a cerebral vein or sinus is a dynamic process with a tendency to propagate forwards or backwards from the point of origin [5]. In some cases thrombosis may occur simultaneously at a number of different sites. If lysis of the red thrombus does not take place immediately, older parts of the thrombus may become organized and attached to the venous wall, with sometimes recanalization, while fresh thrombus may remain free within the lumen.

The effects of venous thrombosis on the cerebral tissue depends upon many parameters such as type of vessel involved, availability of pre-existing collateral channels, and extent of thrombus propagation [2].

Thus, CVT may have no consequence on the brain parenchyma, as in some cases of isolated LS thrombosis. More frequently, elevated cerebral venous pressure due to venous occlusion results in a spectrum of pathophysiological changes including a dilated venous and capillary bed, development of interstitial brain tissue edema, increased CSF production, decreased CSF absorption, and rupture of cerebral veins leading to hemorrhagic lesions [14]. The pathophysiology of venous hemorrhages in CVT has been widely discussed. Some experimental studies have highlighted the importance of extensive occlusion of cortical veins [15–19] whereas others report the possibility of hemorrhagic lesions after induction of SSS thrombosis only [20]. Whatever the site of thrombosis (cortical veins and/or sinuses) hemorrhagic lesions secondary to ruptured veins can present with a huge diversity in size and location. The hemorrhage may be limited to a few petechiae, detectable only on T2*, particularly suggestive of CVT when they are superficial, bilateral, and organized in clots. Sometimes the pattern is that of a "hemorrhagic infarct" consisting of a bleed of variable degree within areas of pure edema or ischemic edema. The most classical presentation is that of bilateral triangular hemorrhagic infarcts, located in the superior and internal part of both hemispheres, due to thrombosis of SSS and its tributary cortical veins [2]. This term "hemorrhagic infarct" has been very misleading because it suggests a similarity with hemorrhagic infarcts of arterial origin and it was one of the reasons why heparin was so long thought to be contraindicated in CVT. It is now well established that the pathophysiology of these two conditions widely

Table 7.2. Frequency of hemorrhagic forms in different series of patients with CVT

References	Milandre *et al.* 1989 [8]	Cantu *et al.* 1993 [9]	Daif *et al.* 1995 [10]	De Bruijn *et al.* 2001 [11]	Ferro *et al.* 2001 [12]	ISCVT 2004 [13]	Authors' series 2007
Number of patients	20	95	40	59	142	624	234
Hemorrhagic CVT	4 (20%)	44 (46%)	5 (12.5%)	21 (36%)	49 (35%)	245 (39%)	58 (25%)

differs so that heparin is indicated in venous hemorrhagic infarcts but contraindicated in arterial hemorrhagic infarcts. Hemorrhagic lesions may also become confluent, particularly in the white matter, leading to a true hematoma. Thus a temporal hematoma, sometimes with a severe mass effect, can complicate LS thrombosis with involvement of its tributary vein, the vein of Labbé [21–23]. Similarly uni- or bilateral thalamic hematoma may occur after internal cerebral vein(s) and/or SS thrombosis [24,25]. When bilateral, thalamic hematoma are highly suggestive of deep venous system thrombosis. Cerebellar hemorrhages due to cerebellar vein thrombosis is extremely rare and, by itself, not distinguishable from other varieties of cerebellar hematoma [2]. Other varieties of intracranial hemorrhages due to CVT are rare. Subarachnoid hemorrhage (SAH) may be associated with ICH or occur in isolation, due to cortical vein thrombosis. It is usually a small cortical SAH highly different from aneurysmal SAH [26,27]. Exceptionally, subdural hematoma can also reveal CVT [28–29].

Incidence

The exact incidence of CVT is unknown but much higher than thought on old autopsy series [3,5,30] as suggested by the publication of large clinical series [7–12] and by the inclusion in three years of 624 cases in the International Study on Cerebral Vein and Dural Sinus Thrombosis (ISCVT), a multicenter prospective cohort of adult patients [13]. It is considered to affect about 5–10 people per million and to account for 0.5% of all stroke [31]. The frequency of hemorrhagic CVT varies according to diagnostic criteria: from nearly 100% in old autopsy series to 12.5–46% in seven recent series based on neuroimaging (Table 7.2). Thus H-CVT roughly accounts for one-third of all CVT. In our own series of 234 patients diagnosed in our institution between 1997 and 2007, 58 patients (25%) had an H-CVT defined as any

parenchymal hemorrhag visible on CT and/or MRI. Eleven of these patients (19%) had associated small localized SAH and three (5%) an associated subdural hematoma. Eleven other patients (5%) had either isolated SAH or subdural hematoma.

All age groups can be affected, with however a slight preponderance in young women because of specific causes such as pregnancy, postpartum, and oral contraceptives. Both in ISCVT and in our series, the same sex-ratio was observed in H-CVT and non-H-CVT. In our series, the female/male ratio was 4/1. In both series, patients were a little older when they had ICH (39.5 years old vs. 35.7 years old in Lariboisière's series).

Cerebral venous thrombosis in neonates is a condition that widely differs from CVT in children and adults because of the frequent association with an acute illness at time of diagnosis and the clinical presentation with seizures and lethargy [32–35]. Parenchymal lesions are frequent, present on neuroimaging in 40–60% of cases [32,35], with a very frequent hemorrhagic component and an intraventricular hemorrhage in 20% of cases [35].

Causes

Numerous causes and risk factors have been identified in CVT. They include all known medical, surgical, gyneco-obstetrical causes of deep vein thrombosis in the legs, as well as a number of local causes either infective or non-infective, such as head trauma, brain tumors, arteriovenous malformations, and local infections such as otitis or sinusitis (Table 7.3). Medical causes and risk factors include congenital or acquired prothrombotic conditions, malignancies, hematological diseases, vasculitis, or other inflammatory systemic disorders. Diagnostic and therapeutic procedures such as surgery, lumbar puncture, jugular catheter and medications in particular oral contraceptives, hormone replacement therapy, steroids, and

Table 7.3. Chief causes and risk factors of CVT

Local causes	
Infectious	Direct septic trauma
	Intracranial infection: abscess, subdural empyema, orbital cellulitis, tonsillitis, cutaneous cellulitis
Non-infectious	Head or neck tumors, neurosurgical procedures
	Head injury
	After lumbar puncture
	Jugular catheterization
General infections	Meningitis, systemic infectious disease
Thrombophilia/ Acquired prothrombotic states	Factor V Leiden mutation, G20210A prothrombin mutation, Hyperhomocysteinemia and methylene tetrahydrofolate reductase (MTHFR) mutation
	Antithrombin, protein S, protein C deficiencies
	Disorders of fibrinolysis
	Antiphospholipid antibodies
	Paroxysmal nocturnal hemoglobinuria
	Disseminated intravascular coagulation
Hematological conditions	Polycythemia, thrombocythemia
	Iron deficiency anemia
	Leukemia, lymphoma
Systemic diseases	Systemic lupus erythematosus, Behcet disease, Wegener granulomatosis, inflammatory bowel disease, sarcoidosis, thyroiditis
	Cancers
Gyneco-obstetrical conditions	Post partum, puerperium
	Oral contraceptives
Medications	Corticoids, L-asparaginase, epsilon aminocaproic acid, tamoxifen
General conditions	Post-surgery
	Severe dehydration (especially in children)
	Nephrotic syndrome
	Cardiac insufficiency

oncology treatments can also cause or predispose to CVT [2]. Various causes and risk factors are often associated in CVT, 28% in our series and 44% in ISCVT. The most frequent association is that of oral contraceptive use and congenital thrombophilia. This means that even when an obvious cause is present, a systematic complete etiological workup should be performed. However, in around 15% of cases, no cause or even risk factor is found, which stresses the need for a long follow-up with repeated investigations.

There are very few data about the distribution of causes according to the presence or absence of ICH in CVT, but the small number of cases due to a given cause makes it unlikely to find significant differences. In ISCVT, the only difference found was a higher frequency of congenital thrombophilia in H-CVT [36]. No difference was found in our series as regards the various causes or risk factors and the frequency of their association. The etiological workup of H-CVT should thus be similar to that of all other CVT.

Clinical presentations

Cerebral venous thrombosis presents with a remarkably wide spectrum of signs and modes of onset, thus potentially mimicking numerous neurological conditions [2,31,37,38]. The most frequent symptoms and signs are headache, seizures, focal neurological deficits, altered consciousness, and papilledema which can present in isolation or in association (Table 7.4). Although they can all be present in H-CVT and non-H-CVT, their respective frequency varies widely (Table 7.5). In our series focal deficits and seizures were both present at admission in 50–60% of cases and disorders of consciousness in 40%. For these three symptoms, the frequency is two to three times that observed in non-H-CVT. By contrast, isolated headache was present in only 1/58 patients with H-CVT

Table 7.4. Chief clinical signs at admission in CVT patients

	ISCVT N = 624 patients (%)	Authors' series N = 234 patients (%)
Headaches	553 89%	229 97%
Papilledema	174 28%	85/230 37%
Motor deficit	232 37%	57 24%
Sensory deficit	34 5%	13 5%
Aphasia	119 19%	31 13%
Altered consciousness/coma	137 22%	47 20%
Seizures before diagnosis	245 39%	81 35%
– Generalized seizures		42 18%
– Focal +/– generalization		43 18%
Other focal cortical signs	21 3%	7 3%
Bilateral signs		8 3%

Table 7.5. Chief clinical data of CVT patients at hospital admission in the authors' series according to the presence of ICH or not

	Hemorrhagic forms N = 58	Non-Hemorrhagic forms N = 176
Headaches	53 (92%)	176 (100%)
Papilledema	16 (28%)	69/172 (40%)
Any focal deficit	44 (76%)	40 (23%)
– *Focal motor deficit*	28 (49%)	29 (16%)
– *Focal sensory deficit*	6 (10%)	7 (4%)
– *Focal motor or sensory deficit*	30 (52%)	30 (17%)
– *Aphasia*	23 (40%)	8 (5%)
Disorders of consciousness	24 (41%)	23 (13%)
Seizures before admission	32 (55%)	49 (28%)
– *Generalized seizures*	20 (34%)	22 (13%)
– *Focal +/– generalization*	16 (28%)	27 (15%)
Mode of onset		
– Acute < 48 h	19 (33%)	29 (16%)
– Subacute (2–30 days)	37 (64%)	135 (77%)
– Chronic (> 30 days)	2 (3%)	12 (7%)
Clinical presentation		
– Isolated headaches	1	51
– Isolated ICH	1	55
– Focal deficit	56	70

compared with 51/176 in non-H-CVT. Papilledema was less frequent in H-CVT (28%) than in non-H-CVT (40%) but this difference was not statistically significant.

The modes of onset were also different with a more frequent acute onset in H-CVT (Table 7.5).

According to the grouping of symptoms and signs, four main patterns have been individualized in CVT [7,37]:

- isolated intracranial hypertension, with headache, papilledema, and sixth nerve palsy
- focal syndrome, defined by focal deficits and/or partial seizures. Any brain symptom such as aphasia, hemiplegia, hemianopia, and so forth can occur in CVT
- subacute encephalopathy mainly characterized by a depressed level of consciousness and sometimes seizures
- cavernous sinus syndrome, with ocular signs dominating the clinical picture as orbital pain, chemosis, proptosis, and oculomotor palsies.

Among the four main patterns of CVT presentation, two (focal deficits and subacute encephalopathy) account for nearly all cases (96%). In our series, isolated cavernous sinus thrombosis never presented

Table 7.6. Clinical outcome in ISCVT and in Lariboisière's series

	ISCVT N = 624		Lariboisière N = 234	
	At discharge	**At last follow-up**	**At discharge**	**At one year (N = 211)**
Complete recovery (mRS 0–1)	410 (66%)	493 (79%)	166 (71%)	191 (91%)
Partial recovery (mRS 2)	96 (15%)	47 (8%)	42 (18%)	11 (5%)
Dependent (mRS 3–5)	91 (15%)	32 (5%)	22 (9%)	5 (2%)
Death (mRS 6)	27 (4%)	52 (8%)	4 (2%)	4 (2%)

Note: mRS, modified Rankin Score.

Table 7.7. Clinical outcome in our series according to the presence of intracranial hemorrhage or not

	Hemorrhagic forms N = 58		Non-hemorrhagic forms N = 176	
	At discharge	**At one year N = 49**	**At discharge**	**At one year N = 162**
Complete recovery (mRS 0–1)	15 (26%)	34 (70%)	151 (86%)	157 (97%)
Partial recovery (mRS 2)	22 (38%)	8 (16%)	20 (11.5%)	3 (2%)
Dependent (mRS 3–5)	18 (31%)	4 (8%)	4 (2%)	1 (0.5%)
Death (mRS 6)	3 (5%)	3 (6%)	1 (0.5%)	1 (0.5%)

with ICH and among our 58 H-CVT, only one presented as progressive isolated intracranial hypertension mimicking idiopathic intracranial hypertension.

Outcome

The outcome of patients with CVT is much better than that of arterial strokes (Table 7.6). A complete recovery is observed in 79% in ISCVT and 91% in our series at one year. Death rates are respectively 4% and 2%. A meta-analysis of recent cohorts, particularly including the data of ISCVT, finds a slightly worse prognosis with a 15% overall deaths or dependency rate [11,13,31,39–43].

Intracerebral hemorrhage has long been recognized a factor of bad prognosis in CVT [11,12]. In ISCVT, the presence of ICH was a predictor of mortality at 30 days [13]. In our series (Table 7.7), patients with ICH had a worse prognosis at both end of hospitalization and at one year of follow-up. The worse outcome in patients with ICH can be explained by the presence of the more frequent occurrence of focal deficits and the presence of large parenchymal lesions. These can be in such case responsible of severe mass effect with transtorial herniation that can lead to death.

Diagnosis

The diagnosis of CVT is based on neuroimaging but, even though some locations of hemorrhages can be suggestive of CVT, brain imaging by itself is of little positive value. The clue to the diagnosis is the imaging of the venous system itself which may show the occluded vessel or even more specifically the presence of the intravascular thrombus. These signs are indispensable to recognize to identify the cause of ICH.

The thrombosed vessel

Computerized tomography scan remains often the first investigation performed on an emergency basis. It is particularly useful in order to rule out many of the conditions that can be mimicked by CVT. Some signs are the direct reflection of the thrombus such as the dense triangle (occlusion of SSS by fresh clot on non-contrast CT), the empty delta sign (filling of collateral veins in the SSS walls after contrast injection, contrasting with the lack of enhancement of the clot inside the thrombosed sinus), the cord sign (visualization of a thrombosed cortical vein on non-contrast CT) and the spontaneous LS hyperdensity (visualization of the thrombosed LS) [44–46] (Fig. 7.2). This last

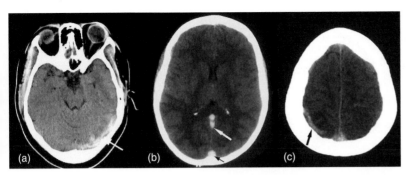

Fig. 7.2 Different aspects of the thrombus on non-contrast-CT. (a) Spontaneous hyperdensity of the lateral sinus; (b) spontaneous hyperdensity of the superior sagittal sinus (= *dense triangle*) and of the straight sinus (arrows); (c) spontaneous hyperdensity of the superior sagittal sinus and of a cortical vein (= *cord sign*, arrow).

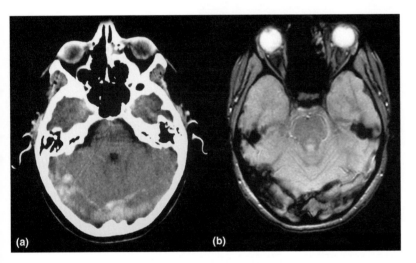

Fig. 7.3 (a) Spontaneous hyperdensity of both lateral sinuses on non-enhanced-CT that was initially misdiagnosed as subarachnoid hemorrhage; (b) lateral sinuses hyposignal on T2* imaging according to the presence of thrombosis.

aspect is important to recognize because it is sometimes difficult to interpret and falsely interpreted as a localized SAH (Fig. 7.3). The current "gold standard" is the combination of MRI to visualize the thrombosed vessel and MRV to detect the non-visualization of the same vessel [31,47,48]. The clot can take different appearances according to the evolution of the thrombosis. At a very early stage (< 5 days), the occluded vessel appears isointense on T1-weighted imaging (WI) and hypointense on T2 and thus very difficult to differentiate from normal veins. Magnetic resonance venography is then necessary to show the absence of flow in the affected sinus. A few days later, because of the conversion of oxyhemoglobin to methemoglobin within the thrombus, the occluded vessel becomes hyperintense first on T1-WI and later on T2-WI. At this stage, diagnosis is thus easy (Fig. 7.4). After the first month, MRI patterns are variable because the thrombosed sinus can either remain totally or partially occluded or can recanalize and return to normal. In the majority of cases, there is an isointensity on T1-WI and

hyperintensity on T2-WI. At 6 months, abnormalities persist in about two-thirds of cases. The signal is often heterogeneous but predominantly isointense on T1-WI and iso- or hyperintense on T2-WI. The combination of MRI/MRV has the best diagnosis yield because with MRI alone, flow artifacts may lead to false-positives and with MRV alone it is difficult and sometimes impossible, as with all other angiographic techniques, to differentiate thrombosis and hypoplasia, a frequent diagnostic dilemma for LSs. Even with the combination of MRI and MRV, the diagnosis may still be difficult, particularly in isolated cortical vein thrombosis which, in the absence of the characteristic "cord sign" on non-contrast CT scan or on MRI, occasionally requires conventional angiography. However, diagnosis remains difficult with indirect signs such as dilated cortical veins with a corkscrew appearance, delayed venous emptying, and collateral circulation. Recently the echo-planar susceptibility weighted images (T2*) have been shown to have a great value for diagnosis of CVT. This sequence, by contrast to T1 and T2, shows the thrombosis as a

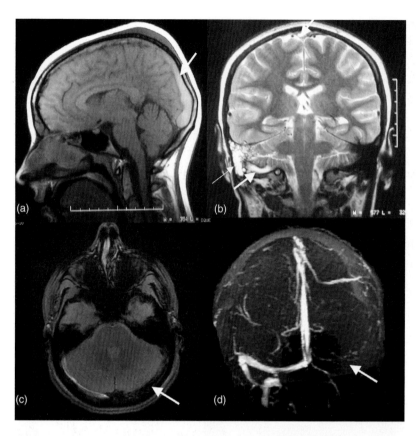

Fig. 7.4 Cerebral venous thrombosis on MRI. (a) Sagittal T1-weighted imaging: superior sagittal sinus hypersignal; (b) Coronal T2-weighted imaging: superior sagittal sinus hypersignal and lateral sinus hypersignal with homolateral increased T2-weighted MRI signal in the mastoid air spaces (thin arrow); (c) T2* imaging: left lateral sinus hyposignal; (d) Magnetic resonance venography: absence of flow in left lateral sinus.

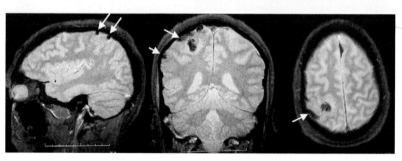

Fig. 7.5 Aspect of isolated cortical venous thrombosis on T2* imaging: venous hypointensities (magnetic susceptibility effect) are observed on the different planes (arrows) corresponding to the cortical vein thrombosis as well as petechial intracerebral hemorrhages.

highly hypointense signal related to the magnetic susceptibility effect and very similar to that observed in ICH [49–51]. The T2* appears to be of additional value for the diagnosis of CVT, particularly during the early days of thrombosis when T1-WI and T2-WI lack sensitivity, and in the case of isolated cortical venous thrombosis [51] (Fig. 7.5).

Parenchymal abnormalities

The detection of hemorrhagic lesions is not different from that of other varieties of ICH: visible on non-contrast CT and MRI, especially on T2* sequence. On CT, in the parenchyma, they appear as hyperdensities, often multifocal and petechial or large (Figs. 7.6 and 7.7). They can be associated with hypodensity corresponding to edema. Brain swelling can be also detected. Contrast-enhanced CT may reveal gyral or ring enhancement in areas of venous infarctions and/or tentorial enhancement [44,48].

On MRI, an increased signal on both T1-WI and T2-WI is typically found in hemorrhagic lesions (Fig. 7.8). These signal changes are frequently surrounded with a large region of edema appearing

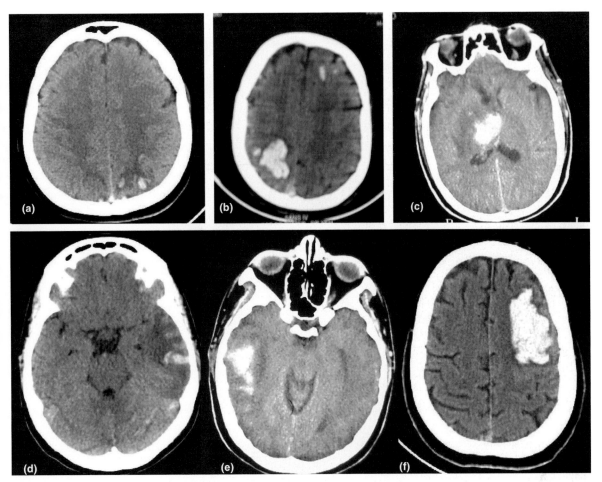

Fig. 7.6 Intracerebral hemorrhages in CVT on non-contrast CT: from petechiae to hematoma. (a, b) superior sagittal sinus thrombosis with cortical or sub cortical, multifocal, sometimes bilateral hyperdensities, presence of spontaneous hyperdensity of superior sagittal sinus = dense triangle; (c) right thalamic hematoma in deep venous system thrombosis; (d) mixture of hypo- and hyperdensity in left temporal lobe in lateral sinus thrombosis; (e) temporal hematoma in right lateral sinus thrombosis; (f) left frontal hematoma due to cortical vein thrombosis.

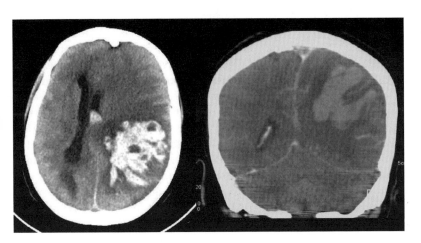

Fig. 7.7 Large hematoma with mass effect in a patient with superior sagittal sinus thrombosis.

93

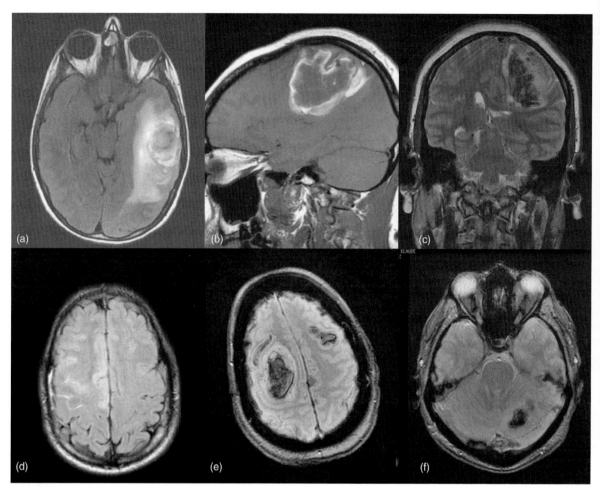

Fig. 7.8 Intracerebral hemorrhages in CVT on MRI. (a) FLAIR imaging: left temporal edema; (b) T1-weighted imaging: large parenchyma hypersignal with adjacent thrombosed vein appearing as a hyperintense spot; (c) T2-weighted imaging: mixture of hyper- and hyposignal in parenchyma due to cortical vein thrombosis; (d) FLAIR imaging: small localized subarachnoid hemorrage associated with frontal edema; (e) T2* imaging: bilateral parenchymal hemorrhages with multiple cortical vein thrombosis; (f) T2* imaging: left intracerebellar hemorrhage in lateral sinus thrombosis.

as hypo- or isosignal on T1-WI and hypersignal on T2-WI. Typically, the hemorrhage in case of CVT is cortical with subcortical extension. The hemorrhagic aspect is particularly well detected on T2* sequence. For instance, this sequence can detect small petechial haemorrhages not visible on other sequences or on non-contrast CT. Flame-shaped irregular zones of lobar hemorrhage in the parasagittal frontal and parietal lobes are very suggestive of SSS thrombosis while occurrence of hemorrhages in temporal or occipital lobes can be due to LS occlusion [48]. However, these signal changes are unspecific and it is their association with signal changes of the thrombus itself that will lead to the diagnosis.

Magnetic resonance imaging diffusion (DWI) shows various patterns [52–60], most frequently heterogeneous signal intensity with normal or increased apparent diffusion coefficient (ADC), suggestive of vasogenic edema combined with some areas of cytotoxic edema. The heterogeneous DWI/ADC pattern of brain lesions in CVT is markedly different from the low ADC of arterial infarcts, probably explaining at least in part the much better recovery observed in CVT than in arterial occlusion. Some studies included patients with hemorrhagic lesions [56,58,59] and showed areas of signal loss corresponding to hematomas. Hemorrhage may occur with both types of edema, with coexistence of various patterns in the same region.

Treatment

As in all CVT, the treatment of CVT with ICH includes:

- Antithrombotic treatment
- Etiological treatment, particularly in the case of septic CVT, underlying malignancies, or connective tissue disease
- Symptomatic treatment, i.e., treatment of intracranial hypertension, seizures, and headache.

Antithrombotic therapy

The use of heparin was first suggested more than half a century ago. Its goals are to limit the spread of thrombus and hence to diminish the intracapillary pressure, to treat the underlying prothrombotic state, in order to prevent other venous thrombosis such as pulmonary embolism, and to prevent the recurrence of CVT [31,61]. Its use has been debated, particularly in H-CVT, for fear of increasing the size of hemorrhage. This risk has, however, been vastly overestimated with very few properly documented cases and there is now good evidence that heparin is safe in CVT, even in patients with hemorrhagic lesions [62–65].

Two randomized trials have been performed to assess the benefit/risk of heparin:

- The first one compared dose-adjusted intravenous heparin and placebo [62]. This study was stopped after the inclusion of 22 patients because of a significant difference in favor of heparin with full recovery in 8 patients contrasting with only 3 in the placebo group. The authors reported an additional retrospective study [62] of 102 patients, including 43 with ICH. Among the 27 patients treated with dose-adjusted intravenous heparin, 14 (52%) patients recovered completely and 4 died (15%) whereas of the 13 patients that did not receive heparin after ICH, 9 died (mortality 69%) and only 3 patients completely recovered.
- The second compared low-molecular-weight heparin (LMWH) and placebo in 60 patients [63]. The difference in "poor outcome" defined as death or a Barthel index score > 15 at 12 weeks was not significant between the two groups (13% in the LMWH vs. 21% in the placebo group). No worsening consequence of new or enlarged cerebral hemorrhages was observed even in the 15 patients with hemorrhagic lesions on initial CT.

A meta-analysis of these two studies has shown that heparin treatment is associated with a 14% absolute risk reduction in mortality and 15% in death or dependency with relative reduction of respectively 70% and 56% [63]. Though not quite statistically significant, these results are clinically relevant and favor heparin treatment which is now widely used. Thus in ISCVT, over 80% of the 624 patients were anticoagulated, with or without ICH [13,36] and in our series, all patients with acute CVT were treated with heparin, whether ICH was present or not.

Very few studies were more specifically devoted to the acute outcome of patients with H-CVT. In a study of 12 patients, 6 anticoagulated and 6 non-anticoagulated, no increase in ICH volume or clinical worsening was observed in the anticoagulated group, whereas in the non-anticoagulated group, 4 had enlarging hematomas with clinical worsening requiring surgery in 2 [64]. In a series of 14 with H-CVT, 11 were treated with heparin, one of them had a minor extension of a very small ($< 1 \, \text{cm}^3$) hemorrhagic transformation within a large venous edema [65]. Three did not receive heparin: two had recurrent ICH with clinical worsening, one of them was then treated with heparin with a good recovery whereas the other died after a third ICH. These data suggest that in CVT, the increase of ICH or the occurrence of a new hemorrhage are much more frequently due to the spontaneous worsening of CVT than to heparin treatment.

In practice, nowadays, according to the European Federation of Neurological Societies (EFNS) recommendations, patients with CVT without contraindications for anticoagulation should be treated either with body weight-adjusted subcutaneous LMWH or dose-adjusted intravenous heparin, and concomitant ICH related to CVT is not a contraindication for heparin treatment [61].

Despite numerous case reports and small series, systematic reviews of thrombolysis in CVT show no good evidence to support the use of either systemic or local thrombolysis in this condition [66,67]. Furthermore, there are a number of potential biases, such as publication bias with possible under-reporting of cases with poor outcome or evaluation bias since treatment and outcome assessment were non-blind. In the meta-analysis of 169 CVT patients, 31% had H-CVT [66] but no detailed data are available about this specific group. In patients with H-CVT who deteriorate despite adequate heparin treatment, mechanical thrombectomy seems more appropriate than *in situ* thrombolysis.

Symptomatic treatment

In the acute phase, increased intracranial pressure (ICP) due to large lesions and/or massive brain edema may be fatal because of transtentorial herniation [68]. This holds particularly true in case of hemorrhagic lesions, sometimes associated with a "malignant" edema uncontrolled by antithrombotic treatment. General recommendations to control acutely increased ICP should therefore be followed, including elevated head bed, mannitol, ICU admission with sedation, hyperventilation to a target $PaCO_2$ of 30–35 mmHg, and ICP monitoring. The use of corticosteroids is not recommended, especially since they promote thrombosis. In patients with impending herniation due to unilateral hemispheric lesion or with temporal herniation due to large temporal hematoma, hemicraniectomy or hematoma evacuation are indicated, even in very severe cases, since first, surgery can be life saving and second, there is a remarkable potential for good recovery [69,70].

Antiepileptic drugs are usually prescribed only in patients who present with seizures (61). Some authors also use them in patients with parenchymal hemorrhagic lesions on admission CT/MRI since they are at higher risk of seizures.

Patients with ICH frequently have severe headaches that may require strong analgesics such as morphine, but these usually rapidly decrease after initiation of heparin treatment.

Management during follow-up

The follow-up of patients with H-CVT is similar to that of patients with non-H-CVT. The aim of continuing anticoagulation after the acute phase is to prevent recurrent CVT and other venous thrombosis, including pulmonary embolism. Following the evidence and recommendations in systemic deep venous thrombosis, anticoagulation with warfarin for 3–12 months is recommended with an INR of 2–3. In patients with inherited or acquired prothrombotic conditions, including patients with the antiphospholipid-antibody syndrome, a more prolonged oral anticoagulation is recommended. Antiepileptic treatment is required in about 11% of patients, mostly those who had seizures in the acute phase

or had a hemorrhagic parenchymal lesion [71,72]. The optimal duration of antiepileptic treatment is unknown. There are no specific data concerning the risk of recurrence in H-CVT versus non-H-CVT.

Summary

- H-CVT accounts for one-third of all CVT. They are due to cortical vein thrombosis. Their clinical presentation differs widely from that of other CVT with a more frequent acute onset, and far more frequent focal signs, seizures, and disorders of consciousness. By contrast, isolated headache or intracranial hypertension as the only manifestation is extremely rare. There is no difference between H-CVT and non-H-CVT as regards causes or risk factors.

- H-CVT have a huge variety of size and location of hemorrhagic lesions on neuroimaging, from small scattered petechiae to huge hematomas. The diagnosis is based, as in other CVT, on the visualization of the thrombus itself by MRI T1, T2, T2*, together with the non-visualization of the occluded venous segment on MR angiography.

- Although the outcome is more severe than in non-H-CVT with a 5% mortality, a complete recovery is observed at one year in three-quarters of cases.

- The medical treatment of H-CVT is similar to that of non-H-CVT, primarily based on heparin (intravenous or LMWH) followed by oral anticoagulants. Only a small minority of cases requires surgery, either hematoma evacuation or hemicraniectomy that can be life saving.

References

1. Ribes MF. Des recherches faites sur la phlébite. *Revue Médicale Française et Etrangère et Journal de Clinique de l'Hôtel-Dieu et de la Charité de Paris.* 1825; **3**: 5–41.

2. Bousser MG, Ross Russell RW. *Cerebral Venous Thrombosis.* 1 Vol. London Saunders, 1997.

3. Barnett HJ, Hyland HH. Non-infective intracranial venous thrombosis. *Brain* 1953; **76**: 36–49.

4. Kalbag RM, Wolf AL. *Cerebral Venous Thrombosis.* Vol 1. London, Oxford University Press, 1967.

5. Garcin R, Pestel M. *Thrombophlébites cérébrales.* Paris, Masson, 1949.

6. Hacker H. Normal supratentorial veins and dural sinuses. In: Newton TH, Potts DG, eds. *Radiology of*

the Skull and Brain. Angiography. St Louis, CV Mosby. 1974; 1851–1877.

7. Ameri A, Bousser MG. Cerebral venous thrombosis. *Neurol Clin* 1992; **10**: 87–111.

8. Milandre L, Gueriot C, Girard N, Ali Cherif A, Khalil R. Les thromboses veineuses cérébrales de l'adulte. *Ann Med Interne (Paris)* 1989; **139**: 544–554.

9. Cantu C, Barinagarrementaria F. Cerebral venous thrombosis associated with pregnancy and puerperium. Review of 67 cases. *Stroke* 1993; **24**: 1880–1884.

10. Daif A, Awada A, Al-Rajeh S, et al. Cerebral venous thrombosis in adults: a study of 40 cases from Saudi Arabia. *Stroke* 1995; **26**: 1193–1195.

11. De Bruijn SFTM, De Haan RJ, Stam J, for the Cerebral Venous Sinus Thrombosis Study Group. Clinical features and prognostic factors of cerebral venous sinus thrombosis in a prospective series of 59 patients. *J Neurol Neurosurg Psychiatry* 2001; **70**: 105–108.

12. Ferro JM, Correia M, Pontes C, Baptista MV, Pita F; Cerebral Venous Thrombosis Portuguese Collaborative Study Group (Venoport). Cerebral vein and dural sinus thrombosis in Portugal: 1980–1998. *Cerebrovasc Dis* 2001; **11**: 177–182.

13. Ferro JM, Canhao P, Stam J, Bousser MG, Barinagarrementeria F. Prognosis of cerebral vein and dural sinus thrombosis: results of the International Study on Cerebral Vein and Dural Sinus Thrombosis (ISCVT). *Stroke* 2004; **35**: 664–670.

14. Schaller B, Graf R. Cerebral venous infarction: the pathophysiological concept. *Cerebrovasc Dis* 2004; **18**: 179–188.

15. Fries G, Wallenfang T, Hennen J, et al. Occlusion of the pig superior sagittal sinus, bridging and cortical veins: multistep evolution of sinus-vein thrombosis. *J Neurosurg* 1992; **77**: 127–133.

16. Ungersbock K, Heimann A, Kempski O. Cerebral blood flow alterations in a rat model of cerebral sinus thrombosis. *Stroke* 1993; **24**: 563–569.

17. Fujita K, Kojima N, Tamaki N, et al. Brain edema in intracranial venous hypertension. In: Inaba Y, Klatzo I, Spatz M, eds. *Brain Edema*. Tokyo, Springer. 1985; 228–234.

18. Sato S, Miyahara Y, Dohmoto Y, et al. Cerebral microcirculation in experimental sagittal sinus occlusion in dogs. In: Auer LM, Lowe F, eds. *The Cerebral Veins*. New York, Springer. 1984; 111–117.

19. Frerichs KU, Deckert M, Kempski O, et al. Cerebral sinus and venous thrombosis in rats induces long-term deficits in brain function and morphology – evidence for a cytotoxic genesis. *J Cereb Blood Flow Metab* 1994; **14**: 289–300.

20. Schaller B, Graf R, Sanada Y, et al. Hemodynamic changes after occlusion of the posterior superior sagittal sinus: an experimental PET study in the cat. *AJNR Am J Neuroradiol* 2003; **24**: 1876–1880.

21. Hatayama T, Ishii M, Oda N, et al. Transverse sinus thrombosis in a patient with colon and rectal double cancers: a case report. *No Shinkei Geka* 1994; **22**: 851–856.

22. Rudolf J, Hilker R, Terstegge K, Ernestus R. Extended hemorrhagic infarction following isolated cortical venous thrombosis. *Eur Neurol* 1999; **41**: 115–116.

23. Jones BV. Case 62: lobar hemorrhage from thrombosis of the vein of Labbé. *Radiology* 2003; **228**: 693–696.

24. Crawford S, Digre KB, Palmer CA, et al. Thrombosis of the deep venous drainage of the brain in adults. *Arch Neurol* 1995; **52**: 1101–1108.

25. Van den Bergh WM, Van der Schaaf I, Van Gijn J. The spectrum of presentations of venous infarctions caused by deep cerebral vein thrombosis. *Neurology* 2005; **65**: 192–196.

26. Chang R, Friedman DP. Isolated cortical venous thrombosis presenting as subarachnoid hemorrhage: a report of three cases. *AJNR Am J Neuroradiol* 2004; **25**: 1676–1679.

27. Oppenheim C, Domigo V, Gaudrit JY, et al. Subarachnoid hemorrhage as the initial presentation of dural sinus thrombosis. *AJNR Am J Neuroradiol* 2005; **26**: 614–617.

28. Matsuda M, Matsuda I, Sato M, Handa J. Superior sagittal sinus thombosis followed by subdural hematoma. *Surg Neurol* 1982; **18**: 206–211.

29. Singh S, Kumar S, Joseph M, Gnanamuthu C, Alexander M. Cerebral venous sinus thrombosis presenting as subdural hematoma. *Australas Radiol* 2005; **49**: 101–103.

30. Ehlers H, Courville CB. Thrombosis of internal cerebral veins in infancy and childhood. Review of literature and report of five cases. *J Pediatr* 1937; **8**: 600–623.

31. Bousser MG, Ferro JM. Cerebral venous thrombosis: an update. *Lancet Neurol* 2007; **6**: 162–170.

32. deVeber G, Andrew M, Adams C, et al. Canadian Pediatric Ischemic Stroke Study Group. Cerebral sinovenous thrombosis in children. *N Engl J Med* 2001; **345**: 417–423.

33. Carvalho KS, Bodensteiner JB, Connolly JP, Garg BP. Cerebral venous thrombosis in children. *J Child Neurol* 2001; **16**: 574–580.

34. Sebire G, Tabarki B, Saunders DE, et al. Cerebral venous sinus thrombosis in children: risk factors, presentation, diagnosis and outcome. *Brain* 2005; **128**: 477–489.

35. Fitzgerald KC, Williams LS, Garg BP, Carvalho KS, Golomb MR. Cerebral sinovenous thrombosis in the neonate. *Arch Neurol* 2006; **63**: 405–409.

36. Girot M, Ferro JM, Canhao P, *et al.* for the ISCVT investigators. Predictors of outcome in patients with cerebral venous thrombosis and intracerebral hemorrhages. *Stroke* 2007; **38**: 337–342.

37. Stam J. Thrombosis of the cerebral veins and sinuses. *N Engl J Med* 2005; **352**: 1791–1798.

38. Cumurciuc R, Crassard I, Sarov M, Valade D, Bousser MG. Headache as the only neurological sign of cerebral venous thrombosis: a series of 17 cases. *J Neurol Neurosurg Psychiatry* 2005; **76**: 1084–1087.

39. Rondepierre P, Hamon M, Leys D, *et al.* Thromboses veineuses cérébrales: étude de l'évolution. *Rev Neurol (Paris)* 1995; **151**: 100–104.

40. Preter M, Tzourio CH, Ameri A, Bousser MG. Long term prognosis in cerebral venous thrombosis: a follow-up of 77 patients. *Stroke* 1996; **27**: 243–246.

41. Ferro JM, Lopes MG, Rosas MJ, Ferro MA, Fontes J. Long-term prognosis of cerebral vein and dural sinus thrombosis: results of the VENOPORT study. *Cerebrovasc Dis* 2002; **13**: 272–278.

42. Breteau G, Mounier-Vehier F, Godefroy O, *et al.* Cerebral venous thrombosis: 3-year clinical outcome in 55 consecutive patients. *J Neurol* 2003; **250**: 29–35.

43. Cakmak S, Derex L, Berruyer M, *et al.* Cerebral venous thrombosis: clinical outcome and systematic screening of prothrombotic factors. *Neurology* 2003; **60**: 1175–1178.

44. Chiras J, Bousser MG, Meder JF, Kouss A, Bories J. CT in cerebral thrombophlebitis. *Neuroradiology* 1985; **27**: 145–154.

45. Goldberg AL, Rosenbaum AE, Wang H, *et al.* Computed tomography of dural sinus thrombosis. *J Comput Assisted Tomogr* 1986; **10**: 16–20.

46. Virapongse C, Cazenave C, Quisling R, Sarvar M, Hunter S. The empty delta sign: frequency and significance in 76 cases of dural sinus thrombosis. *Radiology* 1987; **162**: 779–785.

47. Dormont D, Anxionnat R, Evrard S, *et al.* MRI in cerebral venous thrombosis. *J Neuroradiol* 1994; **21**: 81–89.

48. Leach JL, Fortuna RB, Jones BV, Gaskill-Shipley MF. Imaging of cerebral venous thrombosis: current techniques, spectrum of findings and diagnostic pitfalls. *Radiographics* 2006; **26**: S19–43.

49. Selim M, Fink J, Linfante I, *et al.* Diagnosis of cerebral venous thrombosis with echo-planar T2*-weighted magnetic resonance imaging. *Arch Neurol* 2002; **59**: 1021–1026.

50. Cakmak S, Hermier M, Montavont A, *et al.* T2*-weighted MRI in cortical venous thrombosis. *Neurology* 2004; **63**: 1698.

51. Idbaih A, Boukobza M, Crassard I, *et al.* MRI of clot in cerebral venous thrombosis: high diagnostic value of susceptibility-weighted images. *Stroke* 2006; **37**: 991–995.

52. Corvol JC, Oppenheim C, Manai R, *et al.* Diffusion-weighted magnetic resonance imaging in a case of cerebral venous thrombosis. *Stroke* 1998; **29**: 2649–2652.

53. Keller E, Flacke S, Urbach H, Schild HH. Diffusion-and perfusion-weighted magnetic resonance imaging in deep cerebral venous thrombosis. *Stroke* 1999; **30**: 1144–1146.

54. Manzione J, Newman GC, Shapiro A, Santo-Ocampo R. Diffusion- and perfusion-weighted MR imaging of dural sinus thrombosis. *AJNR Am J Neuroradiol* 2000; **21**: 68–73.

55. Chu K, Kang DW, Yoon BW, Roh JK. Diffusion-weighted magnetic resonance in cerebral venous thrombosis. *Arch Neurol* 2001; **58**: 1569–1576.

56. Doege CA, Tavakolian R, Kerskens CM, *et al.* Perfusion and diffusion magnetic resonance imaging in human cerebral venous thrombosis. *J Neurol* 2001; **248**: 564–571.

57. Ducreux D, Oppenheim C, Vandamme X, *et al.* Diffusion-weighted imaging patterns of brain damage associated with cerebral venous thrombosis. *AJNR Am J Neuroradiol* 2001; **22**: 261–268.

58. Forbes KPN, Pipe JG, Heisermann JE. Evidence for cytotoxic edema in the pathogenesis of cerebral venous infarction. *AJNR Am J Neuroradiol* 2001; **22**: 450–455.

59. Lövblad KO, Bassetti C, Schneider J, *et al.* Diffusion-weighted MR in cerebral venous thrombosis. *Cerebrovasc Dis* 2001; **11**: 169–176.

60. Mullins ME, Grant PE, Wang B, Gilberto Gonzales R, Schaefer PW. Parenchymal abnormalities associated with cerebral venous sinus thrombosis: assessment with diffusion-weighted MR imaging. *AJNR Am J Neuroradiol* 2004; **25**: 1666–1675.

61. Einhäupl K, Bousser MG, de Bruijn SFTM, *et al.* EFNS guideline on the treatment of cerebral venous and sinus thrombosis. *Eur J Neurol* 2006; **13**: 553–559.

62. Einhäupl KM, Villringer A, Meister W, *et al.* Heparin treatment in sinus venous thrombosis. *Lancet* 1991; **338**: 597–600.

63. De Bruijn SFTM, Stam J, for the Cerebral Venous Sinus Thrombosis Study Group. Randomised, placebo-controlled trial of anticoagulant treatment with low-molecular-weight heparin for cerebral sinus thrombosis. *Stroke* 1999; **30**: 484–488.

64. Wingerchuk DM, Wijdicks EF, Fulgham JR. Cerebral venous thrombosis complicated by hemorrhagic infarction: factors affecting the initiation and safety of anticoagulation. *Cerebrovasc Dis* 1998; **8**: 25–30.

65. Fink JN, McAuley DL. Safety of anticoagulation for cerebral venous thrombosis associated with intracerebral hematoma. *Neurology* 2001; **57**: 1138–1139.

66. Canhão P, Falcão F, Ferro JM. Thrombolytics for cerebral sinus thrombosis. A systematic review. *Cerebrovasc Dis* 2003; **15**: 159–166.

67. Ciccone A, Canhão P, Falcão F, Ferro JM, Sterzi R. Thrombolysis for cerebral vein and dural sinus thrombosis (Cochrane Review). In: *The Cochrane Library*, Issue 1, 2004. Oxford: Update Software. © Cochrane Library, John Wiley & Sons Ltd.

68. Canhão P, Ferro JM, Lindgren AG, *et al.* ISCVT Investigators. Causes and predictors of death in cerebral venous thrombosis. *Stroke* 2005; **36**: 1720–1725.

69. Stefini R, Latronico N, Cornali C, Rasulo F, Bollati A. Emergent decompressive craniectomy in patients with fixed and dilated pupils due to cerebral venous and dural sinus thrombosis: a report of three cases. *Neurosurgery* 1999; **45**: 626–629.

70. Petzold A, Smith M. High intracranial pressure brain herniation and death in cerebral venous thrombosis. *Stroke* 2006; **37**: 331–332.

71. Ferro JM, Correia M, Rosas MJ, *et al.* Cerebral Venous Thrombosis Portuguese Collaborative Study Group [Venoport]. Seizures in cerebral vein and dural sinus thrombosis. *Cerebrovasc Dis* 2003; **15**: 78–83.

72. Masühr F, Busch M, Amberger N, *et al.* Risk and predictors of early epileptic seizures in acute cerebral venous thrombosis. *Eur J Neurol* 2006; **13**: 852–856.

8 Clinical presentation of intracerebral hemorrhage

Carlos S. Kase

Intracerebral hemorrhage (ICH) presents clinically in a variety of ways, depending primarily on the location and size of the hematoma. These features determine a set of clinical findings that occur regardless of location, as they reflect the intracranial mass effect that characterizes ICH. These common clinical features will be discussed first, to be followed by the findings that are specific to the various locations of ICH.

General clinical features of intracerebral hemorrhage

Headache is common at the onset of ICH. In the series of Tatu *et al.* [1], headache was reported in 36% of the cases, with similar frequency in the putaminal (37.5%), thalamic (34.5%), and lobar (36.7%) locations; headache was more common (58%) in subjects with cerebellar hemorrhage. A higher frequency of headache at onset of cerebellar and lobar hemorrhage in comparison with the deep varieties (putaminal, thalamic, caudate) has been reported [2,3]. In the latter study [3], female gender, meningeal signs, and signs of transtentorial herniation were features associated with headache at ICH presentation. A recent study by Leira *et al.* [4] correlated headache at onset of ICH not only with the presence of mass effect, but also with features of antecedent infection, as well as markers of inflammation such as higher body temperature, elevated leukocyte count and sedimentation rate, and biochemical markers of inflammation (interleukin-6, tumor necrosis factor-alpha). These findings raise the interesting possibility of an added component of ongoing inflammation in the pathogenesis of headache in ICH.

In terms of headache characteristics, subjects with putaminal hemorrhage frequently report pain in the ipsilateral anterior portion of the head [3]. Other locations of ICH are not associated with specific headache patterns, except for the description of predominantly occipital headache in patients with cerebellar or occipital hematomas [3], although the latter can at times present with periorbital pain [5].

Seizures at onset of ICH are rare, being reported with a frequency below 10% in series of ICH that include all locations [1,6]. However, ICH location determines risk of seizures, as lobar ICH [7–9], especially in the frontal lobe [10], has been associated with increased risk of both immediate (within 24 hours of ICH onset) and early (within 30 days of ICH onset) seizures [11]. In the latter study, no differences were found in 30-day mortality between ICH patients with and without seizures (immediate or early seizures). However, in a study in which continuous EEG monitoring was used, Vespa *et al.* [12] found not only a high frequency of seizures, both convulsive and nonconvulsive, in patients with ICH (28%) in comparison with those with ischemic stroke (6%), but also correlated the presence of seizures in ICH patients with clinical deterioration and midline shift, as well as with a trend towards worse long-term outcome. This study stresses the value of continuous EEG monitoring of stroke patients in the ICU as seizures, both overt and electrographic (which are particularly frequent among ICH patients), appear to correlate with a more severe compromise of neurological function and, possibly, worse outcomes.

Progression of neurological deficits after onset correlates with the common observation of early enlargement of ICH [13]. This course after onset has been observed in both deep (putaminal, thalamic) and lobar ICHs, without a particular site being preferentially associated with early hematoma enlargement [1].

Intracerebral Hemorrhage, ed. J. R. Carhuapoma, S. A. Mayer, and D. F. Hanley. Published by Cambridge University Press.
© J. R. Carhuapoma, S. A. Mayer, and D. F. Hanley 2010.

The studies of Fujii *et al.* [14] and Brott *et al.* [15] documented hematoma enlargement that occurs predominantly within the first six hours of evolution, during which time neurological deterioration is frequently observed. Persistent hypertension has been frequently mentioned as a risk factor for ICH enlargement [16,17], but comparisons of patients with and without hematoma enlargement have failed to confirm the association between elevated blood pressure and ICH enlargement [15]. On occasion, patients with putaminal ICH have a rapid, precipitous enlargement of the hematoma, often leading to clinical deterioration and death [18], as a result of postulated acute rebleeding, rather than gradual continuous leakage at the initial bleeding site.

Clinical features specific to intracerebral hemorrhage location

Putaminal hemorrhage

The spectrum of clinical presentations of putaminal ICH has been clarified since the advent of CT scan [19], as this technique allows the diagnosis of all sizes of acute hemorrhages, in particular the small ones that in the pre-CT scan days may have been misdiagnosed on clinical grounds as infarcts. Early clinico-CT correlations identified syndromes of small (moderate hemiparesis and hemisensory deficits), moderate-size ("classical" syndrome of hemiplegia, hemisensory loss, lateral gaze paresis, homonymous hemianopia, and either aphasia or hemi-inattention), and massive (coma, bilateral Babinski sign, unreactive dilated pupils, and absent extraocular movements) hematomas [19].

Clinical syndromes in relationship to the location of putaminal hemorrhage

Several studies have correlated the anatomical location of putaminal hemorrhages with their clinical presentation. Among these, the studies of Weisberg *et al.* [20] and Chung *et al.* [21] have provided a consistent and comprehensive description of the anatomo-clinical correlations in putaminal ICH. In these studies, the authors described a number of different anatomical sites of origin and patterns of extension of the hemorrhages, and correlated them with the clinical presentation and outcome. Although they used slightly different nomenclatures, an analysis of their studies yields a consistent picture of the clinical correlates of the various anatomical locations of putaminal hemorrhage, as follows:

1. *Medial putaminal hemorrhage*: the ICH originates from rupture of medial branches of the lenticulostriate arteries [21], and extends medially into the genu and posterior limb of the internal capsule, but without extending through it; intraventricular hemorrhage (IVH) occurs rarely. Patients present with contralateral hemiparesis and hemisensory loss, but without abnormalities of ocular motility, visual fields, or level of consciousness. The course is generally benign, as the hematomas tend to be of small size. A posteromedial variety of putaminal hemorrhage, also called "capsular" ICH [21], due to rupture of branches of the anterior choroidal artery, presents with generally small hematomas in the posterior limb of the internal capsule, with hemiparesis, hemisensory loss, and dysarthria. This clinical picture can at times resemble that of the lacunar syndrome of "pure sensorimotor" stroke [22].

2. *Lateral putaminal hemorrhage*: the hematoma is the result of rupture of lateral branches of the lenticulostriate arteries, and it extends anteriorly along the external capsule (Fig. 8.1), leading to contralateral hemiplegia and sensory deficits, often accompanied by either aphasia or hemineglect syndromes in dominant or non-dominant hemisphere hematomas, respectively; it is this type of "lateral" putaminal ICH in the dominant hemisphere that has been associated with the syndrome of conduction aphasia [23], with fluent speech and preserved comprehension but with markedly impaired repetition, as a result of interruption of white matter tracts (arcuate fasciculus, extreme capsule, temporoparietal association areas) in the inferior parietal lobe. These hemorrhages tend to be larger than the medial ones, and are more often associated with neurological deterioration and IVH, as a manifestation of the larger hematoma volume.

3. *Putaminal hemorrhage with extension to internal capsule and subcortical white matter*: these are generally large hematomas that originate from rupture of posterior lenticulostriate branches, and extend medially through the internal capsule (Fig. 8.2) and superiorly into the corona radiata, at times even extending into several cerebral lobes, causing more severe syndromes of hemiplegia

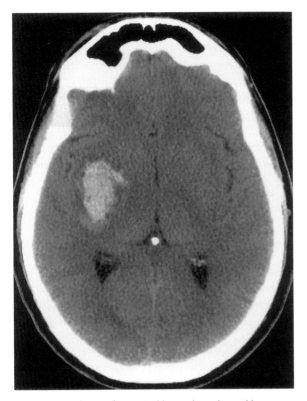

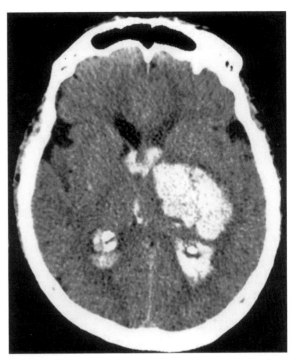

Fig. 8.2 Large posterolateral hematoma with involvement of left putamen and internal capsule, abutting the lateral thalamus, and extending into the ventricular system.

Fig. 8.1 Lateral type of putaminal hemorrhage, located between the right posterior putamen and the insula.

and hemianesthesia, often associated with homonymous hemianopia and conjugate ocular deviation, with variable degrees of depressed consciousness. Intraventricular hemorrhage occurs especially in the large hemorrhages, which often lead to mass effect into the adjacent lateral ventricle. Most patients who survive are left with permanent neurological deficits.

4. *Massive putaminal-thalamic hematoma*: these are the largest hematomas, with extension from the putamen into the thalamus (transecting the internal capsule) (Fig. 8.3) and into the subcortical white matter. They are invariably associated with mass effect on the lateral and third ventricles, IVH is frequent, and mortality can be as high as 80%; in instances with associated obstructive hydrocephalus, prognosis worsens [24] to mortality figures approaching 90% [25]. The clinical picture is characterized by impaired consciousness, hemiplegia, abnormalities of horizontal gaze (ipsilateral conjugate ocular

deviation more often than contralateral deviation), and homonymous hemianopia.

These clinico-CT correlations allowed Weisberg *et al.* [20] to delineate a number of patterns that are clinically useful: IVH and obstructive hydrocephalus, typically present in cases of large hematomas, are associated with high mortality; virtually all putaminal ICH patients present with combined motor and sensory deficits; the best functional outcome occurs in patients with medial or lateral putaminal hematomas that do not involve the internal capsule or the corona radiata; delayed neurological deterioration occurs most often in patients with hematomas that extend into the cerebral hemisphere or the thalamus.

Syndromes due to small putaminal hemorrhages

The availability of CT and MRI have allowed the documentation of a number of unusual presentations of small putaminal ICH. These include:

1. *Pure motor stroke*: rare instances of pure motor stroke due to small putaminal-capsular hemorrhages have been documented [26–29].

103

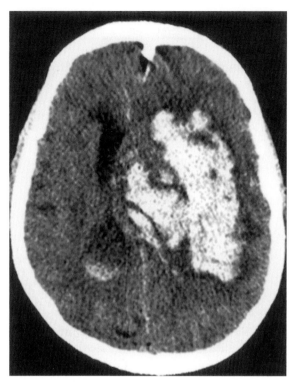

Fig. 8.3 Massive left-sided hemorrhage in the putaminal-capsular area, with medial extension into the thalamus and ventricular system.

The clinical presentation has been with a mild and rapidly improving pure motor syndrome affecting the face and limbs as a result of a small hematoma with origin in the posterior angle of the putamen, with pressure (but generally without extension) into the posterior limb of the internal capsule. In addition, pure "capsular" hemorrhage has rarely been reported as presenting with pure motor stroke and dysarthria [21]. These observations of occasional cases of putaminal ICH that present with an otherwise "typical" syndrome of lacunar infarction stress the importance of imaging in the diagnosis of acute stroke, especially when antithrombotic or thrombolytic treatment is being contemplated.

2. *Pure sensory stroke*: the syndrome of pure sensory stroke has been rarely observed in instances of small putaminal ICH. Kim [30] reported three cases among a group of 152 patients with putaminal ICH, which were the result of a posteriorly located small putaminal hemorrhage that was adjacent to the most posterior portion of the posterior limb of the internal capsule and the

adjacent thalamus. This resulted in a contralateral hemisensory syndrome affecting superficial and deep sensory modalities, with more severe involvement of the leg than the arm and face. The imaging studies suggested compromise of the dorsolateral aspect of the thalamus or the ascending thalamo-cortical projections located in the retro-lenticular portion of the posterior limb of the internal capsule.

3. *Hemichorea-hemiballism*: this unilateral syndrome that has been associated with lacunar infarction in the basal ganglia, thalamus, or subthalamic nucleus [31] is rarely the result of a small putaminal hemorrhage. Jones *et al.* [32] and Altafullah *et al.* [33] reported putaminal hemorrhages of "lateral" [21] location that resulted in transient contralateral chorea and ballism, in the absence of hemiparesis, hemisensory loss, gaze paresis, or hemineglect.

Caudate hemorrhage

Hemorrhage in the head of the caudate nucleus is the least common of the "deep" hemispheric hemorrhages, corresponding to about 2% of ICHs [34]. The bleeding vessels are Heubner's artery and the medial lenticulostriate arteries [21], and the parenchymal hematoma that results is generally small (Fig. 8.4), while the main effects of the hemorrhage are those mediated by the virtually constant IVH, at times complicated with hydrocephalus [35].

Caudate hemorrhage presents with sudden onset of headache, vomiting, and altered level of consciousness, resembling subarachnoid hemorrhage (SAH) from ruptured cerebral aneurysm [34,36]. This presentation is generally associated with imaging evidence of a small hematoma in the head of the caudate nucleus, accompanied by a high frequency (97%) of intraventricular extension [35]. The CT features help to distinguish primary caudate ICH from SAH from a ruptured anterior communicating aneurysm by the absence of subarachnoid blood in the basal cisterns and interhemispheric fissure in caudate hemorrhage [37], a finding that would be expected to occur regularly in SAH due to rupture of an anterior communicating artery aneurysm [34]. Less frequently, the hematoma of the caudate head extends in addition into the internal capsule, and produces transient contralateral hemiparesis and ipsilateral Horner's syndrome [34].

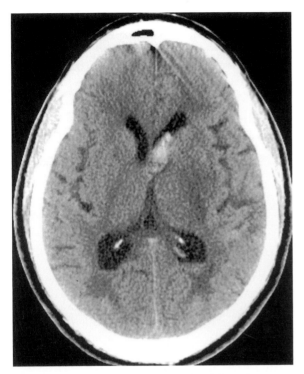

Fig. 8.4 Small hemorrhage in the head of the left caudate nucleus with extension into the adjacent frontal horn of the lateral ventricle.

Behavioral and neuropsychological abnormalities can be a prominent part of the clinical picture of caudate hemorrhage. The neuropsychological abnormalities of caudate hemorrhage involve a combination of abulia (decreased spontaneous motor or verbal initiative, with delayed performance on command), confusion, and disorientation at onset, followed by the development of a prominent amnestic syndrome, at times accompanied by language disturbances [34,37,38]. The latter often corresponds to non-fluent aphasia [38], while occasional examples of transcortical motor aphasia have been reported as well [21]. These deficits are thought to occur as a result of interruption of cortical-subcortical tracts between the caudate nucleus and the frontal cortex [37]. Hematomas in the non-dominant hemisphere only rarely produce unilateral disturbances of attention, such as the patient with visuospatial neglect reported by Kumral *et al.* [38].

The generally small size and localized character of caudate hemorrhage accounts for the relative paucity of focal neurological deficits such as hemiparesis [21]. On the other hand, the virtually constant extension

into the ventricular system results in a high frequency of headache and meningeal signs, resembling the onset of SAH. In rare instances of caudate ICH with IVH and acute hydrocephalus [34], a more dramatic presentation with coma and ophthalmoplegia can occur, the latter likely due to oculomotor nuclei involvement as a result of aqueductal dilatation [39].

Thalamic hemorrhage

Thalamic ICH of moderate to large size presents with the "classical" picture, which includes various combinations of the following features:

1. *Contralateral hemiparesis*: due to the proximity to the posterior limb of the internal capsule, thalamic ICH is associated with hemiparesis in about 95% of the cases, that is in all but the rare cases of lesions that are too small and medial or dorsal to impinge on the internal capsule [40,41]. The hemiparesis or hemiplegia of thalamic ICH involves the face, arm, and leg to a similar degree, and achieves the level of complete hemiplegia in about 70% of patients [42].

2. *Hemisensory syndrome*: patients develop prominent sensory loss, either anesthesia or hypesthesia affecting face, limbs, and trunk, generally for all sensory modalities, in as many as 85% of patients with thalamic ICHs of all sizes and locations within the thalamus [40].

3. *Ophthalmological signs*: these include paresis of upward gaze that often results in a position of downward deviation and convergence of the eyes at rest ("peering at the tip of the nose"), and miotic and unreactive pupils, both due to pressure of the thalamic ICH on the dorsal midbrain [43]; this is often associated with skew deviation and horizontal gaze disturbances; the latter most commonly correspond to the typical conjugate horizontal deviation towards the affected hemisphere, but examples of contralateral deviation ("wrong-way eyes") occasionally occur [44]. The pathogenesis of this phenomenon is controversial, but involvement of descending, crossed oculomotor tracts from the contralateral hemisphere at midbrain level is favored [45]. Other oculomotor phenomena observed in thalamic ICH include "acute esotropia" (markedly adducted eye contralateral to the thalamic hematoma or bilateral convergence spasm, also referred to as "pseudo-sixth" nerve palsy) from

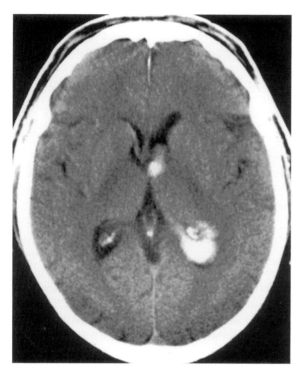

Fig. 8.5 Left anterior thalamic hemorrhage with ventricular extension, presenting with abrupt onset of generalized headache, with preserved alertness but with abulia.

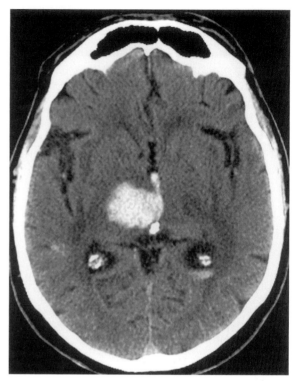

Fig. 8.6 Large right postero medial thalamic hemorrhage with extension into the third ventricle.

involvement at the midbrain level of supranuclear fibers with an inhibitory effect on convergence [46,47].

The clinical syndromes associated with specific areas of involvement of the thalamus by hemorrhage have been analyzed by Kumral *et al.* [42] and Chung *et al.* [41]. These authors divided the thalamic hematomas depending on the topography of the hemorrhage into anterior, posteromedial, posterolateral, dorsal, and global, and Chung *et al.* [41] related these locations to the presumed arterial rupture within the thalamus. The clinical features in these various locations have been described as follows:

1. *Anterior* type: hematoma located in the most anterior portion of the thalamus (Fig. 8.5), presumed from rupture of branches of the "polar" or tuberothalamic artery; these hematomas are often associated with IVH and are clinically characterized by behavioral abnormalities, especially memory impairment and apathy, with preserved alertness, rare and transient sensorimotor deficits, and absent ophthalmological findings.

2. *Posteromedial* type: due to rupture of thalamo-perforating arteries, with hematomas located in the medial thalamus (Fig. 8.6), with frequent rupture into the third ventricle and hydrocephalus, along with extension into the midbrain, results in memory disturbances and behavioral abnormalities in small hematomas, while the larger ones with downward extension into the midbrain lead to early stupor or coma, along with severe motor deficits and oculomotor disturbances.

3. *Posterolateral* type: results from rupture of thalamo-geniculate arteries, producing generally large hemorrhages with extension into the internal capsule (Fig. 8.7) and ventricular space, presenting with severe sensorimotor deficits, as well as aphasia or hemineglect in dominant or non-dominant hemorrhages, respectively; large hematomas can in addition feature ipsilateral Horner's syndrome, depressed level of consciousness, and ophthalmological abnormalities [42]; a substantial proportion of these patients (about one-third) develop the

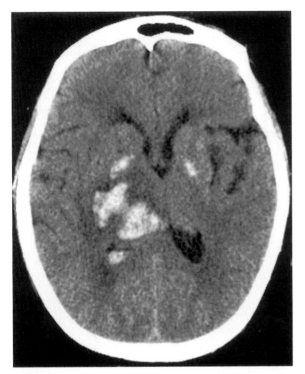

Fig. 8.7 Right postero lateral thalamic hemorrhage with extension into the posterior limb of the internal capsule and ventricular system.

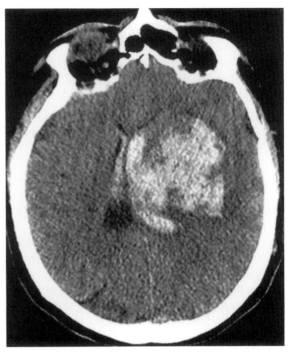

Fig. 8.8 Massive deep hemorrhage with origin in the left thalamus, with extension into the basal ganglia, corona radiata, and ventricular system, with marked shift of the midline.

delayed onset of a "thalamic pain syndrome" [41]. The aphasia of dominant posterolateral thalamic hematomas is often described as "transcortical motor" [42,48], except that in hematomas in the pulvinar nucleus the aphasia is characterized as progressively more paraphasic as the person continues to talk, eventually becoming jargon [49]; the syndromes of hemineglect in non-dominant thalamic hemorrhage can include contralateral auditory inattention [50], anosognosia [48], at times with prominent associated mania [51], as well as examples of motor neglect or "inertia," manifested as lack of use of limbs with normal strength [52]. An intriguing motor phenomenon described as the "pusher syndrome" has been described in patients with thalamic hemorrhage; this refers to a disturbed perception of the patient's sense of own verticality when sitting or standing, resulting in a tendency to use the unaffected limbs to "push" self in the direction of the affected side of the body. This behavior is thought to reflect a disturbance of perception of body posture in relation to gravity [53], and it occurs in posterior thalamic hemorrhages on either the left or right side.

4. *Dorsal* type: due to rupture of branches of the posterior choroidal artery, results in hematomas located high in the thalamus, which often extend into the paraventricular white matter and the ventricular space, with clinical presentation with mild and transient sensorimotor deficits, generally without oculomotor abnormalities, with occasional confusion and memory disturbance in those located most posteriorly (in the area of the pulvinar nucleus).

5. *Global* type: involvement of the whole extent of the thalamus (Fig. 8.8) by large hematomas that enter the ventricular system (with associated hydrocephalus) and extend into the supra-thalamic hemispheric white matter, resulting in stupor or coma, severe sensorimotor deficits, and the "classical" ophthalmological features of paralysis of upward more than downward gaze, skew deviation, and small and unreactive pupils.

Syndromes of small thalamic hemorrhages

In instances of small hemorrhages, a number of different presentations have been described, corresponding to dysfunction of one or a few isolated systems or nuclei within the thalamus. Some of these syndromes include:

1. *Pure sensory stroke*: this syndrome, caused most often by a lacunar thalamic infarction [54], has been rarely described as a result of a small thalamic ICH [55–58] (Fig. 8.9). Abe *et al.* reported a thalamic hematoma of dorsal location depicting a hemisensory syndrome with loss of sensation to pin prick, vibration and joint position sense, with normal motor strength, while coordination in the affected arm was abnormal with eyes closed, reflecting the "sensory" rather than cerebellar character of the ataxia [55]. The two patients reported by Paciaroni and Bogousslavsky [56] had involvement of all sensory modalities affecting the face, arm, and leg contralaterally to a small hemorrhage in the center of the thalamus that affected all the ventral nuclei, the parvocellular and dorsocaudal nuclei, with sparing of the pulvinar. The hemorrhages were thought to have originated from rupture of thalamo-geniculate branches of the posterior cerebral artery. In the study of Shintani *et al.* [57], two patients with sensory loss predominanting in the arm and leg had contralateral hemorrhages in either the ventral-posterior-lateral (VPL) nucleus, or the ventral-posterior-medial (VPM) nucleus, while another patient with a restricted "cheiro-oral" distribution of dysesthesias with "burning" quality in the absence of sensory loss had a small hematoma in the border between VPL and VPM.

2. *Sensory ataxic hemiparesis*: a syndrome similar to the ataxic hemiparesis of lacunar infarction was reported in the setting of small thalamic hemorrhages by Dobato *et al.* [59]. However, the clinical presentation differed from that of lacunar ataxic hemiparesis in that the ataxia of the cases reported by Dobato *et al.* [59] was due to proprioceptive sensory loss (with improvement under visual guidance, worse with eyes closed), as opposed to the cerebellar character of the ataxia in lacunar ataxic hemiparesis. The hematomas were small, all located in the dorsolateral thalamus, associated with markedly impaired

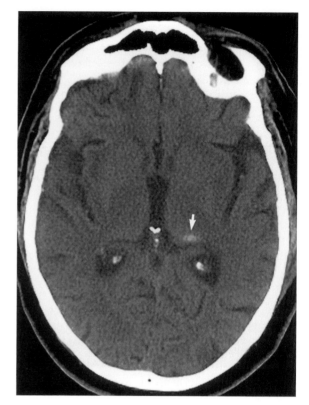

Fig. 8.9 Tiny hemorrhage in the posterior aspect of the left thalamus (arrow) in patient on warfarin anticoagulation, presenting with right "pure sensory" syndrome.

proprioception but with preserved superficial sensory modalities, and the associated hemiparesis was transient and of crural predominance.

3. *Abnormal involuntary movements*: a variety of abnormal motor phenomena has been described in patients with generally small thalamic hemorrhages. These have included a combination of contralateral upper extremity choreiform-dystonic movements along with a pattern of rhythmic alternating movements of low frequency ("myorhythmia") in the setting of a small hemorrhage [60]. A single case of delayed onset (one month) of a contralateral "rubral" tremor in the arm in a patient with a small posterolateral thalamic hemorrhage with subthalamic extension was reported by Mossuto-Agatiello *et al.* [61]. Occasionally, small thalamic hemorrhages are accompanied by contralateral ataxia, hemihypesthesia, hemiparesis (common features of the posterolateral thalamic lesions leading to the

syndrome of Déjérine-Roussy [62]), and a motor disturbance consistent with unilateral asterixis [63]. A case of bilateral facial dystonia and vertical gaze palsy, which in combination led to the facial expression known as "risus sardonicus," resulted from a right thalamic ICH of moderate size [64].

4. *Amnestic syndromes*: in addition to the syndromes of acute and persistent anterograde amnesia in the setting of anterior and posteromedial hematomas [65] and small paramedian hemorrhages [66], a case of transient global amnesia (TGA) has been described in a patient with a dominant hemisphere hematoma that involved the rostral-medial thalamus, with extension into the ventricular system [67]. The basis of TGA in this setting is thought to be due to involvement of the anterior and medial nuclear groups by the ICH, possibly interrupting the mamillothalamic tract or the ventroamygdalofugal pathway.

Lobar hemorrhage

Lobar ICH generally presents suddenly, during activity, like ICH at other sites. The most common symptom, headache, is reported by 50–80% of patients [7,29,68–72]. Vomiting occurs in 26–45% of patients, and is usually present early after the onset of headache. Seizures are reported more frequently in lobar ICH than in other types of brain hemorrhage, with a frequency as low as 11% [29] and as high as 36% [73], although a figure of 6% was reported by Flemming *et al.* [71]. The seizures typically occur at the onset of the ICH [74], they are more often focal than generalized, and status epilepticus can be a common occurrence [73]. Seizures in lobar ICH correlate with the extension of the hematoma into the cerebral cortex, as 26% of patients with this feature seized at onset, in contrast with only 3% of those without cortical extension of the hemorrhage in the series of Berger *et al.* [74]. The occurrence of coma at presentation is less common in patients with lobar ICH than in those with hemorrhage in the deep gray nuclei. The relatively low frequency of 5–19% of coma at presentation likely reflects the peripherally located lobar hematomas that produce less displacement or distortion of diencephalic midline structures concerned with the maintenance of consciousness [75].

Lobar ICHs occur in any of the cerebral lobes, generally favoring the parietal and occipital areas [7,29,68,76,77], although some series have reported a predominance of frontal [72,78,79] or temporal [71] locations. The clinical features have distinctive characteristics depending on the affected lobe.

Frontal hematomas

Frontal hemorrhages present with prominent limb paresis and bifrontal headache, which predominates on the side of the hemorrhage [68]. The weakness tends to be more severe in the contralateral arm, at times as an isolated monoplegia. Leg and face weakness are mild, and conjugate gaze deviation toward the side of the hematoma is uncommon. Different locations of hematomas within the frontal lobe can lead to variations from this clinical presentation. Weisberg [78] and Weisberg and Stazio [69] made the following observations: patients with hemorrhages located superiorly in the frontal lobe, above the frontal horns of the lateral ventricle (Fig. 8.10), present with frontal headache and contralateral leg weakness, while those with inferior frontal hemorrhages, located below

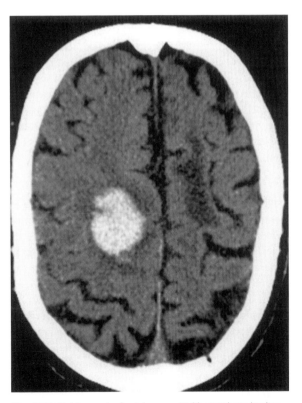

Fig. 8.10 Right superior frontal parasagittal hemorrhage leading to left hemiparesis with predominance in the leg. Scar from old infarct in the distribution in the left anterior cerebral artery is also present.

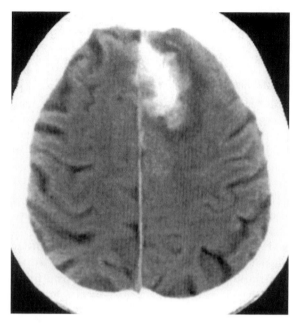

Fig. 8.11 Left anterior, para-falcine frontal hemorrhage due to cerebral amyloid angiopathy in patient who presented with progressive disorientation and headache, in the absence of motor symptoms.

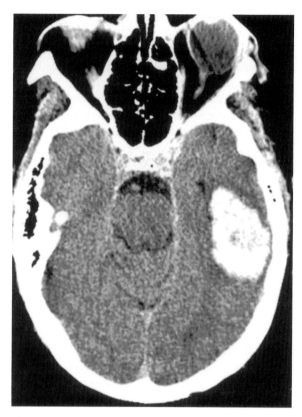

Fig. 8.12 Large left temporal hematoma presenting with features of "amnestic" aphasia and right facial weakness, with intact limb strength and visual fields.

the frontal horn of the lateral ventricle, tend to have more severe clinical presentations, with impaired consciousness, hemiparesis, hemisensory loss, and contralateral horizontal gaze palsy. On rare occasions, patients with frontal hematomas in anterior locations (Fig. 8.11) present without hemiparesis or aphasia, but rather with mental state changes, with prominent abulia [80].

Temporal hematomas

Temporal hematomas present with specific syndromes in relation to their laterality and location within that lobe. Headache is common at onset, and is described as generally centered in front of the ear or around the eye [68]. Dominant hemisphere hematomas produce a fluent aphasia with poor comprehension, and associated paraphasias and anomia [68,78]. A right visual field defect, either hemianopia or inferior quadrantanopia, generally accompanies temporal hematomas of posterior location, which are rarely associated with hemiparesis and hemisensory loss.

In a series of 30 patients with temporal lobe hematomas, Weisberg *et al.* [81] reported seizures at presentation in 23%. Patients with posterior temporal hematomas had retroauricular headache at onset, and those with left-sided lesions (Fig. 8.12) had Wernicke aphasia and right homonymous hemianopia. Patients with right-sided lesions were described as having a confusional state without other neurological signs. Many such patients have an agitated delirium characterized by hyperactivity and pressured speech which goes from one topic to another. Temporal hematomas with extension to adjacent lobes produce less well-defined clinical syndromes that depend on the size of the hematoma and the degree of involvement of structures adjacent to the temporal lobe. In those with medial extension into the basal ganglia area, a combination of hemiplegia, hemisensory abnormalities, aphasia, hemianopia, and horizontal gaze palsy leads to a clinical profile similar to that of large putaminal hemorrhages. Non-dominant temporal hematomas that extend superiorly into the parietal lobe are associated with prominent left-sided hemi-inattention.

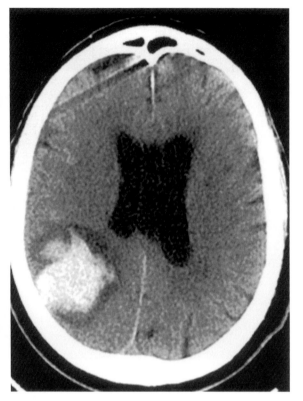

Fig. 8.13 Right lateral parietal hemorrhage with small halo of perihematomal edema.

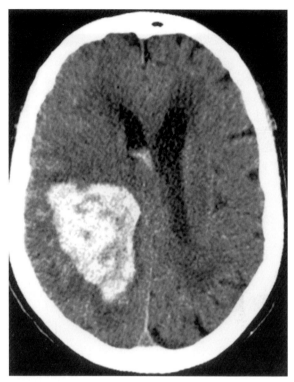

Fig. 8.14 Large right medial parietal hematoma with midline shift and ventricular extension.

Parietal hematomas

Parietal hematomas often present with unilateral headache around the temple area [68]. Hemisensory syndromes dominate the clinical picture, with hypesthesia that involves the limbs and trunk, in combination with hemiparesis of variable severity [7,68,78]. Seizures occurred at the onset in 28% of the patients reported by Weisberg and Stazio [82]. These authors analyzed the clinical features of 25 patients with parietal hemorrhages. In those with lateral hemorrhages (Fig. 8.13), motor and sensory deficits predominated, in addition to homonymous hemianopia in one-half of them. Aphasia or hemi-inattention occurred depending on the laterality of the ICH. Patients with medial hematomas (Fig. 8.14) presented with a similar clinical syndrome, but with more prominent compromise of consciousness as a result of extension into the thalamus, with displacement or distortion of the diencephalic midline. In patients with posterior hematomas, seizures were common at onset, and the clinical features included constructional apraxia, dressing apraxia, and hemi-inattention.

Occipital hematomas

Occipital hemorrhages often lead to severe headache in or around the ipsilateral eye, along with acute awareness of a visual disturbance which on examination corresponds to a contralateral homonymous hemianopia [68]. Hemiparesis does not occur, but contralateral sensory extinction to double simultaneous stimulation, dysgraphia and dyslexia, and the syndrome of "alexia without agraphia" have been reported [68,83].

In the series of Weisberg and Stazio [84] patients with occipital hemorrhages in a medial location (Fig. 8.15) reported headache and "visual blurring," with only homonymous hemianopia on examination, without weakness, memory disturbances, or compromised alertness. Those with laterally located occipital hematomas (Fig. 8.16) reported headache at onset, but had no neurological abnormalities on

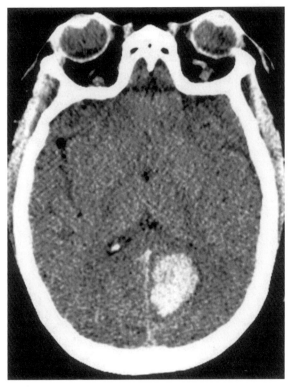

Fig. 8.15 Left medial occipital hematoma, with presentation with isolated right homonymous hemianopia.

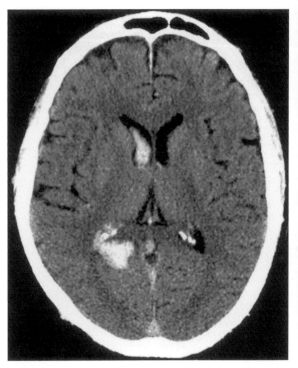

Fig. 8.16 Small right lateral occipital hemorrhage with ventricular extension, clinically presenting with only diffuse headache, without visual field defects or other neurological deficits.

examination, including visual field defects, sensori-motor deficits, or behavioral abnormalities. In patients with large occipital hematomas with extension to adjacent lobes the neurological deficits tend to be more dramatic, with disorientation, agitation, contralateral inattention, and homonymous hemianopia.

Cerebellar hemorrhage

In cerebellar hemorrhage, the hematoma collects around the dentate nucleus and spreads into the hemispheric white matter, often extending into the fourth ventricle as well (Fig. 8.17). The adjacent pontine tegmentum is rarely involved directly by the hematoma, but is often compressed by it, resulting in most of the clinical findings in cerebellar hemorrhage.

Symptoms usually develop during activity, and the most common one is sudden onset of inability to stand or walk, in the absence of hemiparesis. In rare instances patients are able to walk a few steps, but scarcely any patient can walk into the emergency ward or office. Vomiting is very common, with frequencies reported in 75–95% of patients [85,86]. Dizziness, often

corresponding to true vertigo, is a symptom reported in over 75% of patients who are alert on admission [85]. Headache is very common at onset, and is most often of occipital location, although it is occasionally reported in the frontal area or even in a retro-ocular position. Dysarthria, tinnitus, and hiccups can occur, but are less frequently reported. Loss of consciousness at onset is distinctly unusual [85].

The physical findings correspond to a combination of a unilateral cerebellar deficit with variable signs of ipsilateral tegmental pontine involvement. Appendicular ataxia occurs in over two-thirds of the patients who are able to cooperate for cerebellar function testing. Signs of involvement of the ipsilateral pontine tegmentum include peripheral facial palsy, ipsilateral horizontal gaze palsy, sixth cranial nerve palsy, depressed corneal reflex, and miosis. In noncomatose patients, a characteristic triad of ipsilateral appendicular ataxia, horizontal gaze palsy, and peripheral facial palsy has been suggested [85]. Hemiplegia and subhyaloid hemorrhages are uncommon enough in cerebellar hemorrhage that their presence essentially rules out the diagnosis.

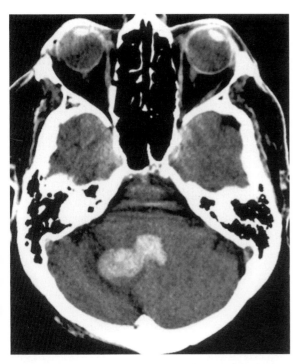

Fig. 8.17 Right cerebellar hemorrhage in the area of the dentate nucleus, with extension into the fourth ventricle.

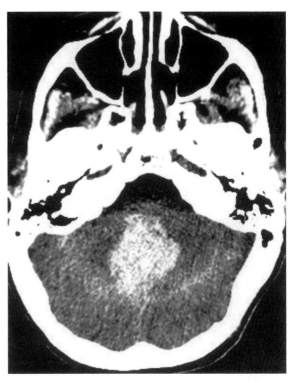

Fig. 8.18 Large midline (vermian) cerebellar hemorrhage with direct extension into the fourth ventricle and pontine tegmentum.

Other findings on neurological examination add little value to the diagnosis: the pupils are small and reactive to light, dysarthria is present in two-thirds of the cases, and the respiratory rhythm is usually normal. Oculomotor abnormalities, such as ocular bobbing, have occasionally been reported in cerebellar hemorrhage [87], but with lower frequency than in pontine hemorrhage or infarction. Along with these focal manifestations on neurological examination, patients with cerebellar hemorrhage may present with variable degrees of decreased alertness. Of the 56 cases reported by Ott *et al*, [85] 14 (25%) were alert, 22 (40%) drowsy, 5 (9%) stuporous, and 15 (26%) comatose. That two-thirds of the patients are responsive (alert or drowsy) on admission justifies the intensive efforts at diagnosing this condition early, as the outcome is largely dependent on the level of consciousness [85,88].

The clinical course in cerebellar hemorrhage is notoriously unpredictable: patients who are alert or drowsy on admission can deteriorate suddenly to coma and death without warning [85,89], while others in a similar clinical status have an uneventful course with complete recovery of function. Although most patients deteriorate early in the course, occasional

ones show fatal decompensations at a later stage [90]. The prediction of the clinical course is difficult when based on clinical parameters on admission; however, St. Louis *et al.* [91] provided useful predictive data from a retrospective analysis of 94 patients with cerebellar hemorrhage. They documented poor outcome in patients with admission systolic blood pressure above 200 mmHg, hematomas larger than 3 cm in diameter, brainstem distortion on brain imaging, and acute hydrocephalus. Fatal outcome was correlated with absence of corneal and oculocephalic reflexes, Glasgow Coma Scale (GCS) score of less than 8, acute hydrocephalus, and IVH.

Computerized tomography scan in cerebellar hemorrhage is a useful indicator of subsequent course. Hematomas of ≥ 3 cm in diameter, accompanied by obstructive hydrocephalus and ventricular extension of the hemorrhage, are often followed by neurological deterioration, and require emergency surgical drainage in order to prevent brainstem compression and death [92].

The midline variant of cerebellar hemorrhage originates from the vermis (Fig. 8.18), and accounts for only about 5% of the cases [89]. It virtually always communicates with the fourth ventricle through its roof, and frequently extends into the pontine tegmentum bilaterally. The bleeding vessel in this form of cerebellar hemorrhage corresponds to distal branches of the superior or the posterior-inferior cerebellar artery. This variety of cerebellar hematoma represents a serious diagnostic challenge, and its outcome is generally poor. A common presentation is with acute onset of coma, ophthalmoplegia, and respiratory abnormalities, with variable degrees of bilateral limb weakness, at times indistinguishable from primary pontine hemorrhage [93], with which it shares its poor prognosis. Occasionally, small vermian hematomas have presented with isolated positional vertigo, resembling benign paroxystic positional vertigo, in the absence of cerebellar ataxia or tegmental pontine signs [94].

Midbrain hemorrhage

Spontaneous, nontraumatical primary midbrain hemorrhage is rare. In most instances the hemorrhage in the midbrain represents dissection from a hemorrhage with primary origin in the thalamus or, less commonly, in the pons. When truly a primary hemorrhage in the midbrain (Fig. 8.19), it most commonly arises from a ruptured arteriovenous malformation (AVM) or blood dyscrasia, although occasional examples are attributed to hypertension [95].

Midbrain hemorrhage generally evolves with a stepwise course, with onset of either ipsilateral ataxia or contralateral hemiparesis in combination with ophthalmoplegia, typically an ipsilateral partial or complete third cranial nerve palsy. A presentation with features of the dorsal midbrain syndrome (vertical gaze palsy, nystagmus retractorius, eyelid retraction, and light-near pupillary dissociation) has been described in cases of midbrain hemorrhage [96]. In rare instances, small hemorrhages lead to more restricted syndromes, such as: contralateral hemisensory deficits with ipsilateral partial involvement of oculomotor (third nerve) function [97]; features of Weber's syndrome with ipsilateral third nerve palsy and contralateral hemiparesis [98], and even the rare occurrence of isolated ipsilateral third nerve palsy, without hemiparesis, as a result of a small hematoma located between the red nucleus and the cerebral peduncle, causing a "fascicular" third nerve palsy [99]; and the combination of the

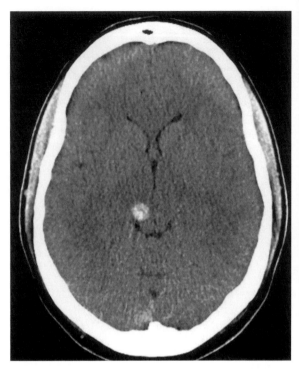

Fig. 8.19 Midbrain hemorrhage, to the right of the midline and ventral to the aqueduct, causing isolated right third nerve palsy.

features of the dorsal midbrain syndrome with associated bilateral fourth nerve palsy [100]. Larger hematomas can lead to bilateral third nerve palsy, bulbar weakness, and extensor plantar responses [95]. In rare occasions, a movement disorder has developed with a latency of several months after the acute hemorrhage; the main features have been contralateral limb dystonia and a tremor with "rubral" characteristics [101].

Pontine hemorrhage

The clinical spectrum of pontine hemorrhage is quite wide, as the hematomas may vary a great deal in terms of size and location within the pons. The "classical" form of massive bleeding into the pontine base and tegmentum is associated with a uniformly dismal prognosis, while smaller hematomas with partial involvement of either basal or tegmental structures are compatible with survival, at times with surprisingly mild persistent neurological deficits [102]. Due to their distinctive clinical features, these anatomically different forms of pontine hemorrhage will be discussed separately.

Large paramedian pontine hemorrhage

Massive pontine hemorrhage results from rupture of parenchymal midpontine branches originating from the basilar artery. The bleeding vessel is thought to be a paramedian perforator in its distal portion, causing initial hematoma formation at the junction of tegmentum and basis pontis, with subsequent growth into its final round or oval shape that involves most of the basis and tegmentum of the pons [103]. The hematoma generally begins in the mid-pons and extends along the longitudinal axis of the brainstem rostrally into the lower midbrain, and caudally as far as the pontomedullary junction. This process of rapid hematoma expansion leads to destruction of tegmental and ventral pontine structures, resulting in the classical combination of involvement of cranial nerve nuclei, long tracts, autonomic centers, and structures responsible for maintenance of consciousness. Large pontine hematomas also regularly rupture into the fourth ventricle.

Patients with this type of bilateral and massive pontine hemorrhage often present with acute onset of occipital headache and vomiting, rapidly followed by the development of coma. At times, seizures have been described during this rapidly progressive brainstem syndrome, probably representing a combination of true convulsive phenomena in rare instances, along with seizure "mimics" represented primarily by episodic decerebrate posturing, in combination with the sometimes violent shivering associated with autonomic dysfunction and rapidly evolving hyperthermia. In some patients, prior to the development of coma, there may be a brief period with symptoms of focal pontine involvement, including facial or limb "numbness," deafness, diplopia, bilateral leg weakness, or progressive hemiparesis. Physical examination often reveals an abnormal respiratory rhythm with hypoventilation or apnea [104]. Hyperthermia frequently coexists, with temperatures above 39 °C in more than 80% of the cases, in some patients reaching levels of 42–43 °C, usually in the preterminal stages [105]. Neurological examination characteristically shows quadriplegia with decerebrate posturing, bilateral Babinski signs, absent corneal reflexes, pupillary abnormalities, and various forms of ophthalmoplegia. The spectrum of oculomotor and pupillary changes includes:

1. Miotic pinpoint pupils of about 1 mm in diameter, reactive to light (if a strong light source is used) with a tiny constriction that may require a magnifying lens to be detected. This pupillary abnormality is the result of bilateral interruption of descending sympathetic pupillodilator fibers [44].

2. Absent horizontal eye movements. Their voluntary and reflex absence is due to bilateral injury to the paramedian pontine reticular formation. Small and lateralized hematomas can lead to variants such as the "one-and-a-half syndrome" [44] from a combination of ipsilateral horizontal gaze palsy plus internuclear ophthalmoplegia, the only remaining horizontal eye movement being abduction of the eye contralateral to the hematoma.

3. Ocular bobbing, corresponding to brisk movements of conjugate ocular depression, followed by a slower return to midposition, occurring either spontaneously, or following noxious stimuli, or upon attempted voluntary horizontal eye deviation in the awake patient [106]. Typically, it affects both eyes simultaneously and is accompanied by bilateral paralysis of horizontal gaze, but atypical varieties include unilateral or markedly asymmetric forms, and those occurring when horizontal eye movements are still present [107]. The atypical form is less strictly localizing to pontine disease, as it can be seen in cerebellar hemorrhage, SAH, and even in coma of non-vascular mechanism.

Weakness of pontine and bulbar musculature is invariable with large median hemorrhages; its detection in the comatose patient is facilitated by the observation of puffing of the cheeks with expiration, diminished eyelid tone, and pooling of secretions in the oropharynx. Facial weakness is often asymmetric and may be associated with a crossed hemiplegia at the time the patient is first seen [108].

Limb weakness is always present in large hemorrhages involving the basis pontis and tegmentum, usually as quadriplegia with occasional and minor asymmetries noted in decerebrate posturing, deep tendon reflexes, or clonus. Shivering and decerebrate posturing are characteristic in patients with rapidly deteriorating motor function.

Unilateral basal or basotegmental hemorrhages

The unilateral basotegmental hemorrhages (Fig. 8.20) are less common than the large paramedian lesions. Reports of basal unilateral hematomas diagnosed by CT scan or MRI have shown more restricted clinical

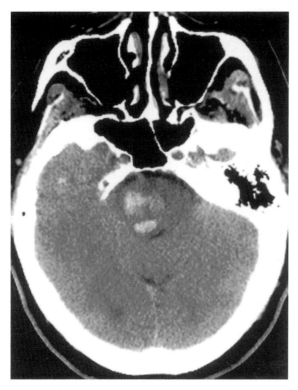

Fig. 8.20 Basotegmental pontine hemorrhage, predominating on the right side, with partial compression and displacement of the fourth ventricle.

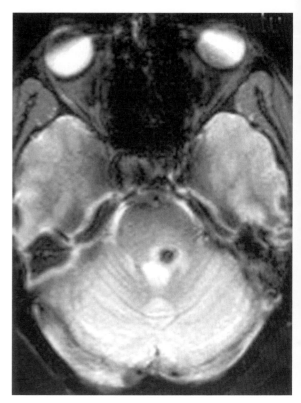

Fig. 8.21 Magnetic resonance imaging (gradient echo sequence) with small hemorrhage on the left side of the tegmentum, presenting with left "one-and-a-half" syndrome, peripheral facial palsy, and facial hypesthesia.

presentations [109], including the syndromes of pure motor stroke [110] and "ataxic hemiparesis" [111], clinically indistinguishable from lacunar infarction in the basis pontis. Further examples of restricted clinical expression of small unilateral basal hematomas include rare instances of isolated abducens nerve palsy [112], in which a tiny unilateral basal hematoma led to a "fascicular" abducens palsy from interruption of the intrapontine nerve fibers at a distance from the origin from the sixth nerve nucleus.

Lateral tegmental hematomas

Lateral tegmental pontine hematomas usually originate from rupture of penetrating branches of long circumferential arteries, as they enter the tegmentum laterally and course medially. Small hematomas remain confined to the lateral tegmentum (Fig. 8.21), while larger lesions spread across to the opposite side and can destroy the entire tegmentum. Neurological examination reveals a predominantly unilateral tegmental lesion with variable degrees of basal involvement [113,114]. Oculomotor abnormalities, especially

the "one-and-a-half syndrome," horizontal gaze palsy, internuclear ophthalmoplegia, partial involvement of vertical eye movements, and ocular bobbing have been described [113–115]. Ataxia, either unilateral or bilateral, may accompany the oculomotor signs, and an action tremor has been described as a result of involvement of the red nucleus or its connections [114]. Facial numbness, ipsilateral miosis, and hemiparesis have also been noted. Palatal myoclonus has been described as a persistent sequela, with onset after a latency from the acute event, and is thought to be due to damage to the dentato-rubro-olivary pathway, with eventual development of olivary hypertrophy contralateral to the original hemorrhage [116].

Medullary hemorrhage

Primary hemorrhage into the medulla oblongata is the least common of all brain hemorrhages. Single case reports have delineated a range of clinical presentations and mechanisms, the latter for the most part corresponding to ruptured AVMs, bleeding due to anticoagulant treatment, or rare instances of hemorrhagic transformation of an ischemic infarct that presented with the features of Wallenberg's lateral medullary syndrome [117–119].

The most consistent clinical profile in medullary hemorrhage has been with sudden onset of headache, vertigo, dysphagia, dysphonia or dysarthria, and limb incoordination. Findings on physical examination have included palatal weakness, nystagmus, cerebellar ataxia, limb weakness, and hypoglossal nerve palsy. Less common signs have been facial palsy and Horner's syndrome. As expected, medullary hemorrhage patients have had clinical features generally extending beyond those that characterize the lateral medullary syndrome due to infarction. Due to the mass effect and/or medial extension of the hematoma, elements of medial (hypoglossal nerve palsy) and ventral (pyramidal tract involvement) medullary involvement are added to those restricted to the dorsolateral medullary infarction of Wallenberg's.

References

1. Tatu L, Moulin T, El Mohamad R, *et al.* Primary intracerebral hemorrhages in the Besançon stroke registry: initial clinical and CT findings, early course and 30-day outcome in 350 patients. *Eur Neurol* 2000; **43**: 209–214.

2. Hier DB, Babcock DJ, Foulkes MA, *et al.* Influence of site on course of intracerebral hemorrhage. *J Stroke Cerebrovasc Dis* 1993; **3**: 65–74.

3. Melo TP, Pinto AN, Ferro JM. Headache in intracerebral hematomas. *Neurology* 1996; **47**: 494–500.

4. Leira R, Castellanos M, Álvarez-Sabín J, *et al.* Headache in cerebral hemorrhage is associated with inflammatory markers and higher residual cavity. *Headache* 2005; **45**: 1236–1243.

5. Mitsias P, Jensen TS. Ischemic stroke and spontaneous intracerebral hematoma. In: Olesen J, Goadsby PJ, Ramadan NM, Tfelt-Hansen P, Welch KMA, eds. *The Headaches.* 3rd edn. New York, Lippincott Williams & Wilkins. 2006; 885–892.

6. Anderson CS, Chakera TMH, Stewart-Wynne EG, Jamrozik KD. Spectrum of primary intracerebral haemorrhage in Perth, Western Australia, 1989–90: incidence and outcome. *J Neurol Neurosurg Psychiatry* 1994; **57**: 936–940.

7. Kase CS, Williams JP, Wyatt DA, Mohr JP. Lobar intracerebral hematomas: clinical and CT analysis of 22 cases. *Neurology* 1982; **32**: 1146–1150.

8. Lipton RB, Berger AR, Lesser ML, Lantos G, Portenoy RK. Lobar vs thalamic and basal ganglion hemorrhage: clinical and radiographic features. *J Neurol* 1987; **234**: 86–90.

9. Bladin CF, Alexandrov AV, Bellevance A, *et al.* Seizures after stroke: a prospective multicenter study. *Arch Neurol* 2000; **57**: 1617–1622.

10. De Reuck J, Hemelsoet D, Van Maele G. Seizures and epilepsy in patients with a spontaneous intracerebral haematoma. *Clin Neurol Neurosurg* 2007; **109**: 501–504.

11. Passero S, Rocchi R, Rossi S, Ulivelli M, Vatti G. Seizures after spontaneous supratentorial intracerebral hemorrhage. *Epilepsia* 2002; **43**: 1175–1180.

12. Vespa PM, O'Phelan K, Shah M, *et al.* Acute seizures after intracerebral hemorrhage: a factor in progressive midline shift and outcome. *Neurology* 2003; **60**: 1441–1446.

13. Broderick JP, Brott TG, Tomsick T, *et al.* Ultra-early evaluation of intracerebral hemorrhage. *J Neurosurg* 1990; **72**: 195–199.

14. Fujii Y, Tanaka R, Takeuchi S, *et al.* Hematoma enlargement in spontaneous intracerebral hemorrhage. *J Neurosurg* 1994; **80**: 51–57.

15. Brott T, Broderick J, Kothari R, *et al.* Early hemorrhage growth in patients with intracerebral hemorrhage. *Stroke* 1997; **28**: 1–5.

16. Kelley RE, Berger JR, Scheinberg P, *et al.* Active bleeding in hypertensive intracerebral hemorrhage: computed tomography. *Neurology* 1982; **32**: 852–856.

17. Bae HC, Lee K, Yun I, *et al.* Rapid expansion of hypertensive intracerebral hemorrhage. *Neurosurgery* 1992; **31**: 35–41.

18. Wijdicks EFM, Fulgham JR. Acute fatal deterioration in putaminal hemorrhage. *Stroke* 1995; **26**: 1953–1955.

19. Hier DB, Davis KR, Richardson ER, Mohr JP. Hypertensive putaminal hemorrhage. *Ann Neurol* 1977; **1**: 152–159.

20. Weisberg LA, Stazio A, Elliot D, Shamsnia M. Putaminal hemorrhage: clinical-computed tomographic correlations. *Neuroradiology* 1990; **32**: 200–206.

21. Chung C, Caplan LR, Yamamoto Y, *et al.* Striatocapsular haemorrhage. *Brain* 2000; **123**: 1850–1862.

22. Mohr JP, Kase CS, Meckler RJ, Fisher CM. Sensorimotor stroke due to thalamocapsular ischemia. *Arch Neurol* 1977; **34**: 734–741.

23. D'Esposito M, Alexander MP. Subcortical aphasia: distinct profiles following left putaminal hemorrhage. *Neurology* 1995; **45**: 38–41.

24. Diringer MN, Edwards DF, Zazulia AR. Hydrocephalus: a previously unrecognized predictor of poor outcome from supratentorial intracerebral hemorrhage. *Stroke* 1998; **29**: 1352–1357.

25. Phan TG, Koh M, Vierkant RA, Wijdicks EFM. Hydrocephalus is a determinant of early mortality in putaminal hemorrhage. *Stroke* 2000; **31**: 2157–2162.

26. Tapia JF, Kase CS, Sawyer RH, Mohr JP. Hypertensive putaminal hemorrhage presenting as pure motor hemiparesis. *Stroke* 1983; **14**: 505–506.

27. Weisberg LA, Wall M. Small capsular hemorrhages: clinico-computed correlations. *Arch Neurol* 1984; **41**: 1255–1257.

28. Kim JS, Lee JH, Lee MC. Small primary intracerebral hemorrhage: clinical presentation of 28 cases. *Stroke* 1994; **25**: 1500–1506.

29. Arboix A, Manzano C, García-Eroles L, *et al.* Determinants of early outcome in spontaneous lobar cerebral hemorrhage. *Acta Neurol Scand* 2006; **114**: 187–192.

30. Kim JS. Lenticulocapsular hemorrhages presenting as pure sensory stroke. *Eur Neurol* 1999; **42**: 128–131.

31. Kase CS, Maulsby GO, Mohr JP, DeJuan E. Hemichorea-hemiballism and lacunar infarction in the basal ganglia. *Neurology* 1981; **31**: 452–455.

32. Jones HR, Baker RA, Kott HS. Hypertensive putaminal hemorrhage presenting with hemichorea. *Stroke* 1985; **16**: 130–131.

33. Altafullah I, Pascual-Leone A, Duvall K, Anderson DD, Taylor S. Putaminal hemorrhage accompanied by hemichorea-hemiballism. *Stroke* 1990; **27**: 1093–1094.

34. Stein RW, Kase CS, Hier DB, *et al.* Caudate hemorrhage. *Neurology* 1984; **34**: 1549–1554.

35. Liliang PC, Liang CL, Lu CH, *et al.* Hypertensive caudate hemorrhage: prognostic predictor, outcome, and role of external ventricular drainage. *Stroke* 2001; **32**: 1195–1200.

36. Weisberg LA. Caudate hemorrhage. *Arch Neurol* 1984; **41**: 971–974.

37. Fuh JL, Wang SJ. Caudate hemorrhage: clinical features, neuropsychological assessments and radiological findings. *Clin Neurol Neurosurg* 1995; **97**: 296–299.

38. Kumral E, Evyapan D, Balkir K. Acute caudate vascular lesions. *Stroke* 1999; **30**: 100–108.

39. Caplan LR. Caudate hemorrhage. In: Kase CS, Caplan LR, eds. *Intracerebral Hemorrhage.* Boston, Butterworth-Heinemann. 1994; 329–340.

40. Steinke W, Sacco R, Mohr JP, *et al.* Thalamic stroke: presentation and prognosis of infarcts and hemorrhages. *Arch Neurol* 1992; **49**: 703–710.

41. Chung CS, Caplan LR, Han W, *et al.* Thalamic haemorrhage. *Brain* 1996; **119**: 1873–1886.

42. Kumral E, Kocaer T, Ertubey NO, Kumral K. Thalamic hemorrhage: a prospective study of 100 patients. *Stroke* 1995; **26**: 964–970.

43. Fisher CM. The pathologic and clinical aspects of thalamic hemorrhage. *Trans Am Neurol Assoc* 1959; **84**: 56–59.

44. Fisher CM. Some neuro-ophthalmological observations. *J Neurol Neurosurg Psychiatry* 1967; **30**: 383–392.

45. Tijssen CC. Contralateral conjugate eye deviation in acute supratentorial lesions. *Stroke* 1994; **25**: 1516–1519.

46. Hertle RW, Bienfang DC. Oculographic analysis of acute esotropia secondary to a thalamic hemorrhage. *J Clin Neuroophthalmol* 1990; **10**: 21–26.

47. Scoditti U, Colonna F, Bettoni L, Lechi A. Acute esotropia from small thalamic hemorrhage. *Acta Neurol Belg* 1993; **93**: 290–294.

48. Karussis D, Leker RR, Abramsky O. Cognitive dysfunction following thalamic stroke: a study of 16 cases and review of the literature. *J Neurol Sci* 2000; **172**: 25–29.

49. Mohr JP, Watters WC, Duncan GW. Thalamic hemorrhage and aphasia. *Brain Lang* 1975; **2**: 3–17.

50. Wester K, Irvine DRF, Hugdahl K. Auditory laterality and attentional deficits after thalamic haemorrhage. *J Neurol* 2001; **248**: 676–683.

51. Liebson E. Anosognosia and mania associated with right thalamic haemorrhage. *J Neurol Neurosurg Psychiatry* 2000; **68**: 107–108.

52. Manabe Y, Kashibara K, Ota T, Shohmori T, Abe K. Motor neglect following left thalamic hemorrhage: a case report. *J Neurol Sci* 1999; **171**: 69–71.

53. Karnath H-O, Johannsen L, Broetz D, Küker W. Posterior thalamic hemorrhage induces "pusher syndrome". *Neurology* 2005; **64**: 1014–1019.

54. Fisher CM. Pure sensory stroke involving face, arm and leg. *Neurology* 1965; **15**: 76–80.

55. Abe K, Yorifuji S, Nishikawa Y. Pure sensory stroke resulting from thalamic haemorrhage. *Neuroradiology* 1992; **34**: 205–206.

56. Paciaroni M, Bogousslavsky J. Pure sensory syndromes in thalamic stroke. *Eur Neurol* 1998; **39**: 211–217.

57. Shintani S, Tsuruoka S, Shiigai T. Pure sensory stroke caused by a cerebral hemorrhage: clinical-radiologic correlations in seven patients. *AJNR Am J Neuroradiol* 2000; **21**: 515–520.

58. Arboix A, Rodriguez-Aguilar R, Oliveres M, *et al.* Thalamic haemorrhage vs. internal capsule-basal

ganglia haemorrhage: clinical profile and predictors of in-hospital mortality. *BMC Neurology* 2007; **7**: 32.

59. Dobato JL, Villanueva JA, Gimenez-Roldán S. Sensory ataxic hemiparesis in thalamic hemorrhage. *Stroke* 1990; **21**: 1749–1753.

60. Lera G, Scipione O, Garcia S, *et al.* A combined pattern of movement disorders resulting from posterolateral thalamic lesions of a vascular nature: a syndrome with clinico-radiologic correlation. *Mov Disord* 2000; **15**: 120–126.

61. Mossuto-Agatiello L, Puccetti G, Castellano AE. "Rubral" tremor after thalamic haemorrhage. *J Neurol* 1993; **241**: 27–30.

62. Déjérine J, Roussy G. Le syndrome thalamique. *Rev Neurol (Paris)* 1906; **14**: 521–532.

63. Kim JS. Asterixis after unilateral stroke: lesion location in 30 patients. *Neurology* 2001; **56**: 533–536.

64. Sibon I, Burbaud P. Risus sardonicus after thalamic haemorrhage. *Mov Disord* 2004; **19**: 829–831.

65. Kawahara N, Sato K, Muraki K, *et al.* CT classification of small thalamic hemorrhages and their clinical implications. *Neurology* 1986; **36**: 165–172.

66. Saez de Ocariz MDM, Nader JA, Santos JA, Bautista M. Thalamic vascular lesions: risk factors and clinical course for infarcts and hemorrhages. *Stroke* 1996; **27**: 1530–1536.

67. Chen WH, Liu JS, Wu SC, Chang YY. Transient global amnesia and thalamic hemorrhage. *Clin Neurol Neurosurg* 1996; **98**: 309–311.

68. Ropper AH, Davis KR. Lobar cerebral hemorrhages: acute clinical syndromes in 26 cases. *Ann Neurol* 1980; **8**: 141–147.

69. Weisberg LA, Stazio A. Nontraumatic frontal lobe hemorrhages: clinical-computed tomographic correlations. *Neuroradiology* 1988; **30**: 500–505.

70. Massaro AR, Sacco RL, Mohr JP, *et al.* Clinical discriminators of lobar and deep hemorrhages: the Stroke Data Bank. *Neurology* 1991; **41**: 1881–1885.

71. Flemming KD, Wijdicks EFM, St Louis EK, Li H. Predicting deterioration in patients with lobar haemorrhages. *J Neurol Neurosurg Psychiatry* 1999; **66**: 600–605.

72. Ohtani R, Kazui S, Tomimoto H, Minematsu K, Naritomi H. Clinical and radiographic features of lobar cerebral hemorrhage: hypertensive versus non-hypertensive cases. *Intern Med* 2003; **42**: 576–580.

73. Sung CY, Chu NS. Epileptic seizures in intracerebral haemorrhage. *J Neurol Neurosurg Psychiatry* 1989; **52**: 1273–1276.

74. Berger AR, Lipton RB, Lesser ML, Lantos G, Portenoy RK. Early seizures following intracerebral hemorrhage: implications for therapy. *Neurology* 1988; **38**: 1363–1365.

75. Ropper AH. Lateral displacement of the brain and level of consciousness in patients with an acute hemispheral mass. *N Engl J Med* 1986; **314**: 953–958.

76. Schütz H, Bödeker RH, Damian M, Krack P, Dorndorf W. Age-related spontaneous intracerebral hematoma in a German community. *Stroke* 1990; **21**: 1412–1418.

77. Iwasaki Y, Kinoshita M. Subcortical lobar hematomas: clinico-computed tomographic correlations. *Comput Med Imaging Graph* 1989; **13**: 195–198.

78. Weisberg LA. Subcortical lobar intracerebral haemorrhage: clinical-computed tomographic correlations. *J Neurol Neurosurg Psychiatry* 1985; **48**: 1078–1084.

79. Loes DJ, Smoker WRK, Biller J, Cornell SH. Nontraumatic lobar intracerebral hemorrhage: CT/angiographic correlation. *AJNR Am J Neuroradiol* 1987; **8**: 1027–1030.

80. Kase CS. Lobar hemorrhage. In: Kase CS, Caplan LR, eds. *Intracerebral Hemorrhage*. Boston, Butterworth-Heinemann. 1994; 363–382.

81. Weisberg LA, Stazio A, Shamsnia M, Elliott D. Nontraumatic temporal subcortical hemorrhage: clinical computed tomographic analysis. *Neuroradiology* 1990; **32**: 137–141.

82. Weisberg LA, Stazio A. Nontraumatic parietal subcortical hemorrhage: clinical-computed tomographic correlations. *Comput Med Imaging Graph* 1989; **13**: 355–361.

83. Weisberg LA, Wall M. Alexia without agraphia: clinical-computed tomographic correlations. *Neuroradiology* 1987; **29**: 283–286.

84. Weisberg LA, Stazio A. Occipital lobe hemorrhages: clinical-computed tomographic correlations. *Comput Med Imaging Graph* 1988; **12**: 353–358.

85. Ott KH, Kase CS, Ojemann RG, Mohr JP. Cerebellar hemorrhage: diagnosis and treatment. *Arch Neurol* 1974; **31**: 160–167.

86. Brennan RW, Bergland RM. Acute cerebellar hemorrhage: analysis of clinical findings and outcome in 12 cases. *Neurology* 1977; **27**: 527–532.

87. Bosch EP, Kennedy SS, Aschenbrener CA. Ocular bobbing: the myth of its localizing value. *Neurology* 1975; **25**: 949–953.

88. Salvati M, Cervoni L, Raco A, Delfini R. Spontaneous cerebellar hemorrhage: clinical remarks on 50 cases. *Surg Neurol* 2001; **55**: 156–161.

89. Fisher CM, Picard EH, Polak A, *et al.* Acute hypertensive cerebellar hemorrhage: diagnosis and surgical treatment. *J Nerv Ment Dis* 1965; **140**: 38–57.

119

90. Brillman J. Acute hydrocephalus and death one month after non-surgical treatment for acute cerebellar hemorrhage. *J Neurosurg* 1979; **50**: 374–376.

91. St. Louis EK, Wijdicks EFM, Li H, Atkinson JD. Predictors of poor outcome in patients with spontaneous cerebellar hematoma. *Can J Neurol Sci* 2000; **27**: 32–36.

92. Little JR, Tubman DE, Ethier R. Cerebellar hemorrhage in adults: diagnosis by computerized tomography. *J Neurosurg* 1978; **48**: 575–579.

93. Kase CS, Mohr JP, Caplan LR. Intracerebral hemorrhage. In: Mohr JP, Choi DW, Grotta JC, Weir B, Wolf PA, eds. *Stroke: Pathophysiology, Diagnosis, and Treatment*. Philadelphia, Churchill Livingstone. 2004; 327–376.

94. Johkura K. Central paroxysmal positional vertigo: isolated dizziness caused by small cerebellar hemorrhage. *Stroke* 2007; **38**: e26–27 (letter).

95. Durward QJ, Barnett HJM, Barr HWK. Presentation and management of mesencephalic hematoma. *J Neurosurg* 1982; **56**: 123–127.

96. Lee AG, Brown DG, Diaz PJ. Dorsal midbrain syndrome due to mesencephalic hemorrhage. *J Neuroophthalmol* 1996; **16**: 281–285.

97. Roig C, Carvajal A, Illa I, *et al.* Hémorragies mésencéphaliques isolées. *Rev Neurol* 1982; **138**: 53–61.

98. Morel-Maroger A, Metzger J, Bories J, *et al.* Les hématomes benins du tronc cérébral chez les hypertendus artériels. *Rev Neurol (Paris)* 1982; **138**: 437–445.

99. Mizushima H, Seki T. Midbrain hemorrhage presenting with oculomotor nerve palsy: case report. *Surg Neurol* 2002; **58**: 417–420.

100. Bhola R, Olson RJ. Dorsal midbrain syndrome with bilateral superior oblique palsy following brainstem hemorrhage. *Arch Ophthalmol* 2006; **124**: 1786–1788.

101. Walker M, Kim H, Samii A. Holmes-like tremor of the lower extremity following brainstem hemorrhage. *Mov Disord* 2007; **22**: 272–274.

102. Wessels T, Möller-Hartmann W, Noth J, Klötzsch C. CT findings and clinical features as markers for patient outcome in primary pontine hemorrhage. *AJNR Am J Neuroradiol* 2004; **25**: 257–260.

103. Dinsdale HB. Spontaneous hemorrhage in the posterior fossa: a study of primary cerebellar and pontine hemorrhage with observations on the pathogenesis. *Arch Neurol* 1964; **10**: 200–217.

104. Steegmann AT. Primary pontile hemorrhage. *J Nerv Ment Dis* 1951; **114**: 35–65.

105. Okudera T, Uemura K, Nakajima K, *et al.* Primary pontine hemorrhage: correlations of pathologic features with postmortem microangiographic and vertebral angiography studies. *Mt Sinai J Med* 1978; **45**: 305–321.

106. Fisher CM. Ocular bobbing. *Arch Neurol* 1964; **11**: 543–546.

107. Susac JO, Hoyt WF, Daroff DB, Lawrence W. Clinical spectrum of ocular bobbing. *J Neurol Neurosurg Psychiatry* 1970; **33**: 771–775.

108. Goto N, Kaneko M, Koga H. Primary pontine hemorrhage: clinicopathologic correlations. *Stroke* 1980; **11**: 84–90.

109. Zuccarello M, Iavicoli R, Pardatscher K, *et al.* Primary brain stem hematomas: diagnosis and treatment. *Acta Neurochir (wien)* 1980; **54**: 45–52.

110. Gobernado JM, Fernandez de Molina AR, Gimeno A. Pure motor hemiplegia due to hemorrhage in the lower pons. *Arch Neurol* 1980; **37**: 393.

111. Schnapper RA. Pontine hemorrhage presenting as ataxic hemiparesis. *Stroke* 1982; **13**: 518–519.

112. Sherman SC, Saadatmand B. Pontine hemorrhage and isolated abducens palsy. *Am J Emerg Med* 2007; **25**: 104–105.

113. Kase CS, Maulsby GO, Mohr JP. Partial pontine hematomas. *Neurology* 1980; **30**: 652–655.

114. Caplan LR, Goodwin JA. Lateral tegmental brainstem hemorrhages. *Neurology* 1982; **32**: 252–260.

115. Lhermitte F, Pagès M. Abducens nucleus syndrome due to pontine haemorrhage. *Cerebrovasc Dis* 2006; **22**: 284–285.

116. Moon SY, Park SH, Hwang JM, Kim JS. Oculopalatal tremor after pontine hemorrhage. *Neurology* 2003; **61**: 1621.

117. Mastaglia FL, Edis B, Kakulas BA. Medullary hemorrhage: a report of two cases. *J Neurol Neurosurg Psychiatry* 1969; **32**: 221–225.

118. Barinagarrementeria F, Cantú C. Primary medullary hemorrhage: report of four cases and review of the literature. *Stroke* 1994; **25**: 1684–1687.

119. Jung HH, Baumgartner RW, Hess K. Symptomatic secondary hemorrhagic transformation of ischemic Wallenberg's syndrome. *J Neurol* 2000; **247**: 463–464.

Computerized tomography and CT angiography in intracerebral hemorrhage

Rush H. Chewning and Kieran P. Murphy

Introduction

When patients present with acute onset of focal neurological deficits urgent neuroimaging is essential. The initial diagnostic question in these cases is whether or not the deficits are caused by intracerebral hemorrhage (ICH). The answer is of utmost importance in determining the direction of treatment. Non-contrast CT is the first-line imaging modality in this setting.

Computerized tomography

Computerized tomography scans are rapid, readily available, and relatively inexpensive. Most importantly they have exquisite sensitivity and specificity, approaching 100%, in the detection of acute blood [1]. Owing to its high protein concentration and high mass density, acute hematoma appears as hyperdense on non-contrast CT (Figs. 9.1, 9.2a, b). However, there are some rare cases where acute blood may appear isodense on CT, such as in patients with coagulation disorders or very low hemoglobin concentrations [2].

The relative density seen on CT varies in accordance with the evolution of the hematoma, and thus is connected to the timing of the scan. In the hyperacute phase (less than 12 hours) the bleed appears as hyperdense, though the exact boundaries of the hemorrhage may be difficult to define given that fresh blood has similar density to the surrounding brain parenchyma. As the clot evolves in the acute (12 hours to 2 days) and early subacute (2 to 7 days) phases the density of the hematoma increases, as serum is extruded and globin protein concentration rises. The late subacute phase (8 days to 1 month) displays declining density due to red blood cell lysis

and globin protein proteolysis. Hematomas in the chronic phase (greater than 1 month) progress to a hypodense appearance as they are phagocytosed [3].

In addition to detecting acute blood, non-contrast CT scans carry the added benefit of revealing worrisome complications that may be associated with the hemorrhage. These include extension of the hemorrhage into the intraventricular space, hydrocephalus, edema, mass effect, and herniation. Early discovery of a complication is paramount to initiating emergent treatment in an effort to reduce morbidity and mortality.

Volume of hemorrhage on CT is an important predictor of mortality and functional ability after ICH [4]. Using non-contrast CT, volume of a hematoma can be easily calculated using the formula ($A \times B \times C$)/2, where A is the largest diameter (in cm) of the hematoma on axial CT; B is the diameter perpendicular to A on the same slice; and C is the slice thickness multiplied by the number of slices showing the hemorrhage [5]. Expansion of the hematoma, an important cause of neurological decline, is detectable on repeat CT and is an indication for intervention [6].

The initial non-contrast CT scan may provide clues as to the origin of the bleed, particularly when combined with the clinical history of the patient. Primary ICH caused by chronic hypertension should top the differential in elderly hypertensives whose scans demonstrate blood in the pons, basal ganglia, thalamus, or cerebellum. Arteriovenous malformation (AVM) should be suspected in cases of ICH in association with perilesional or intralesional large vessels. Ruptured aneurysm may be the cause when subarachnoid blood is in the Sylvian fissure in association with temporal lobe ICH, or in the intrahemispheric fissure in association with frontal lobe ICH.

Hemorrhage from a neoplasm or cavernous angioma should be suspected when calcification is seen [1]. Determination of the source is of great importance in guiding initial management and treatment. Of particular concern in identifying the source of the

bleed is assessing the risk for rebleeding. Hemorrhages from vascular abnormalities, such as aneurysm or AVM, carry a high likelihood of recurrence, often with devastating outcomes [7].

The emerging role of CT angiography

Though non-contrast CT may provide clues as to the source of bleeding, further study is usually required. Cerebral digital subtraction angiography (DSA) is the gold standard for locating and assessing vascular abnormalities [8]. However, advances in CT angiography (CTA) (Figs. 9.3, 9.4), coupled with its clinical advantages, have enabled this modality to gain acceptance and widespread use in cases of ICH.

Computerized tomography angiography offers many clinical advantages over DSA for the evaluation of intracranial vascular abnormalities in cases of ICH. As all patients with suspected intracerebral bleeds get a non-contrast CT as an initial diagnostic study, patients are already in place for CTA to be performed. Injection of contrast via a peripheral intravenous catheter immediately after the patient has undergone non-contrast CT enables CTA to be conducted rapidly and without having to move the patient to another location, such as a dedicated angiography suite. Moreover, not all hospitals have the resources to supply physicians trained in cerebral angiography at all hours, nor do all hospitals have dedicated angiography suites. The relative ubiquity of CT scanners and their ease of operation convey a great advantage to CTA over DSA. Additionally, CTA is much less expensive and less invasive than DSA. While CTA does carry very small risks, such as radiation exposure, contrast reaction,

Fig. 9.1 Head CT demonstrating SAH around the brainstem and the left side of the tentorium cerebellum and sylvian region. This distribution of blood is suspicious for a posterior communication artery or posterior cerebral artery or superior cerebellar aneurysm bleed. It is a good idea to look for the cause of the bleed. Often the aneurysm is apparent as a filling defect or low attenuation area in the high attenuation blood.

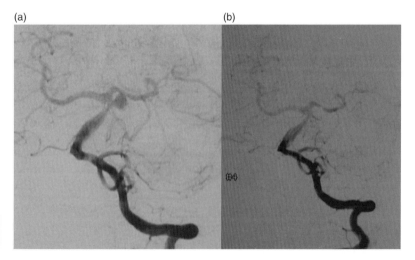

(a)   (b)

Fig. 9.2 (a and b) The patient with the head CT in Fig. 9.1 went on to cerebral angiogram and that demonstrated the left superior cerebellar artery aneurysm we see here. It was narrow necked, posterior fossa in a difficult place for open surgical repair so we decided to treat it by endovascular technique. (b) Demonstrates the successful coiling of the aneurysm following Guglielmi detachable coil (GDC) embolization.

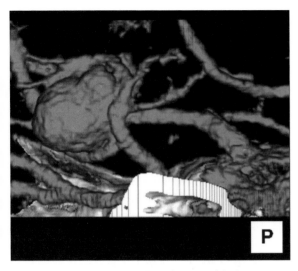

Fig. 9.3 This is bone subtracted 256 slice CTA of the brain in a patient with a large aneurysm. This technique allows dynamic CT to be performed over several cardiac cycles and thus nipples or rupture points can be seen pulsating allowing differentiation of ruptured from unruptured aneurysms. As the whole brain is covered the bone of the skull can be subtracted easily allowing visualization of the skull base region and in particular better visualization of posterior communicating artery aneurysms. See plate section for color version.

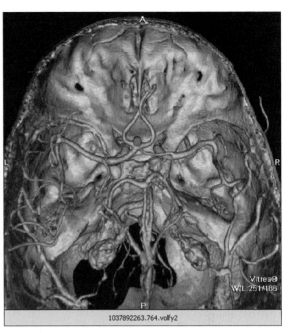

Fig. 9.4 This is a 32 slice CTA of the head reconstructed on a 3-D work station. The beautifully demonstrated anterior communicating artery aneurysm can be seen easily and has been color-coded (Gray). See plate section for color version.

and even rebleeding [9], risks are much lower and less severe than the risks of DSA, which include permanent neurological damage and death from stroke [10].

For CTA to supplant DSA in the evaluation of vascular abnormalities in cases of ICH, it is not enough for CTA to have clinical advantages over DSA. Computerized tomography angiography must be shown to have similar sensitivity and specificity as DSA in the detection of secondary causes of ICH, such as aneurysms and vascular malformations. Meta-analysis of early studies of three-dimensional computed tomography angiography (3D-CTA) for the detection of intracranial aneurysms revealed a sensitivity of 93% [8]. Many of these studies demonstrated that CTA sensitivity was equal to DSA except in cases of small aneurysms (less than 4 mm) [11,12]. More recent studies have found 3D-CTA to have sensitivity approaching 100%, and equivalent to that of DSA [13]. As technological advances in both scanning equipment and software image processing improve, increasing sensitivity of CTA for diagnosing aneurysms may obviate the need for DSA. Though at this time CTA is also quite good at detecting AVMs, the inferiority of this modality compared with DSA in demonstrating the intricate vascular detail of

the lesion make DSA a requirement, particularly for pre-procedural planning [14,15].

As mentioned previously, detection of hematoma expansion is of critical importance in cases of ICH, as it can lead to neurological deterioration and death. Computerized tomography angiography may be of benefit in predicting such expansion. One study described the presence of a focus of enhancement within an acute ICH, called the "spot sign," as a reliable and early predictor of hematoma expansion [16]. Another study noted that contrast extravasation on CTA was also an independent predictor of hematoma expansion [17]. Findings such as these on CTA may serve as a more rapid method of discovering hematoma expansion as compared with repeat CT. Reducing time to detection allows for earlier intervention and may improve outcomes.

Conclusion

The use of non-contrast CT in the initial evaluation of patients presenting with suspected ICH is well established and universally accepted. Recently, advances in CTA have enabled this modality to gain wide acceptance in evaluating possible secondary causes of ICH, such as aneurysm or vascular malformation. As scanner technology and software rendering capabilities continue to improve, CTA appears poised to replace DSA and become the new gold standard for such evaluations.

References

1. Hsieh PC, Awad IA, Getch CC, *et al.* Current updates in perioperative management of intracerebral hemorrhage. *Neurol Clin* 2006; **24**: 745–764.

2. Wanke FJ, Forsting M. Imaging of intracranial hemorhage: a review article. *Iran J Radiol* 2007; **4**: 65–76.

3. Huisman TAGM. Intracranial hemorrhage: ultrasound, CT, and MRI findings. *Eur Radiol* 2005; **15**: 434–440.

4. Broderick JP, Brott TG, Duldner JE, *et al.* Volume of intracerebral hemorrhage. A powerful and easy-to-use predictor of 30-day mortality. *Stroke* 1993; **24**: 987–993.

5. Kothari RU, Brott T, Broderick JP, *et al.* The ABCs of measuring intracerebral hemorrhage volumes. *Stroke* 1996; **27**: 1304–1305.

6. Mayer SA, Brun NC, Begtrup K, *et al.* Recombinant activated factor VII for acute intracerebral hemorrhage. *N Engl J Med* 2005; **352**: 777–785.

7. Kassell NF, Torner JC, Haley EC, *et al.* The international cooperative study on the timing of aneurysm surgery. Part 1: overall management results. *J Neurosurg* 1990; **73**: 18–36.

8. Chappell ET, Moure FT, Good MC. Comparison of computed tomographic angiography with digital subtraction angiography in the diagnosis of cerebral aneurysms: a meta-analysis. *Neurosurgery* 2003; **52**: 624–631.

9. Hashiguchi A, Mimata C, Ichimura H, *et al.* Rebleeding of ruptured cerebral aneurysms during three-dimensional computed tomographic angiography: report of two cases and literature review. *Neurosurg Rev* 2007; **30**: 151–154.

10. Cloft HJ, Joseph GJ, Dion JE. Risk of cerebral angiography in patients with subarachnoid hemorrhage, cerebral aneurysm, and arteriovenous malformation: a meta-analysis. *Stroke* 1999; **30**: 317–320.

11. Dammert S, Krings T, Moller-Hartmann W, *et al.* Detection of intracranial aneurysms with multislice CT: comparison with conventional angiography. *Neuroradiology* 2004; **46**: 427–434.

12. Tipper G, U-King-Im JM, Price SJ, *et al.* Detection and evaluation of intracranial aneurysms with 16-row multislice CT angiography. *Clin Radiol* 2005; **60**: 565–572.

13. Papke K, Kuhl CK, Fruth M, *et al.* Intracranial aneurysms: role of multidetector CT angiography in diagnosis and endovascular therapy planning. *Radiology* 2007; **244**: 532–540.

14. Friedlander R. Arteriovenous malformations of the brain. *N Engl J Med* 2007; **356**: 2704–2712.

15. Sasiadek M, Hendrich B, Turek T, *et al.* Our own experience with CT angiography in early diagnosis of cerebral vascular malformations. *Neurol Neurochir Pol* 2000; **34**: 48–55.

16. Wada R, Aviv RI, Fox AJ, *et al.* CT angiography "spot sign" predicts hematoma expansion in acute intracerebral hemorrhage. *Stroke* 2007; **38**: 1257–1262.

17. Goldstein JN, Fazen LE, Snider R, *et al.* Contrast extravasation on CT angiography predicts hematoma expansion in intracerebral hemorrhage. *Neurology* 2007; **68**: 889–894.

Chapter 1

MRI of intracerebral hemorrhage

Ken Butcher and Stephen M. Davis

Diagnosis of intracerebral hemorrhage with MRI

Stroke clinicians have been somewhat reluctant to consider MRI a reliable tool for the clinical assessment of intracerebral hemorrhage (ICH). This is based on the ease of identification of blood on CT scans and the perceived difficulty associated with visualization of acute hemorrhage on MRI. We will review the evidence that blood is readily identifiable on MRI and describe how the use of multiple sequences provides additional information regarding the age of blood products. Magnetic resonance imaging also makes it possible to diagnose, or rule out, many underlying etiologies of secondary ICH and should ideally be considered a routine investigation in all acute stroke patients. Finally, we will review studies utilizing MRI to investigate the pathophysiological sequelae of primary ICH.

MRI signal acquisition review

The following is an extremely simplified summary of basic MRI principles, intended only to provide the reader with information relevant to the remainder of the chapter. Interested readers are referred to more comprehensive MRI texts for additional information [1,2]. Magnetic resonance imaging signal acquisition can be summarized in four basic steps. Protons are initially aligned in a magnetic field. The protons have a natural magnetic spin, which results in precession about the longitudinal axis of this magnetic field. Protons are then excited with a radiofrequency (RF) pulse. This is followed by proton relaxation (two types), resulting in an RF signal that is "read out" by the receiver coil, which is essentially an antenna, of the MRI. The fourth step is construction of an image through spatial and frequency encoding of this signal.

In spin echo (SE) imaging, protons are initially excited with an RF pulse transmitted at 90° to the alignment of the protons in the magnetic field. These protons are now in a higher energy state and no longer aligned with the magnetic field axis. In addition, the precession of the protons is synchronized or "in phase," but this is only temporary. Proton relaxation takes two forms: longitudinal or spin-lattice and transverse or spin-spin (phase) relaxation, which are the basis of the T1 and T2 signals respectively. These two forms of relaxation occur concurrently, although T1 effects are seen earlier after excitation. Therefore, T1 signals are maximized by reducing the time between excitation and signal readout (echo time; TE). Conversely, T2-weighted images are generated using a longer TE.

Normally, SE images also utilize a second 180° re-phasing RF pulse, which serves to "re-focus" images, making them less susceptible to field inhomogeneities which occur at the interface between tissues with different susceptibilities, such as bone and air or even Cerebrospinal Fluid (CSF) and gray matter. It is this second RF pulse which produces the relaxation "echo," for which SE images are named. This second RF pulse preserves the MRI signal, improving image contrast, but also makes detection of magnetic inhomogeneities more difficult. T2-weighted images which are acquired without a 180° re-phasing pulse are known as T2* sequences and these are very susceptible to any inhomogeneities in the magnetic field. Field inhomogeneities also result from any substances with unpaired electrons, which are referred to as paramagnetic. T2* images are therefore sensitive to the presence of any paramagnetic materials and are an example of susceptibility-weighted sequences.

Intracerebral Hemorrhage, ed. J. R. Carhuapoma, S. A. Mayer, and D. F. Hanley. Published by Cambridge University Press.
© J. R. Carhuapoma, S. A. Mayer, and D. F. Hanley 2010.

Gradient recalled echo (GRE), sometimes referred to simply as gradient echo, images are generated in a different manner to the conventional SE technique described above. Protons are excited with an RF pulse of less than 90°, which permits more frequent excitations (decreased repetition time; TR). Unlike SE, an echo is generated using a biphasic magnetic gradient, which first de-phases and then re-phases protons, and gives the sequence its name. The primary advantage of this sequence is that image acquisition time is shorter. In addition, as GRE sequences lack the 180° re-phasing pulse, T2* images are also obtained. In fact, GRE T2* images are the most common susceptibility-weighted sequences in clinical use.

Conventional SE and GRE images rely on multiple RF excitations to produce numerous echoes, which are used to generate images. Echo-planar imaging (EPI) is a technique which allows sampling of an entire volume of tissue with a single RF pulse excitation. This is accomplished through high performance gradients, which are cycled on and off during a single period of proton relaxation. This ultra fast technique therefore allows imaging of physiological phenomenon, including water diffusion and blood flow. The EPI technique can be applied to conventional SE or GRE images. The decrease in acquisition time is associated with some increase in artifacts, due primarily to mismatched timing of echoes as well as currents (eddy) caused by the gradients themselves.

MRI and blood

Intravascular blood is normally visible on routine SE sequences only due to the effects of flow, which disrupt signal acquisition, resulting in the "voids" familiar to most clinicians. Four factors have been identified with the potential to alter MRI signal intensity in the presence of extravascular blood. These are increased red cell density, clot matrix formation, decreasing cellular hydration, and finally blood deoxygenation and breakdown [3]. While all of these ultimately affect the MRI signal, it is the latter which is most important, due to the susceptibility properties of these blood components as well as their effects on relaxivity of adjacent water molecules (protons). Paramagnetic blood constituents and metabolic products include deoxyhemoglobin, methemoglobin and hemosiderin. In contrast, oxyhemoglobin is diamagnetic and therefore does not result in changes in MRI signal. In addition to oxyhemoglobin and deoxyhemoglobin, acute blood also contains significant amounts of water in the form of plasma, which is heavily T2-weighted. Thus, acute intraparenchymal blood has a mixed signal on traditional T2-weighted images [3,4].

Studies of hyperacute ICH indicate that the susceptibility effects are first observed at the periphery of the hematoma (Fig. 10.1) [5]. This is related to formation of deoxyhemoglobin and magnetic field inhomogeneities at the interface with surrounding normal diamagnetic tissue. This is useful in delineating the boundary of the hematoma, from the rim of perihematomal edema, as the latter is always hyperintense on T2-weighted images. It is important to recognize that measurements of hematoma volume made on MRI will tend to over estimate the true volume [6]. This is most marked on susceptibility-weighted images and results from the fact that the paramagnetic effects of deoxyhemoglobin extend beyond the physical limits of the hematoma (Fig. 10.1). This is a relevant consideration, given the well-known prognostic value of acute hematoma volume [7]. The hypointensity associated with increasing amounts of deoxyhemoglobin progressively spreads into the hematoma core over time.

The paramagnetic effects of acute blood increase with the strength of the magnetic field. In addition, susceptibility-weighted sequences including GRE T2*, which are more sensitive to the paramagnetic effects of deoxyhemoglobin, make acute blood even more obvious on MRI (Fig. 10.1) [3,8–10]. As described above, the absence of a second pulse on the T2* images results in increased sensitivity to field inhomogeneities. Gradient recalled echo T2* images generated using EPI are equally sensitive to blood products, relative to non-EPI sequences, although they generally contain more artifacts (Figs. 10.1 and 10.2). Both of these susceptibility-weighted sequences are particularly useful in the diagnosis of both acute and remote ICH.

Magnetic resonance imaging signal changes on GRE, T1- and T2-weighted images can be used to estimate the age of intracranial blood. In addition to the increasingly hypointense T2 signals seen with progressive deoxygenation, after 72 hours, T1 signal intensity increases due to the presence of methemoglobin (Table 10.1). After approximately seven days, the T2 signal intensity will also increase, as red blood cells are lysed. Eventually, both T1 and T2 signals are significantly decreased, as only hemosiderin is left as a remnant of the hematoma. Depending on the size

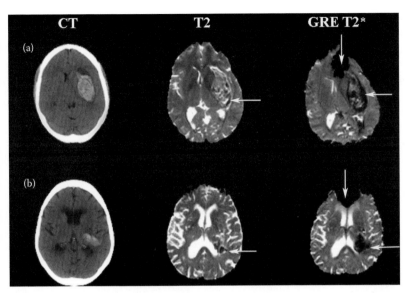

Fig. 10.1 Examples of primary intracerebral hemorrhage (ICH) imaged with CT, echo-planar T2-weighted (T2) and susceptibility-weighted gradient recalled echo (GRE T2*) MRI. (a) Putamenal ICH (57 ml on CT) imaged at 2 (CT) and 4.5 hours (MRI) after symptom onset. (b) Thalamic ICH (13 ml on CT) imaged at 1 (CT) and 4.5 hours (MRI) after symptom onset. Blood appears hypointense on both MRI sequences, due to the paramagnetic effects of deoxyhemoglobin, which forms initially at the margin of the hematoma (arrows), and are more marked on the GRE T2* images. Edema and fluid components of the hematoma appear bright on the T2-weighted images. The paramagnetic effects of the deoxyhemoglobin extend beyond the physical limits of the hematoma, particularly on the GRE T2* images, an effect sometimes referred to as "bloom." The GRE T2* images also demonstrate magnetic field inhomogeneities occurring at CSF/bone/air interfaces (vertical arrows).

of the hematoma, a CSF filled cavity, which is heavily T2-weighted, may also be evident.

Comparative studies: MRI and CT

Computerized tomography has long been considered the gold standard for diagnosis of acute primary ICH. Conversely, MRI has been shown to have superior sensitivity for detection of early cerebral ischemia [11]. In order to avoid unnecessary delays in acute stroke assessment, which decrease the efficacy of therapies such as thrombolysis, a single imaging investigation is certainly preferable. In cases of suspected ischemic stroke, the most common differential diagnosis is primary ICH.

Although early studies indicated that MRI was insensitive to the presence of acute intraparenchymal blood, this appears to be a reflection of the low field strengths (0.5–0.6 Tesla) and the lack of susceptibility-weighted imaging sequences available [12]. Since that time, 1.5 Tesla scanners have become the standard clinical tool. In the course of investigating the use of MRI as an assessment tool for ischemic stroke, it has become clear that acute ICH can be readily diagnosed

and differentiated from ischemia. An early report found that 6 of 35 stroke patients imaged within six hours were found with subsequent CT to have ICH [8]. In all cases, a peripheral hypointense rim was evident at the site of ICH on SE T1- and T2-weighted images. Susceptibility-weighted images including GRE and T2* images demonstrated the hematomas as unequivocally hypointense regions.

Two prospective studies have confirmed that MRI can be used to reliably diagnose acute ICH and differentiate it from ischemic infarction. One study evaluated 200 acute stroke patients imaged with CT and MRI within six hours of symptom onset (median time to MRI 2 hours, 13 minutes; CT 3 hours, 3 minutes) [13]. Patients with symptoms suggestive of subarachnoid hemorrhage were excluded. All patients were imaged with GRE and diffusion-weighted (DWI) sequences, using standard 1.5 Tesla MRI scanners. The MRI scans were evaluated by four independent and blinded investigators, including two stroke neurologists and two neuroradiologists. Acute intracranial blood was detected in 28 patients with CT. In 25 patients, the diagnosis of acute hemorrhage was confirmed by MRI. In the remaining three patients,

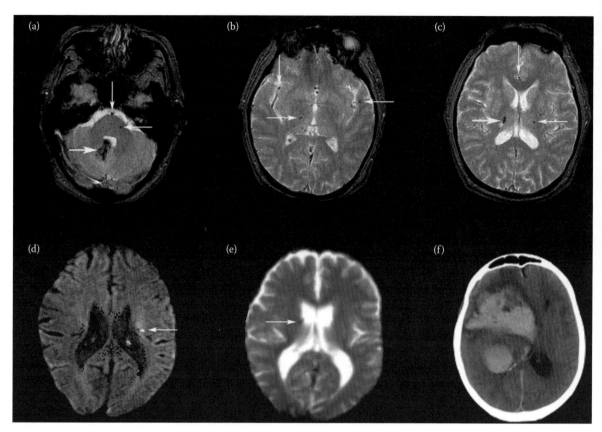

Fig. 10.2 Examples of patients with cerebral microbleeds (CMB). (a–c) Gradient recalled echo (GRE T2*) images of a patient who suffered a primary intracerebral hemorrhage in the right cerebellar hemisphere. The superior, medial limit of this hemorrhage can be seen in (a) (thick arrow). The patient also has multiple cerebral microbleeds (CMBs; thin arrows; note not all of the CMBs are indicated). The hypointense signal at the lateral aspect of the right thalamus, (c) (thick arrow) was also visible on T2-weighted images and was 0.57 cm in diameter. This also represents hemosiderin secondary to remote ICH, but the criteria for CMB are not met, making it a "macrobleed." (d) Diffusion-weighted image showing acute left hemispheric ischemia (arrow). (e) An incidental CMB was found on this GRE T2* image, generated using an echoplanar imaging sequence. Note the lower clarity of the image relative to the GRE images from the patient shown in a–c. After early anticoagulation for atrial fibrillation, the patient suffered an ICH, the center of which appears to be related to the site of the CMB (f).

Table 10.1. Appearance of intracerebral hemorrhage on MRI sequences

Time from onset	Hematoma constituents	T1	T2	SWI (GRE/T2*)
Hyperacute (< 24 hours)	Oxyhemoglobin, deoxyhemoglobin, plasma	$\leftrightarrow$	Mixed: $\downarrow$ (rim) $\uparrow$ (center)	$\downarrow$†
Acute (1–3 days)	Deoxyhemoglobin (increased), plasma	$\leftrightarrow$	$\downarrow$	$\downarrow$
Early subacute (3–7 days)	Intracellular methemoglobin, plasma	$\uparrow$	$\downarrow$	$\downarrow$
Late subacute (7–14 days)	Extracellular methemoglobin	$\uparrow$	$\uparrow$	$\downarrow$
Chronic (> 2 weeks)	Hemosiderin±CSF cavity	$\downarrow$	$\downarrow$	$\downarrow$

Notes: $\leftrightarrow$ = isointense appearance; $\uparrow$ = hyperintense appearance; $\downarrow$ = hypointense appearance (relative to normal gray matter).
†SWI (susceptibility weighted images): gradient recalled echo (GRE) and T2* images are more sensitive than T1 and T2 sequences for magnetic field inhomogeneities produced by paramagnetic deoxyhemoglobin. SWI images will therefore demonstrate ICH prior to any observed signal changes on T1/T2 sequences.

blood was evident on MRI, but interpreted as chronic. In another four patients, acute hemorrhagic transformation of ischemic infarcts was seen on MRI, but not on CT. Thus, MRI and CT appeared to have equivalent sensitivity for the detection of acute hemorrhage. The misclassification of acute as chronic hemorrhage in three patients may have been improved if the raters had been given access to T1-weighted images. These sequences would be expected to have demonstrated an absence of either hyperintense signal, indicating methemoglobin and subacute hemorrhage, or hypointense signal associated with hemosiderin and chronic blood (Table 10.1). In contrast to the similar diagnostic accuracy between the two imaging modalities for acute blood, MRI was markedly superior for the detection of chronic blood. Evidence of prior intracerebral bleeding was found in 49 patients on MRI, with no changes seen on CT scan. The majority of theses cases (41) included at least one microbleed, evident on GRE sequences (see below).

A second similar study evaluated a total of 124 acute stroke patients imaged within 6 hours of symptom onset with MRI and CT, which were performed in random order [14]. A total of 62 patients had an acute primary ICH diagnosed by CT. Using T1, T2, DWI and T2* images, three experienced stroke neurologists/radiologists correctly identified the acute hematomas on MRI scan. In addition, three medical students with minimal training were able to differentiate hemorrhage from ischemia with a diagnostic accuracy of 97%.

Secondary intracerebral hemorrhage

The majority of elderly patients presenting with intracerebral blood have suffered a primary ICH resulting from spontaneous rupture of an intraparenchymal blood vessel which has been rendered less compliant by the chronic effects of hypertension and/or amyloid deposition [15]. Although studies are limited, approximately 10–18% of patients above the age of 45 will have experienced bleeding secondary to a structural lesion [16]. The probability of secondary ICH decreases with age and a previous diagnosis of hypertension. Lobar ICH is more often secondary than those located in the basal ganglia or brainstem [16]. Determination of the need for further radiological assessment including invasive cerebral angiography is a major challenge for the managing physician.

Magnetic resonance imaging is the initial diagnostic procedure of choice for investigation of underlying structural causes of secondary ICH, including vascular malformations and neoplasms [17]. Although cerebral angiography remains the gold standard for the diagnosis of aneurysms and arteriovenous malformations (AVMs), the low prevalence and small complication rate make this an impractical initial investigation in every case of ICH. Following the diagnosis of intraparenchymal bleeding on CT, we advise an initial MRI and proceed directly to angiography only when the volume of subarachnoid blood is large and/or the hematoma is in proximity to the circle of Willis. Magnetic resonance imaging combined with MRA will reveal most aneurysms greater than 3 mm in diameter as well as larger AVMs [18–20]. It has superior sensitivity to angiography in the diagnosis of cavernomas [21,22]. In younger and normotensive patients, we repeat the MRI in 6–8 weeks to assess regions which may have been obscured by the paramagnetic effects of the acute blood.

Subarachnoid hemorrhage

It is generally recognized that MRI is superior to CT in the evaluation of subarachnoid space diseases of an inflammatory or neoplastic origin [23]. Acute subarachnoid hemorrhage (SAH) has been viewed differently, due to the inability to image blood in the CSF filled spaces with traditional SE images. Fortunately, FLAIR images have been shown to be much more sensitive for the presence of acute subarachnoid blood. The FLAIR sequence has a long echo (readout) time, making it heavily T2-weighted, but the normally high CSF signal is effectively nulled by a second RF pulse, timed to match the longitudinal relaxation properties of CSF [24]. Edema related to cerebral pathology has different relaxation properties and is therefore not suppressed by the FLAIR sequence. Acute subarachnoid blood also appears hyperintense on FLAIR images (Fig. 10.3). Although the exact mechanism of this high signal appearance is unknown, it may be related to elevated protein concentrations, which alter the magnetization properties of CSF. Indeed proteinaceous exudates also result in high FLAIR signal within the subarachnoid space.

An early systematic analysis of the utility of MRI in the diagnosis of SAH included only patients more than three days after symptom onset. In patients imaged within two weeks of onset, FLAIR detected

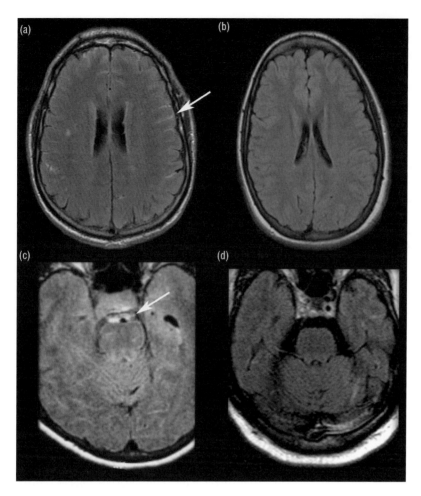

Fig. 10.3 Examples of acute subarachnoid hemorrhage (< 24 hours after symptom onset) demonstrated with FLAIR sequences. (a) High signal corresponding to acute hemorrhage in the cortical sulci (arrow) secondary to anterior communicating artery aneurysmal rupture. (b) Normal FLAIR at the same level with low signal corresponding to CSF in the cortical sulci. (c) High signal indicating acute hemorrhage in the pre-pontine cistern (arrow) of another patient found to have an anterior communicating artery aneurysm. (d) Normal FLAIR at the level of the pons demonstrating the normally low signal of CSF in the cisterns.

100% of bleeds and was superior to T1 and T2 SE sequences as well as CT [25]. After 14 days, the sensitivity of FLAIR images dropped to 62%, which was still superior to CT (17%). Another small retrospective study in the acute phase demonstrated that SAH evident on CT, performed less than 12 hours prior to MRI, was correctly identified on FLAIR images with 100% sensitivity [23]. In addition, FLAIR images have been shown to demonstrate extremely small amounts of subarachnoid blood not visible on CT. Traumatic and aneurysmal SAH can be detected with equal sensitivity by FLAIR. Acute intraventricular blood is also easily detectable as high signal on FLAIR images [26].

Magnetic resonance imaging can also be useful in the delayed diagnosis of SAH. This often occurs when thunderclap headache is not investigated immediately with a CT scan. The hyperdense appearance of subarachnoid blood on CT becomes progressively less dense in the acute stage. An isodense appearance, relative to CSF, has been reported as early as 24 hours after symptom onset and the sensitivity of CT for subarachnoid blood decreases to 50% after one week [27,28]. It has been shown in aneurysmal SAH patients that susceptibility-weighted images demonstrate hemosiderin deposition within the subarachnoid space in 72% of patients [29]. In addition, the hemosiderin was deposited preferentially near the site of the ruptured aneurysm.

Cerebral microbleeds

Cerebral microbleeds (CMBs) have been defined as hypointensities, less than 5 mm in diameter, most easily identified on susceptibility-weighted sequences [30–33]. These foci of MR signal loss represent deposits of hemosiderin within macrophages, resulting from past bleeding episodes. Histopathological analysis demonstrates a strong association with microangio-pathy secondary to lipo/fibrohyalinosis and amyloid deposition [31].

The incidence of CMBs in populations without neurological disease has been estimated to be between 4% and 6% [34,35]. In the first of these studies involving 280 healthy elderly individuals, CMBs were seen more frequently in patients with advancing age, hypertension, and leukoaraiosis [35]. A large prospective MRI investigation (n = 472), performed as part of the Framingham risk study, reported the prevalence of CMBs was 4.7% in a cohort with a mean age of 64 [34]. The frequency of CMBs was 12.6% in patients over 75 and only 2.2% in those below this age. They were also more common in men (7%) than women (2.7%). The majority of patients had only a single lesion and the most common location was the cerebral cortex or subcortical white matter. No associations could be identified with cardiovascular risk factors including blood pressure, diabetes, smoking, cholesterol. Although leukoaraiosis and CMBs appeared to be correlated in the crude analysis, the relationship was no longer significant after adjusting for age and sex.

The frequency of CMBs appears to be elevated in patients with both ischemic stroke and previous ICH [36–42]. As many as 71% of patients presenting with ICH have been found to have CMBs [41]. Estimates for the prevalence of CMBs in patients presenting with ischemic stroke range from 20% to 68% [39,42]. This likely reflects the common risk factors for ischemic stroke and ICH. Two studies have indicated a positive correlation between lacunar stroke and CMB lesion load, which is suggestive of common pathophysiology, specifically small-vessel vasculopathy [37,41]. Despite these shared pathological mechanisms and correlations, the development of hemorrhagic versus ischemic stroke in individual patients is likely more complex. This seems the most probable explanation for the inconsistent studies assessing the correlation between CMBs and small-vessel ischemic changes.

Despite a predilection for lobar location, no association between CMBs and Apolipoprotein E genotype was identified in the Framingham study [34]. This was somewhat surprising, given the increased risk for lobar ICH recurrence in patients with the Apolipoprotein E ϵ2 and ϵ4 alleles [43]. Thus, it has been hypothesized that CMBs may be a marker of cerebral amyloid angiopathy-related lobar ICH [44]. Indeed, a serial MRI investigation of survivors of lobar ICH indicated that the development of *new* CMBs was associated with Apolipoprotein E ϵ2 and ϵ4 genotypes [38]. Regardless of genotype, the total hemorrhage burden detected by MRI, including previous CMBs as well as larger bleeds, was strongly predictive of ICH recurrence. Thus, MRI may be useful as a tool for risk stratification for future ICH in stroke survivors.

The prognostic value of CMBs in therapeutic decision making remains unclear. It has been proposed that CMBs may be predictors of symptomatic hemorrhagic transformation following thrombolytic therapy for acute ischemic stroke. Indeed, there have been reports of increased rates of ICH following both intra-arterial and intravenous therapy in patients with CMBs [45,46]. This association has been particularly compelling in cases where the focus of hemorrhage has occurred at the site of a CMB, sometimes remote from the ischemic region [46]. Cerebral microbleeds may also be useful in stratifying risk–benefit ratios for patients being considered for long-term anti coagulation. We have observed hemorrhage co-localized with a CMB in a patient aggressively anticoagulated in the subacute phase of stroke (Fig. 10.2). At this point, however, the evidence that CMBs predict hemorrhagic complications of thrombolytic or anticoagulant therapy is restricted to case reports such as this. Indeed, another study demonstrated that the presence of CMBs independently predicted hemorrhagic transformation of ischemic infarcts, irrespective of treatment with recombinant tissue plasminogen activator (t-PA) [39]. Thus, while CMBs are likely to be associated with increased risk of early hemorrhage after ischemic stroke, it is not clear that thrombolysis necessarily significantly adds to this risk. Indeed, a preliminary report from an ongoing trial assessing the ability of MRI to predict the response to ischemic stroke thrombolysis 3–6 hours after onset indicated no increased risk of symptomatic or asymptomatic hemorrhage in patients with CMBs [47]. In this study, CMBs were found in 11 of 70 consecutive patients treated with rt-PA, none of whom experienced symptomatic hemorrhagic transformation. Assessing the absolute risk that CMBs represent to potential thrombolysis candidates will require a very large number of patients, but at this point it does not appear to be excessive.

Role of MRI in acute stroke assessment

It has been clearly demonstrated that MRI is the investigation of choice for patients presenting with acute ischemic stroke symptoms. The studies summarized above have conclusively demonstrated that concerns about the ability of MRI to detect ICH or SAH are now unwarranted. In addition, MRI is much more likely than CT to reveal a secondary cause of ICH. Magnetic resonance imaging can generally be performed earlier and with less risk to the patient than angiography, allowing specific surgical or other management to begin earlier in cases of secondary ICH. Finally, MRI is the only diagnostic procedure that makes it possible to definitively diagnose previous bleeding episodes. This information is useful in risk stratification of patients for future ICH and may alter therapy. Thus, where available and feasible, we advocate the use of MRI as the preferred hyperacute investigation for patients presenting with acute focal neurological deficits.

Pathophysiological investigations of intracerebral hemorrhage with MRI

The existence and nature of the penumbra in ICH is arguably the most pressing outstanding information required by clinicians to make rational management decisions in ICH patients. The recognition that hematoma volume is not static in a significant proportion of patients has revolutionized the approach to ICH management [48]. In addition to the promising treatment effects of hemostatic therapy, there is increasing evidence that clot expansion is correlated with acute systolic blood pressure [49,50]. Furthermore, there is some limited evidence from retrospective studies that higher systolic blood pressure is associated with poor clinical outcome [51,52]. The hypothesis that blood pressure reduction may attenuate hematoma expansion is therefore an intriguing possibility. It has also been postulated, however, that compression of the microvasculature surrounding the hematoma may result in decreased regional cerebral blood flow [53]. Therefore, many clinicians remain concerned that acute blood pressure reduction may aggravate, or even precipitate, cerebral ischemia within the perihematomal region and/or more globally. These two theories therefore lend themselves to opposing blood pressure management strategies and the clinical dilemma will only be resolved with randomized controlled trials, which are currently underway [54,55]. Of course, proponents of the ischemic hypothesis consider such a trial potentially dangerous. A number of MRI investigations of regional cerebral blood flow and

ischemia in ICH have been performed, which support the safety of such a trial.

Blood flow changes in ICH: perfusion-weighted imaging

The most commonly used MRI perfusion imaging technique is the dynamic susceptibility contrast method. This perfusion-weighted MRI (PWI) sequence allows the visualization of areas of decreased cerebral blood flow via bolus tracking of intravascular gadolinium contrast media as it transits through the cerebral circulation. Plotting the change in MRI ($T2^*$) signal intensity over time, the tissue response curve, allows an estimate of regional cerebral blood flow. More accurate measures can be obtained by generating an impulse response curve, using the technique of deconvolution [56,57]. The impulse response curve can be used to estimate regional cerebral blood flow, proportional to the peak amplitude and regional cerebral blood volume, which is proportional to the area under the curve. Commonly, other measures of flow are used, including the time to peak of the impulse response curve (Tmax) and mean transit time, calculated as a ratio of regional cerebral blood volume to regional cerebral blood flow.

Perfusion-weighted MRI sequences have been utilized in an effort to assess blood flow in ICH. A total of 59 acute ICH patients in three separate studies have been studied with PWI (Table 10.2). The first study of six patients with acute ICH demonstrated no evidence of focally decreased blood flow in the perihematomal region [58]. More consistently, these authors observed a relative hypoperfusion of the cerebral hemisphere ipsilateral to the hematoma. The two largest PWI studies in ICH reported mild hypoperfusion in the perihematomal region and/or more diffusely throughout the ipsilateral hemisphere in approximately half (29/53) of the patients studied (Fig. 10.4) [6,59]. The severity of these changes appears to be inversely correlated to the time of imaging [59]. We have also observed that both perihematomal and diffuse hemispheric perfusion changes occur only in larger hematomas, generally larger than 15 ml. Furthermore, repeat imaging demonstrated that hypoperfusion is transient, resolving completely within 3–5 days [6]. Finally, this study also included an analysis of relative cerebral blood flow and cerebral blood volume in the perihematomal region. Although relative cerebral blood flow was decreased moderately, commensurate with a prolongation of

Table 10.2. MRI investigations of blood flow/perihematomal edema etiology in ICH

Investigator/ Study	Number of patients	Location of ICH	Time of study/ studies from symptom onset	Primary findings
Carhuapoma et al. [70] (DWI)	9	Basal ganglia (5) Thalamus (1) Lobar (3)	1–9 days	Increased perihematomal ADC in 8/9 patients' voxels with decreased ADC in 1 patient (80 ml hematoma)
Kidwell et al. [58] (PWI and DWI)	12 (DWI) 6 (PWI)	Putamen (5) Thalamus (4) Lobar (3)	<5 h	Perihematomal Tmax delay (hypoperfusion) in 2/6 patients. Rim of peri hematoma decreased ADC values in 3 patients with large hematoma volumes and mass effect
Schellinger et al. [59] (PWI and DWI)	32	Subcortical (27) Lobar (5)	1.3–5.75 h	Perihematomal (4/32) and diffuse ipsilateral hemispheric (14/32) MTT delay (hypoperfusion) MTT was inversely correlated with time to imaging. Perihematomal ADC was decreased (7/32), increased or normal (25/32) and unrelated to perfusion or outcome
Butcher et al. [6] (PWI and DWI)	21 acute 12 subacute	Putamen (14) Thalamus (3) Caudate (1) Lobar (2)	Scan 1: 4.5–110 h (50% < 21 h) Scan 2: 3–5 days (median 4.5 d)	Transient perihematomal (11/21) and diffuse ipsilateral hemispheric (9/21) MTT delay (hypoperfusion) in patients with larger hematoma volumes, all of which resolved by scan 2. Elevated ADC values positively correlated with perihematomal edema volumes acutely and subacutely

Notes: DWI, diffusion-weighted imaging; PWI, perfusion-weighted imaging; ADC, apparent diffusion coefficient; Tmax, time to peak of the impulse residue; MTT, mean transit time.

MTT, no changes in relative cerebral blood volume were observed (Fig. 10.4). This is inconsistent with the traditional hypothesis that perihematomal oligemia results from compression of the local microvasculature by the hematoma mass effect. Furthermore, maintenance of relative cerebral blood volume is incompatible with cerebral ischemia.

The inability to demonstrate significant hypoperfusion in patients with small hematomas may be a limitation of studying blood flow with MRI. The paramagnetic effects of deoxyhemoglobin extend beyond the hematoma itself, making determination of blood flow immediately adjacent to the clot impossible (Fig. 10.1) [6]. It is therefore possible that smaller hematomas are associated with a more restricted zone of perihematomal hypoperfusion, below the resolution of PWI. Nonetheless, nuclear medicine, xenon CT and perfusion CT studies have all been consistent with the results of MRI studies [60–68]. All of these studies indicate that hypoperfusion occurs in the region surrounding the hematoma acutely in some, but not all, patients. Hypoperfusion is seen most commonly in the hyperacute stages and in association with larger clot volumes. All investigations reveal a pattern of spontaneous resolution of the blood flow deficits subacutely.

Edema etiology: diffusion-weighted imaging

Magnetic resonance imaging also provides another tool useful in identification of ischemic tissue. Diffusion-weighted imaging is based on the principle of detection of spontaneous water molecule movement within the brain. This is accomplished using diffusion gradients, which successively de-phase and then re-phase protons [69]. In tissue where water is freely diffusing, the MRI signal will be attenuated due to the movement of protons in the intervening period between the de-phasing and re-phasing of protons.

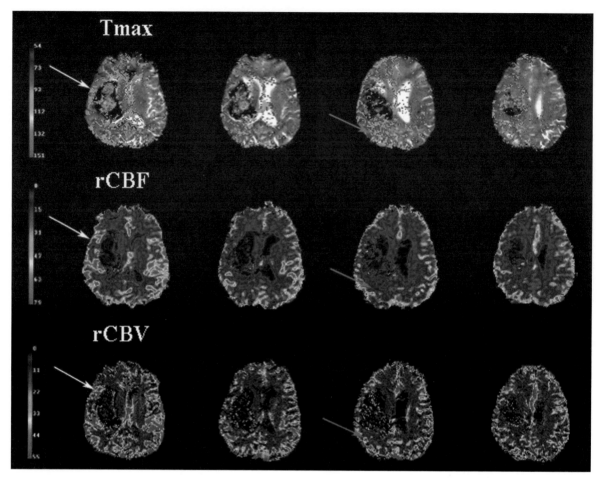

Fig. 10.4 Example of perihematomal blood flow changes in a patient with a putaminal ICH (6 hour after onset). Blood appears black due to the paramagnetic effects of deoxyhemoglobin. Time to peak of the impulse response curve (Tmax) is delayed > 2 seconds (colored voxels) in regions of decreased blood flow (units are 1/10 second). This patient had perihematomal (white arrows) and diffuse ipsilateral hemispheric Tmax delay (gray arrows). Relative cerebral blood volume (rCBV; arbitrary units) in the perihematomal region and ipsilateral hemisphere is maintained however, which is inconsistent with ischemia. See plate section for color version.

In contrast, areas of restricted diffusion will have a relatively enhanced signal, as there has been little or no change in spatial position during the application of the diffusion gradients, resulting in a greater number of these protons being in phase. Areas of diffusion restriction are thought to represent cytotoxic edema, which occurs as ATPase-dependent sodium-potassium exchange pumps fail, resulting in an influx of sodium and water into both neurons and glia. This results in a sequestration of water within cells and a constriction of the extracellular space, both of which restrict the diffusion of water. The degree of bio energetic compromise can be quantified by the apparent diffusion coefficient (ADC), which is most decreased in regions where ATP levels are lowest and

diffusion restriction is greatest. The ADC values are calculated on a voxel-wise basis using the Stejskal-Tanner equation, which is essentially an inverse natural log regression of the ratio of signal intensities observed at varying diffusion gradient strengths.

Four DWI studies in a total of 71 acute ICH patients have been reported (Table 10.2) [6,58,59,70]. Perihematomal diffusion restriction was reported in 11 patients from two studies [58,59]. The degree and volume of the diffusion restriction regions were moderate in all cases. Most patients have been observed to have elevated ADC values in the perihematomal region and this has been interpreted as evidence that edema is plasma derived or vasogenic [70]. In a serial study of diffusion changes in ICH, we

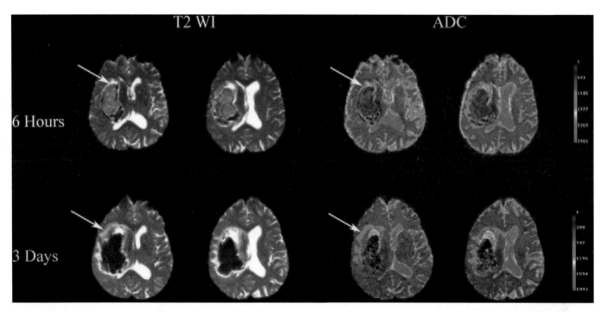

Fig. 10.5 Echoplanar T2-weighted MRI (T2WI; left) demonstrating a large acute putaminal hematoma imaged 6 hours after onset and perihematomal edema (arrows; same patient as Fig. 10.4), which expands over 72 hours. Blood appears hypointense (black) due to the paramagnetic effects of the deoxyhemoglobin, and edema is bright on the acute T2-weighted images. The visibly contracted hematoma contains methemoglobin at 3 days, making it more hypointense. Diffusion-weighted images also demonstrate the hypointense hematoma, as well as perihematomal high signal intensity. This is not diffusion restriction, but an effect known as "shine through" resulting from the heavily T2-weighted edema. The apparent diffusion coefficient (ADC; right) maps indicate elevated rates of water movement in the perihematomal region (arrows; units are 10–6 mm²/s), which are strongly correlated to edema volume both acutely and subacutely. This is consistent with edema of plasma origin and not ischemia. See plate section for color version.

found that ADC values were consistently elevated in the perihematomal region [6]. Furthermore, the ADC was directly correlated to the volume of edema, independent of hematoma size, at both the acute and subacute time points. In essence, higher rates of water movement in the perihematomal region were associated with larger edema volumes. This was highly consistent with edema of plasma origin and not ischemia (Fig. 10.5) [6].

In the three studies of concurrent DWI and PWI in acute ICH, none have reported ischemic signatures, i.e. a reduction of ADC, in association with perfusion changes. In one study, a limited number of voxels with ADC decreases were observed in a single patient, but this was not associated with any focal change in cerebral blood flow in the same region [58]. This suggests that any perihematomal diffusion restriction changes resulted from failure of energy metabolism that is not related to ischemia. Similarly, prolongation of contrast transit time, consistent with relative hypoperfusion, is not associated with any reduction in ADC (Fig. 10.4) [6,59].

Therefore, although hypoperfusion occurs in the same region as perihematomal edema, the two do not appear to be causally related. Edema appears to be plasma derived, rather than cytotoxic. There is little evidence for cellular ischemia in most patients, the possible exceptions occurring in those with extremely large hematomas.

Summary and conclusions

Magnetic resonance imaging has been definitively demonstrated to be as sensitive as CT for the detection of acute ICH. In addition, it is much more sensitive for detection of previous bleeding events. Magnetic resonance imaging may also allow the diagnosis of underlying etiologies in secondary ICH. Given the proven benefits of MRI in assessment of ischemic stroke, this should be considered the initial imaging investigation of choice in centers where it is readily available. In addition, MRI is a valuable tool for investigating the pathophysiology of acute and chronic ICH.

References

1. Atlas SW. *Magnetic Resonance Imaging of the Brain and Spine*. Philadelphia, Lippincott Williams & Wilkins, 2002.

2. Hashemi RH, Bradley WG, Lisanti CJ. *MRI: The Basics*. Philadelphia, Lippincott Williams & Wilkins, 2004.

3. Hayman L, Taber K, Ford J, Bryan R. Mechanisms of MR signal alteration by acute intracerebral blood: old concepts and new theories. *AJNR Am J Neuroradiol* 1991; **12**: 899–907.

4. Zamani AA. Imaging of intracranial hemorrhage. In: Rumbaugh CL, Wang A, Tsai FY, eds. *Cerebrovascular Disease Imaging and Interventional Treatment Options.* New York, Igaku-Shoin. 1995; 232–247.

5. Linfante I, Llinas RH, Caplan LR, Warach S. MRI features of intracerebral hemorrhage within 2 hours from symptom onset. *Stroke* 1999; **30**: 2263–2267.

6. Butcher KS, Baird T, MacGregor L, *et al.* Perihematomal edema in primary intracerebral hemorrhage is plasma derived. *Stroke* 2004; **35**: 1879–1885.

7. Broderick JP. Volume of intracerebral hemorrhage: a powerful and easy-to-use predictor of 30-day mortality. *Stroke* 1993; **24**: 987–993.

8. Patel MR, Edelman RR, Warach S. Detection of hyperacute primary intraparenchymal hemorrhage by magnetic resonance imaging. *Stroke* 1996; **27**: 2321–2324.

9. Lin DD, Filippi CG, Steever AB, Zimmerman RD. Detection of intracranial hemorrhage: comparison between gradient-echo images and b(0) images obtained from diffusion-weighted echo-planar sequences. *AJNR Am J Neuroradiol* 2001; **22**: 1275–1281.

10. Hardy PA, Kucharczyk W, Henkelman RM. Cause of signal loss in MR images of old hemorrhagic lesions. *Radiology* 1990; **174**: 549–555.

11. Barber PA, Darby DG, Desmond PM, *et al.* Identification of major ischemic change. Diffusion-weighted imaging versus computed tomography. *Stroke.* 1999; **30**: 2059–2065.

12. Weingarten K, Zimmerman RD, Cahill PT, Deck MD. Detection of acute intracerebral hemorrhage on MR imaging: ineffectiveness of prolonged interecho interval pulse sequences. *AJNR Am J Neuroradiol* 1991; **12**: 475–479.

13. Kidwell CS, Chalela JA, Saver JL, *et al.* Comparison of MRI and CT for detection of acute intracerebral hemorrhage. *JAMA* 2004; **292**: 1823–1830.

14. Fiebach JB, Schellinger PD, Gass A, *et al.* Kompetenznetzwerk Schlaganfall B5. Stroke magnetic resonance imaging is accurate in hyperacute intracerebral hemorrhage: a multicenter study on the validity of stroke imaging. *Stroke* 2004; **35**: 502–506.

15. Butcher K, Laidlaw J. Current intracerebral haemorrhage management. *J Clin Neurosci* 2003; **10**: 158–167.

16. Zhu XL, Chan MS, Poon WS. Spontaneous intracranial hemorrhage: which patients need diagnostic cerebral angiography? A prospective study of 206 cases and review of the literature. *Stroke* 1997; **28**: 1406–1409.

17. Atlas SW, Grossman RI, Gomori JM, *et al.* Hemorrhagic intracranial malignant neoplasms: spin-echo MR imaging. *Radiology* 1987; **164**: 71–77.

18. Atlas SW, Sheppard L, Goldberg HI, *et al.* Intracranial aneurysms: detection and characterization with MR angiography with use of an advanced postprocessing technique in a blinded-reader study. *Radiology* 1997; **203**: 807–814.

19. Atlas SW. Intracranial vascular malformations and aneurysms. Current imaging applications. *Radiol Clin North Am* 1988; **26**: 821–837.

20. Adams WM, Laitt RD, Jackson A. The role of MR angiography in the pretreatment assessment of intracranial aneurysms: a comparative study. *AJNR Am J Neuroradiol* 2000; **21**: 1618–1628.

21. Gomori JM, Grossman RI, Goldberg HI, *et al.* Occult cerebral vascular malformations: high-field MR imaging. *Radiology* 1986; **158**: 707–713.

22. Rigamonti D, Hadley MN, Drayer BP, *et al.* Cerebral cavernous malformations. Incidence and familial occurrence. *N Engl J Med* 1988; **319**: 343–347.

23. Singer M, Atlas S, Drayer B. Subarachnoid space disease: diagnosis with fluid-attenuated inversion-recovery MR imaging and comparison with gadolinium-enhanced spin-echo MR imaging–blinded reader study. *Radiology* 1998; **208**: 417–422.

24. Zimmerman RA. Recent advances in MR imaging: FLAIR imaging. *Crit Rev Neurosurg* 1998; **8**: 188–192.

25. Noguchi K, Ogawa T, Seto H, *et al.* Subacute and chronic subarachnoid hemorrhage: diagnosis with fluid-attenuated inversion-recovery MR imaging. *Radiology* 1997; **203**: 257–262.

26. Bakshi R, Ariyaratana S, Benedict RH, Jacobs L. Fluid-attenuated inversion recovery magnetic resonance imaging detects cortical and juxtacortical multiple sclerosis lesions. *Arch Neurol* 2001; **58**: 742–748.

27. Ohta T, Kuroiwa T. Timing of CT scanning after SAH. *J Neurosurg* 1985; **63**: 817.

28. van Gijn J, van Dongen KJ. The time course of aneurysmal haemorrhage on computed tomograms. *Neuroradiology* 1982; **23**: 153–156.

29. Imaizumi T, Chiba M, Honma T, Niwa J. Detection of hemosiderin deposition by T2*-weighted MRI after subarachnoid hemorrhage. *Stroke* 2003; **34**: 1693–1698.

30. Greenberg S, Finklestein S, Schaefer P. Petechial hemorrhages accompanying lobar hemorrhage:

detection by gradient-echo MRI. *Neurology* 1996; **46**: 1751–1754.

31. Fazekas F, Kleinert R, Roob G, *et al.* Histopathologic analysis of foci of signal loss on gradient-echo T2*-weighted MR images in patients with spontaneous intracerebral hemorrhage: evidence of microangiopathy-related microbleeds. *AJNR Am J Neuroradiol* 1999; **20**: 637–642.

32. Roob G, Lechner A, Schmidt R, *et al.* Frequency and location of microbleeds in patients with primary intracerebral hemorrhage. *Stroke* 2000; **31**: 2665–2669.

33. Roob G, Kleinert R, Seifert T, *et al.* [Indications of cerebral micro-hemorrhage in MRI. Comparative histological findings and possible clinical significance]. *Nervenarzt* 1999; **70**: 1082–1087.

34. Jeerakathil T, Wolf PA, Beiser A, *et al.* Cerebral microbleeds: prevalence and associations with cardiovascular risk factors in the Framingham Study. *Stroke* 2004; **35**: 1831–1835.

35. Roob G, Schmidt R, Kapeller P, *et al.* MRI evidence of past cerebral microbleeds in a healthy elderly population. *Neurology* 1999; **52**: 991–994.

36. Fan YH, Zhang L, Lam WW, Mok VC, Wong KS. Cerebral microbleeds as a risk factor for subsequent intracerebral hemorrhages among patients with acute ischemic stroke. *Stroke* 2003; **34**: 2459–2462.

37. Fan YH, Mok VC, Lam WW, Hui AC, Wong KS. Cerebral microbleeds and white matter changes in patients hospitalized with lacunar infarcts. *J Neurol* 2004; **251**: 537–541.

38. Greenberg SM, Eng JA, Ning M, Smith EE, Rosand J. Hemorrhage burden predicts recurrent intracerebral hemorrhage after lobar hemorrhage. *Stroke* 2004; **35**: 1415–1420.

39. Nighoghossian N, Hermier M, Adeleine P, *et al.* Old microbleeds are a potential risk factor for cerebral bleeding after ischemic stroke: a gradient-echo T2*-weighted brain MRI study. *Stroke* 2002; **33**: 735–742.

40. Tanaka A, Ueno Y, Nakayama Y, Takano K, Takebayashi S. Small chronic hemorrhages and ischemic lesions in association with spontaneous intracerebral hematomas. *Stroke* 1999; **30**: 1637–1642.

41. Kato H, Izumiyama M, Izumiyama K, Takahashi A, Itoyama Y. Silent cerebral microbleeds on T2*-weighted MRI: correlation with stroke subtype, stroke recurrence, and leukoaraiosis. *Stroke* 2002; **33**: 1536–1540.

42. Kinoshita T, Okudera T, Tamura H, Ogawa T, Hatazawa J. Assessment of lacunar hemorrhage associated with hypertensive stroke by echo-planar gradient-echo T2*-weighted MRI. *Stroke* 2000; **31**: 1646–1650.

43. O'Donnell HC, Rosand J, Knudsen KA, *et al.* Apolipoprotein E genotype and the risk of recurrent lobar intracerebral hemorrhage. *N Engl J Med* 2000; **342**: 240–245.

44. Greenberg SM, O'Donnell HC, Schaefer PW, Kraft E. MRI detection of new hemorrhages: potential marker of progression in cerebral amyloid angiopathy. *Neurology* 1999; **53**: 1135–1138.

45. Chalela JA, Kang DW, Warach S. Multiple cerebral microbleeds: MRI marker of a diffuse hemorrhage-prone state. *J Neuroimaging* 2004; **14**: 54–57.

46. Kidwell CS, Saver JL, Villablanca JP, *et al.* Magnetic resonance imaging detection of microbleeds before thrombolysis: an emerging application. *Stroke* 2002; **33**: 95–98.

47. Kakuda W, Thijs VN, Lansberg MG, *et al.* Clinical importance of microbleeds in patients receiving IV thrombolysis. *Neurology* 2005; **65**: 1175–1178.

48. Brott T, Broderick J, Kothari R, *et al.* Early hemorrhage growth in patients with intracerebral hemorrhage. *Stroke* 1997; **28**: 1–5.

49. Kazui S, Minematsu K, Yamamoto H, Sawada T, Yamaguchi T. Predisposing factors to enlargement of spontaneous intracerebral hematoma. *Stroke* 1997; **28**: 2370–2375.

50. Takizawa K, Suzuki A, Nagate K, *et al. Blood Pressure Control in Acute Stages of Hypertensive Intracerebral Hemorrhage to Prevent Growth of Hematoma.* Tokyo, NEURON publishing, 2002.

51. Willmot M, Leonardi-Bee J, Bath PM. High blood pressure in acute stroke and subsequent outcome: a systematic review. *Hypertension* 2004; **43**: 18–24.

52. Fogelholm R, Avikainen S, Murros K. Prognostic value and determinants of first-day mean arterial pressure in spontaneous supratentorial intracerebral hemorrhage. *Stroke* 1997; **28**: 1396–1400.

53. Mendelow AD. Mechanisms of ischemic brain damage with intracerebral hemorrhage. *Stroke* 1993; **24**: I115–117.

54. Anderson CS, Huang Y, Wang JG, *et al.* INTERACT Investigators Intensive blood pressure reduction in acute cerebral haemorrhage trial (INTERACT): a randomised pilot trial. *Lancet Neurol* 2008; **7**(5): 391–399.

55. Qureshi AI, Mohammad YM, Yahia AM, *et al.* A prospective multicenter study to evaluate the feasibility and safety of aggressive antihypertensive treatment in patients with acute intracerebral hemorrhage. *J Intensive Care Med* 2005; **20**: 34–42.

56. Ostergaard L, Weisskoff RM, Chesler DA, Gyldensted C, Rosen BR. High resolution measurement of cerebral blood flow using intravascular tracer bolus passages.

Part I: Mathematical approach and statistical analysis. *Magn Reson Med* 1996; **36**: 715–725.

57. Ostergaard L, Sorensen AG, Kwong KK, *et al.* High resolution measurement of cerebral blood flow using intravascular tracer bolus passages. Part II: Experimental comparison and preliminary results. *Magn Reson Med* 1996; **36**: 726–736.

58. Kidwell CS, Saver JL, Mattiello J, *et al.* Diffusion-perfusion MR evaluation of perihematomal injury in hyperacute intracerebral hemorrhage. *Neurology* 2001; **57**: 1611–1617.

59. Schellinger PD, Fiebach JB, Hoffmann K, *et al.* Stroke MRI in intracerebral hemorrhage: is there a perihemorrhagic penumbra? *Stroke* 2003; **34**: 1674–1679.

60. Gebel JM, Brott TG, Sila CA, *et al.* Decreased perihematomal edema in thrombolysis-related intracerebral hemorrhage compared with spontaneous intracerebral hemorrhage. *Stroke* 2000; **31**: 596–600.

61. Rosand J, Eskey C, Chang Y, *et al.* Dynamic single-section CT demonstrates reduced cerebral blood flow in acute intracerebral hemorrhage. *Cerebrovasc Dis* 2002; **14**: 214–220.

62. Sills C, Villar-Cordova C, Pasteur W, *et al.* Demonstration of hypoperfusion surrounding intracerebral hematoma in humans. *J Stroke Cerebrovasc Dis* 1996; **6**: 17–24.

63. Mayer SA, Lignelli A, Fink ME, *et al.* Perilesional blood flow and edema formation in acute intracerebral hemorrhage: a SPECT study. *Stroke* 1998; **29**: 1791–1798.

64. Siddique MS, Fernandes HM, Arene NU, *et al.* Changes in cerebral blood flow as measured by HMPAO SPECT in patients following spontaneous intracerebral haemorrhage. *Acta Neurochir Suppl* 2000; **76**: 517–520.

65. Uemura K, Shishido F, Higano S, *et al.* Positron emission tomography in patients with a primary intracerebral hematoma. *Acta Radiol Suppl* 1986; **369**: 426–428.

66. Videen TO, Dunford-Shore JE, Diringer MN, Powers WJ. Correction for partial volume effects in regional blood flow measurements adjacent to hematomas in humans with intracerebral hemorrhage: implementation and validation. *J Comput Assisted Tomogr* 1999; **23**: 248–256.

67. Zazulia AR, Diringer MN, Videen TO, *et al.* Hypoperfusion without ischemia surrounding acute intracerebral hemorrhage. *J Cereb Blood Flow Metab* 2001; **21**: 804–810.

68. Powers WJ, Zazulia AR, Videen TO, *et al.* Autoregulation of cerebral blood flow surrounding acute (6 to 22 hours) intracerebral hemorrhage. *Neurology* 2001; **57**: 18–24.

69. Baird AE, Warach S. Magnetic resonance imaging of acute stroke. *J Cereb Blood Flow Metab* 1998; **18**: 583–609.

70. Carhuapoma JR, Wang PY, Beauchamp NJ, *et al.* Diffusion-weighted MRI and proton MR spectroscopic imaging in the study of secondary neuronal injury after intracerebral hemorrhage. *Stroke* 2000; **31**: 726–732.

Cerebral angiography

Rush H. Chewning and Kieran P. Murphy

Introduction

Patients presenting with acute onset of focal neurological deficits must be evaluated for intracerebral hemorrhage (ICH). First-line imaging in these cases is non-contrast CT of the head. In cases where ICH is detected and no underlying cause is seen on initial CT, further evaluation is necessary to determine the source of the bleed. Advances in CT angiography (CTA) and magnetic resonance angiography (MRA) have enabled these modalities to be employed in the secondary evaluation of patients presenting with ICH. These non-invasive imaging modalities offer several clinical advantages over cerebral digital subtraction angiography (DSA), principally cost savings ($400 for a CTA vs. $8000 for a four-vessel cerebral angiogram) and more rapid availability. Computerized tomography angiography has evolved beyond MRA now with the advent of whole head volumetric imaging and 320 slice CTA. However, due to its superior sensitivity and specificity, DSA remains the gold standard in the detection and evaluation of intracranial vascular abnormalities and has a greater temporal and spatial resolution than CT (0.325 mm isotropic voxels), and far greater than MRA (1 mm range voxel size) [1,2].

There is a trend towards CT being chosen as the primary modality for diagnosis but there have as yet been no prospective larger randomized series showing even equivalence let alone superiority. There is often an institutional practice pattern towards a patient workup for subarachnoid hemorrhage (SAH). In Baltimore at Johns Hopkins University we always go with CT (Fig.11.1), followed by lumbar puncture if negative, followed by DSA catheter cerebral angiography if positive. In the same city, at University of Maryland equally intelligent committed and scientific physicians have replaced DSA cerebral angiography with CTA.

Role of cerebral angiography

In patients with non aneurysmal intraparenchymal hemorrhage (IPH) or intraventricular hemorrhage (IVH), the vascular anomalies that can cause these are usually easily seen on CT, post-contrast CT, CTA, or MRI. Where there is doubt or an atypical appearance or combination of SAH and IVH, or IPH, a catheter angiogram is sometimes performed to identify a possible vascular structural abnormality responsible for the hemorrhage. Vascular abnormalities presenting as hemorrhage are at great risk for rebleeding, which typically leads to severe neurological dysfunction or death [3]. It is therefore of great concern to rapidly diagnose an underlying vascular structural abnormality so that urgent treatment may be initiated to minimize the risks of recurrent bleed. Common vascular abnormalities causing ICH include aneurysm, arteriovenous malformation (AVM), cavernous malformation, and dural arteriovenous fistula. More rare causes include vasculitis, moyamoya disease, and rare hypertensive- or drug-related vasculopathy hemorrhage. If intracranial clot thrombolysis is to be performed these possible causes must be absolutely excluded.

The traditional literature statement is that in 85% of cases of non-traumatic SAH, ruptured aneurysm is the underlying cause [4]. Digital subtraction angiography is the most definitive method of identifying the aneurysmal source (Figs. 11.2a,b). Three-dimensional rotational angiography (3DRA) is capable of providing exquisite characterization of the aneurysm, and is even more sensitive than planar DSA and has increased

Intracerebral Hemorrhage, ed. J. R. Carhuapoma, S. A. Mayer, and D. F. Hanley. Published by Cambridge University Press. © J. R. Carhuapoma, S. A. Mayer, and D. F. Hanley 2010.

the sensitivity of DSA beyond 85%. The big advantage of this technique is in detection of aneurysms that project posteriorly off the A 1 segment of the anterior cerebral artery [5]. In spite of this, angiograms will be

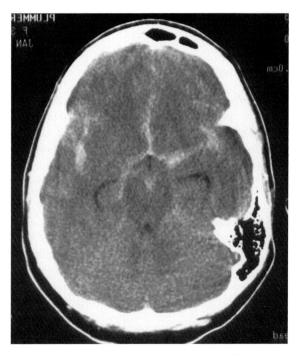

Fig. 11.1 Head CT without contrast demonstrates diffuse subarachnoid bleed as high attenuation material in the subarachnoid space.

negative in 10–20% of cases of SAH [4]. Some of these patients do, in fact, have aneurysms that are missed by initial DSA. Vasospasm, thrombosis of the aneurysm, compression by adjacent hematoma, or poor angiographic technique may account for these false negatives [4]. Repeat DSA should be performed in 7–10 days but if there is any suspicion of a false negative then repeat study in 2–5 days is indicated.

Non-aneurysmal perimesencephalic hemorrhage (PMH), a benign condition with a characteristic cisternal pattern of blood being visible on CT, is responsible for approximately 10% of cases of SAH. Some have argued that recognition of this pattern is sufficient for diagnosis of PMH and that DSA is not necessary [6,7]. However, others have noted that ruptured posterior fossa aneurysms may present with PMH pattern on CT in up to 10% of cases [8]. Therefore, DSA should be considered even when suspicion of aneurysm based on CT is low. Aneurysms can sometimes defy text books, and dogma. Posterior communicating artery, basilar tip, and superior cerebellar artery aneurysms can give pure PMH. The threshold for catheter angiography should be low.

The remaining 5% of cases of SAH are caused by a variety of conditions, including AVM, dural arteriovenous fistula, septic aneurysm, cocaine abuse, and arterial dissection [4]. In some communities, drug use will be the most common cause of IVH and IPH. Digital subtraction angiography plays an important

(a) (b)

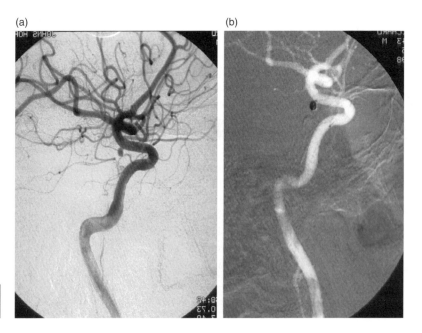

Fig. 11.2 (a and b) This lateral internal carotid artery cerebral angiogram shows a patient after endovascular coiling of a posterior communicating artery aneurysm with no flow in the aneurysm.

role in the diagnosis of these conditions. However, most cases of AVM will be seen on initial CT or CTA. In these cases, the role of DSA is one of pre-procedural analysis and characterization of the malformation and its nidus, including identifying specific feeding vessels and patterns of venous drainage [9].

Patients presenting with a CT pattern of hemorrhage in the putamen, thalamus, or posterior fossa, with no visible abnormality on initial scan most likely have primary hypertensive ICH. Older age (greater than 45) and a history of hypertension increase this likelihood [10]. However, DSA is still indicated in these cases, as 9–18% of these patients will have an underlying AVM or aneurysm detected by angiography [10].

When children present with spontaneous ICH, developmental malformations, such as AVM, and vein of Galen aneurysmal malformation or dilatation (VGAM or VGAD, respectively) are typically the cause. Evaluation with DSA should be conducted when CTA or MRA fail to uncover a vascular abnormality. Digital subtraction angiography in children has been demonstrated to be safe when conducted by an experienced interventional neuroradiologist [11].

Risks of cerebral angiography

While DSA offers advantages over CTA and MRA, it does so at the expense of greater risk. It carries a 1.3–1.8% risk of neurological complication and a 0.2–0.3% risk of permanent deficit [12,13]. Patient factors, such as age and hypertension, long procedure times, and relative inexperience of the angiographer have all been demonstrated to increase rates of neurological complications [13]. In addition to neurological adverse outcomes, contrast reactions (including nephrotoxicity), femoral artery dissection, and hematoma can occur. Computerized tomography contrast accounts for 15% of in-hospital renal failure.

Current management of intracranial aneurysms

The International Subarachnoid Aneurysm Trial (ISAT) [14] and the International Study of Unruptured Intracranial Aneurysms (ISUIA) [15,16] are two landmark studies of intracranial aneurysm therapy. Neither is perfect but both are changing how we manage this disease. They cast doubt on well-developed medical practices and challenge the livelihood of leaders of medical communities all over the world. Naturally they were interpreted differently by the coiling (Fig. 11.3), clipping, and watchful waiting groups depending on how their "team" did. So where is the signal in the noise?

ISAT, The International Subarachnoid Aneurysm Trial

The ISAT was a multicenter randomized trial that compared the safety and efficacy of endovascular coil treatment versus surgical clipping for the treatment of ruptured brain aneurysms. To be eligible for enrollment in the ISAT, each patient had to be deemed

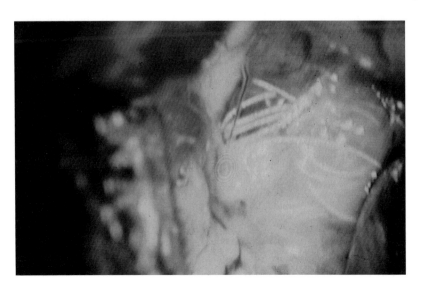

Fig. 11.3 Intra-operative image obtained of a stable coiled aneurysm while another uncoilable aneurysm was being clipped. See plate section for color version.

equally suitable for either coiling or clipping. The investigators used the term "clinical equipoise" to describe this balance. The treatment was on average performed on 1.7 days after aneurysm rupture. Two thousand one hundred and forty-three patients were randomized in 43 centers worldwide. One thousand and seventy nine patients underwent coiling, 1073 underwent clipping. The ISAT's primary goal was to determine which procedure had better patient outcomes as defined by Rankin scores, a functional scoring system. The study was ended early by the Medical Research Council (MRC), because the one-year post-treatment scores showed 31% of the surgical patients were disabled or died compared to 24% of coiled patients. There was a 22.3% overall improvement in the coiled patients. The response to ISAT in Europe was different to that in America. Our European colleagues accepted the results as recognition of technological progress (medical evolution?) and confirmation of established European medical practice. Approximately 60–70% of all ruptured cranial aneurysms are coiled in Europe.

In the USA, however, the study was attacked by neurosurgeons as being fundamentally flawed. Many arguments were put forth. It was said that American neurosurgeons were more skillful than the European counterparts, more experienced in dealing with ruptured aneurysms. We, at Johns Hopkins, were the only US site in the study, and though we randomized very few patients, we are very proud of our membership of this study. We entered because the relationship we had as a group of neurovascular specialists in interventional neuroradiology, neurosurgery, and neurology was strong enough to let us randomize. Such randomization fundamentally requires honesty about one's own technical weakness, and is not possible in combative politicized environments. Neither participation in, nor the results of this study represented a change in our daily practice. It has always been our standard practice to obtain informed consent by offering both options when they are available, or if not to explain the benefit of one over the other when equipoise does not exist. We have always documented these conversations in the permanent medical record.

ISUIA, The International Study of Unruptured Intracranial Aneurysms

There have been two ISUIA studies; the first reported in 1998 was very controversial and widely attacked.

It reported a 0.05% yearly rupture rate for intracranial aneurysms. The results were clearly affected by the inclusion of giant skull base aneurysms in elderly women, which have a very low rupture rate. The more recently reported ISUIA paper from July 2003 in the *Lancet* is a more significant work and represents a softening of the previous position of the authors. In this study, unruptured aneurysms were randomized to coiling versus clipping, or observation. Once again, amongst the aneurysm randomized in the treatment arm an endovascular approach had a 22% relative risk reduction over conventional surgery, reinforcing the results of the ISAT.

In the ISUIA study, patients with aneurysms of the anterior circulation (defined as middle cerebral artery [MCA] or anterior communicating artery) had better outcomes when they were clipped rather then coiled. Very few of these aneurysms were randomized in the ISAT study, a weakness in that study. This is consistent with our practice where in the past eight years we have very rarely treated MCA aneurysms. We have found it difficult to control coil position in these clipable aneurysms. In the hands of our five neurovascular surgeons clips can be placed to remodel an MCA allowing all branches to be kept open in a way that would be impossible by coiling. It must be said, however, that sometimes the clip is not in the right location (Fig. 11.4). The use of multiple neuroform stents is being popularized for these lesions but the published stroke rate exceeds the surgical complication rate so we do not do this in our practice.

Despite the many criticisms leveled at the ISUIA prospective data, it is a helpful study and must make us reflect on its implications. They conclude that patients with no history of SAH and an asymptomatic anterior circulation aneurysm less than 7 mm do not require treatment on a simple analysis of risk–benefit ratio alone. For other sizes or sites, ISUIA provides robust information for rupture risk analysis. If treatment is indicated on an individual risk–benefit analysis which treatment should be provided? The ISUIA study failed to resolve one of the fundamental clinical problems, which is the discrepancy between their reported extremely low rupture risk in asymptomatic aneurysms under 7 mm at 0.7% per year compared to the large proportion of ruptured aneurysms in this same category. In our practice, we see an average of 172–180 aneurysms a year, and, as in ISAT, 61% of aneurysms that ruptured are 5 mm or less. The ISUIA

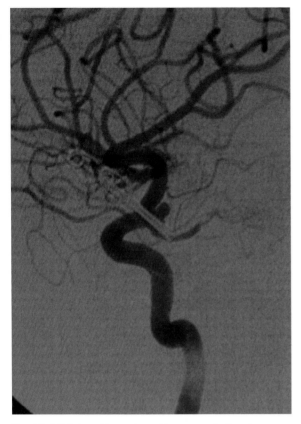

Fig. 11.4 This lateral internal carotid artery cerebral angiogram shows a patient status post-clipping of a posterior communicating artery aneurysm with residual flow in the aneurysm.

rupture risk is higher for larger aneurysms. How can this be reconciled with the ISUIA position that these lesions, the very ones we see most often, have the lowest rupture rate? The ISUIA investigators (led by neurologists who have focused on this area for many years) state posterior circulation aneurysms (which includes by definition aneurysms of the posterior communicating artery and the vertebral basilar system) have a higher rupture rate and appear to be more appropriate for coiling than for clipping. Patients with a prior history of SAH have a higher risk of bleeding from any intracranial aneurysm.

Overall, looking at the results of ISUIA and ISAT, when the anatomy is favorable an endovascular approach seems to be the treatment of choice in patients over 50 years of age and in those with posterior circulation aneurysms. For those patients aged under 50 with anterior circulation aneurysms, the situation is not so clear. However, in those patients,

treatment options and relative benefits and risks including post-craniotomy epilepsy must be discussed carefully with patient and relatives before elective treatment and conformed consent can be obtained.

On a daily basis, we struggle with the balance of rupture risk per year versus patient's life-expectancy. When the patient is greater than 70 years of age, we counsel the patient about risks/benefits. In our series, the risk of death from an endovascular approach in an unruptured aneurysm is well below 1%, but the risk of stroke is approximately 5%. The risk of death in an endovascular approach to a ruptured aneurysm is approximately 5%. The risk of stroke is also 5%, and any attempt at thrombolysis in this setting is usually fatal.

It is critical not to overlook anesthesia in this mix as their ability to harm your patient during the procedure far exceeds that of your fellow, but is harder to identify. The most common anesthesia error is to keep the patient's blood pressure too low (mistakenly applying open operating room traditions to endovascular procedures), thus resulting in watershed hypoperfusion stroke in these often elderly patients.

We believe that there are three types of intracranial aneurysms. Ones that should be coiled (posterior circulation), ones that should be clipped (middle cerebral and some if not most anterior communicating artery aneurysms), and a third group that can be treated in either way. This third group relates to the ISAT study data. It is clear that ISAT represents an evolutionary technological trend towards an endovascular or more minimal approach to aneurysms when they are amenable to coiling. A collaborative multidisciplinary team that has trust at its center is essential to a successful outcome for any patient.

The Center for Medicare and Medicaid Services (CMS) has prudently mandated there must be biannual national reporting of individual and site complication rates for carotid stenting. This approach mirrors the standard for coronary artery bypass graft and cardiac surgery. We must adopt the same approach for intracranial aneurysm therapy. Informed consent on the morning of a coiling or clipping cannot be based on the complication rates from peer-reviewed research performed in centers of excellence. For that patient it can only be obtained based on the experience in that center. This data should be available on the Web so the patient/consumer can make an informed decision and the truth be told. After the ISAT study was published many fine seasoned interventional neuroradiologists confronted aggressive actions to replace them with less trained neurosurgeons. This kind of political, tribal behavior has no place in medicine practiced in the pursuit of quality. The patient must be equally safe in all hands.

Current management of cerebral arteriovenous malformations (AVMs) and dural arteriovenous fistula (DAVF)

The incidence and prevalence of cerebral AVMs cannot be precisely established, because of the relative rarity of the disease and the existence of asymptomatic patients [17]. The best available estimate of AVM incidence is based on a single population-based study, and shows an overall detection rate of 1.11 per 100 000 person-years, and a rate of 0.94 per 100 000 person-years for symptomatic lesions [17,18]. These values are lower than the commonly quoted prevalence rates derived from autopsy series (0.14–0.5%), which probably represent overestimates due to selection bias [17]. The prevalence of detected AVMs is unknown, but it is lower than approximately 10 per 100 000 population [17]. Despite their congenital nature, cerebral AVMs can become symptomatic in any age category, with a mean presentation age of 31.2 years [19]. More than 50% of AVMs present with intracranial hemorrhage [19,20], which are predominantly intracerebral, but may also be of subarachnoid or intraventricular location. The overall annual risk of rupture ranges between 2% and 4% [21,22]. However, the risk of hemorrhage in patients who initially presented with a rupture is as high as 17% during the first year following the event, before decreasing to a baseline level after three years [23,24,25]. After a second hemorrhage, this risk further increases to 25% within the first year [23]. The overall rate of re-hemorrhage after a first event reaches up to 67% [10]. Besides prior rupture, risk factors for intracranial hemorrhage include deep nidus location, impairment of the AVM venous drainage, and the presence of intra/extranidal aneurysms. Contrary to a commonly held view, the rupture of an AVM is as devastating as that of an aneurysm: if the latter has a higher mortality rate, AVM rupture tends to result in more neurological disability due to the high occurrence of lobar cerebral hematoma [11]. Mortality rates of the first AVM-related hemorrhage range between 17.6% and 40.5%, and can be as high as 66.7% for posterior fossa

AVMs [20,26]. Other types of AVM presentation include general or focal seizures (40%), chronic headache (14%), and persistent or progressive neurological deficit (12%) [19].

The basic pathophysiological element of a cerebral AVM is an abnormal connection (or shunt) between a feeding artery and a draining vein. The capillary bed is congenitally absent in AVMs. As opposed to a cortical AVF, which is made of one or a few arteriovenous shunts, an AVM contains a large number of shunts, entangled in a central tumor-like component called the AVM nidus. The AVM nidus can have a complex angioarchitecture that combines various types of arteriovenous shunts. Superselective angiographic studies performed prior to embolization frequently document nidus features that are most often not detected by other imaging modalities, such as intranidal aneurysms or high-flow "fistula-like" connections hidden among more typical moderate-to-fast arteriovenous shunts.

A DAVF is a rarer entity than an AVM. These are the most interesting type of vascular malformation. They are a challenge to understand and treat, but when deciphered they can be cured. They represent a pathological response to clotting of a venous pathway secondary to a mysterious inciting event, usually some long forgotten episode of infection. After a period of hypervascularization shunts develop between arteries and veins of varying size. Issues arise when arterial pressure is deployed against the walls of thin walled cerebral veins for prolonged periods. The same sequence of events that occur with spinal vascular malformation occur in the brain. The effect of venous hypertension is to impair venous drainage of normal brain tissue. This results in stagnation and sometimes hemorrhage. The treatment is to reduce the venous pressure. This can be done by closing the shunt or increasing venous drainage.

Diagnostic imaging

Although DSA remains the most accurate technique for the diagnosis of cerebral vascular disorders, CT and MRI now play a significant part in the diagnosis and management of cerebral AVMs. Fast and widely available, CT is the first-line imaging technique for patients presenting with a suspicion of acute intracranial hemorrhage. Contrast-enhanced CT can confirm the presence of abnormal blood vessels around the hematoma. The role of CTA in the characterization

(a) (b)

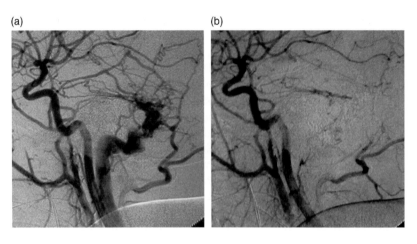

Fig. 11.5 (a and b) Lateral common carotid artery injection showing a complex dural arteriovenous fistula of the left transverse sinus. (a) Shows the lesion prior to embolization, (b) shows the lesion after glue embolization and near complete occlusion of the shunt.

(a) (b)

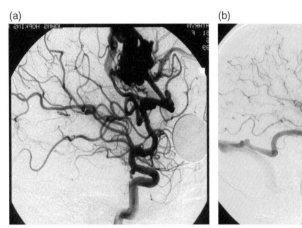

Fig. 11.6 (a and b) Patient with a large AVM and a concomitant small aneurysm that had bleed. (a) This could have been missed by a CTA through the phenomenon of satisfaction of search by the CTA reviewer and early venous overlap at the cavernous sinus from the AVM shunt. We coiled the aneurysm and glued the AVM at one setting (b).

of cerebral AVMs and AVFs remains undefined (Figs. 11.5 and 11.6). Non-ruptured AVMs may be apparent on non-enhanced CT, in particular when associated with large draining veins. Magnetic resonance imaging is a sensitive modality for the detection, localization, and sizing of the AVM nidus. It plays an important role in radiosurgery planning, where it is used in conjunction with catheter angiography [27], as well as for the follow-up of treated AVMs. Magnetic resonance angiography provides limited information on the nature of the feeding arteries and draining veins, the dynamic characteristics of the arteriovenous shunts, or the presence of associated vascular lesions such as extra- and intranidal aneurysms and AVFs [28]. The diffusion of modern non-invasive cerebral imaging has increased the detection rate and apparent prevalence of intracranial vascular malformations, including AVMs [2]. It is important to remember that compression of the nidus by a hematoma may lead to underestimation of the actual size of an AVM by any imaging technique, and may even sometimes completely prevent its detection. Such mass effect therefore represents a pitfall for both accurate diagnosis and treatment planning of AVM. Digital subtraction angiography remains the gold standard imaging technique for the evaluation of cerebral AVMs. Modern DSA carries extremely low risks of complications, and offers precise information about the nidus configuration, the number, size, location, and morphology of arterial feeders and draining veins. Digital subtraction angiography also documents associated vascular anomalies with significant management and prognostic implications, such as arterial and/or venous stenoses or occlusions, extranidal and intranidal aneurysms, or the presence of surrounding moyamoya-like vasculature that may simulate AVM nidus. Critical hemodynamic characteristics of the AVM are also better analyzed by DSA, including the presence of intranidal AVFs.

Dural arteriovenous fistulae can only be definitively identified and understood with catheter angiography. They are routinely missed on MRI and CT. Often the only suggestion of their presence on axial imaging is some asymmetry in venous flow voids. In the presence of asymmetric tinnitus that can be heard on examination on auscultation, we consider angiography essential.

The role of endovascular therapy

The modern management of AVMs and AVFs is based on three therapeutic modalities, microneurosurgery, endovascular embolization, and stereotactic radiosurgery [29–32]. Multimodality has been shown to improve overall patient outcomes in both the adult and pediatric populations, and has in particular opened the door to successful therapy of giant and deeply seated AVMs. Combined AVM therapy by embolization and surgery has even proved superior to surgery alone in cost-effectiveness analyses. When not primarily curative, embolization facilitates subsequent radiosurgery by reducing the volume of the nidus (in particular for AVMs larger than 10 ml), prepares the resection of surgically accessible AVMs, and immediately addresses the risks related to associated intra/extranidal aneurysms and AVFs. Embolization can also supplement radiosurgery for AVMs that have not responded to initial radiotherapy. It is essential for the interventional neuroradiologist to understand the role of alternative treatment options and balance the desire to achieve curative embolization in a careful risk and benefit analysis. Although many AVMs can, from a technical standpoint, be totally embolized, partial embolization followed by surgery or radiosurgery may be ultimately more satisfying in terms of functional outcome. Lesions safely curable by embolization alone principally consist of small AVMs with one or a few arterial feeder(s).

Intracranial aneurysms are frequently associated with AVMs. When they are found in typical aneurysmal locations (i.e., circle of Willis), they should be treated as independent lesions either endovascularly or surgically. In such cases, the presence of AVM feeders and draining veins renders surgical access more challenging. It is usually suggested to treat the aneurysm(s) before the AVM itself, although the large series of Meisel et al. [33] did not document rupture of untreated proximal aneurysms after partial AVM treatment. Arteriovenous malformation-related hemodynamic stress plays at least a partial role in the growth of aneurysms in typical proximal location, as may be inferred from the progressive shrinkage of these aneurysms sometimes observed after treatment of the AVM. Aneurysms located either on the arteries feeding the nidus or within the nidus itself are, on the other hand, directly dependent on the AVM-related increase of flow. Embolization is effective for the treatment of these intranidal aneurysms, which represent a likely site for AVM rupture, and should constitute a primary target of endovascular therapy.

Conclusion

Cerebral DSA is the gold standard in the detection and evaluation of intracranial vascular abnormalities when patients present with spontaneous ICH. Aneurysms and AVM are the most typical causes of ICH uncovered by DSA. The procedure is invasive and carries a small but real amount of risk. However, the potential for detecting a vascular abnormality with a high likelihood of rebleeding, causing significant neurological damage or death, makes DSA a necessity in the majority of cases where the source of the bleed is not apparent on initial CT.

References

1. Chappell ET, Moure FT, Good MC. Comparison of computed tomographic angiography with digital subtraction angiography in the diagnosis of cerebral aneurysms: a meta-analysis. *Neurosurgery* 2003; **52**: 624–631.

2. Hill MD, Demchuk AM, Frayne R. Noninvasive imaging is improving but digital subtraction angiography remains the gold standard. *Neurology* 2007; **68**: 2057–2058.

3. Kassell NF, Torner JC, Haley EC, *et al.* The international cooperative study on the timing of aneurysm surgery. Part 1: overall management results. *J Neurosurg* 1990; **73**: 18–36.

4. van Gijn J, Rinkel GJ. Subarachnoid hemorrhage: diagnosis, causes and management. *Brain* 2001; **124**: 249–278.

5. Ishihara H, Kato S, Akimura T, *et al.* Angiogram-negative subarachnoid hemorrhage in the era of three dimensional rotational angiography. *J Clin Neurosci* 2007; **14**: 252–255.

6. Rinkel GJ, Wijdicks EF, Vermeulen M, *et al.* Nonaneurysmal perimesencephalic subarachnoid hemorrhage: CT and MR patterns that differ from

aneurysmal rupture. *AJNR Am J Neuroradiol* 1991; **12**: 829–834.

7. Velthuis BK, Rinkel GJ, Ramos L, *et al*. Perimesencephalic hemorrhage: exclusion of vertebrobasilar aneurysms with CT angiography. *Stroke* 1999; **30**: 1103–1109.

8. Kallmes DF, Clark HP, Dix JE, *et al*. Ruptured vertebrobasilar aneurysms: frequency of the nonaneurysmal perimesencephalic pattern of hemorrhage on CT scans. *Radiology* 1996; **201**: 657–660.

9. Friedlander, RM. Arteriovenous malformations of the brain. *N Engl J Med* 2007; **356**: 2704–2712.

10. Zhu XL, Chan MSY, Poon WS. Spontaneous intracranial hemorrhage: which patients need diagnostic cerebral angiography? *Stroke* 1997; **28**: 1406–1409.

11. Burger IM, Murphy KJ, Jordan LC, *et al*. Safety of cerebral digital subtraction angiography in children: complication rate analysis in 241 consecutive diagnostic angiograms. *Stroke* 2006; **37**: 2535–2539.

12. Cloft HJ, Joseph GJ, Dion JE. Risk of cerebral angiography in patients with subarachnoid hemorrhage, cerebral aneurysm, and arteriovenous malformation: a meta-analysis. *Stroke* 1999; **30**: 317–320.

13. Willinsky RA, Taylor S, TerBrugge K, *et al*. Neurological complications of cerebral angiography: prospective analysis of 2,899 procedures and review of the literature. *Radiology* 2003; **227**: 522–528.

14. Molyneux A, Kerr R, Stratton I, *et al*. International Subarachnoid Aneurysm Trial (ISAT) Collaborative Group. International Subarachnoid Aneurysm Trial (ISAT) of neurosurgical clipping versus endovascular coiling in 2143 patients with ruptured intracranial aneurysms: a randomised trial. *Lancet* 2002; **360** (9342): 1267–1274.

15. Wiebers DO, Whisnant JP, Huston J 3rd, *et al*. International Study of Unruptured Intracranial Aneurysms Investigators. Unruptured intracranial aneurysms: natural history, clinical outcome, and risks of surgical and endovascular treatment. *Lancet* 2003; **362**(9378): 103–110.

16. Wiebers DO Piepgras DG, Thielen K, *et al*. Unruptured intracranial aneurysms–risk of rupture and risks of surgical intervention. International Study of Unruptured Intracranial Aneurysms Investigators. *N Engl J Med* 1998; **339M**(24): 1725–1733. Erratum in: *N Engl J Med* 1999; **340**(9): 744.

17. Berman MF, Sciacca RR, Pile-Spellman J, *et al*. The epidemiology of brain arteriovenous malformations. *Neurosurgery* 2000; **47**: 389–396; discussion 397.

18. Brown RD Jr, Wiebers DO, Torner JC, O'Fallon WM. Incidence and prevalence of intracranial vascular malformations in Olmsted County, Minnesota, 1965 to 1992. *Neurology* 1996; **46**: 949–952.

19. Hofmeister C, Stapf C, Hartmann A, *et al*. Demographic, morphological, and clinical characteristics of 1289 patients with brain arteriovenous malformation. *Stroke* 2000; **31**: 1307–1310.

20. Brown RD Jr, Wiebers DO, Torner JC, O'Fallon WM. Frequency of intracranial hemorrhage as a presenting symptom and subtype analysis: a population-based study of intracranial vascular malformations in Olmsted Country, Minnesota. *J Neurosurg* 1996; **85**: 29–32.

21. Kondziolka D, McLaughlin MR, Kestle JR. Simple risk predictions for arteriovenous malformation hemorrhage. *Neurosurgery* 1995; **37**: 851–855.

22. Ondra SL, Troupp H, George ED, Schwab K. The natural history of symptomatic arteriovenous malformations of the brain: a 24-year follow-up assessment. *J Neurosurg* 1990; **73**: 387–391.

23. Forster DM, Steiner L, Hakanson S. Arteriovenous malformations of the brain. A long-term clinical study. *J Neurosurg* 1972; **37**: 562–570.

24. Mast H, Young WL, Koennecke HC, *et al*. Risk of spontaneous hemorrhage after diagnosis of cerebral arteriovenous malformation. *Lancet* 1997; **350**: 1065–1068.

25. Graf CJ, Perret GE, Torner JC. Bleeding from cerebral arteriovenous malformations as part of their natural history. *J Neurosurg* 1983; **58**: 331–337.

26. Fults D, Kelly DL Jr. Natural history of arteriovenous malformations of the brain: a clinical study. *Neurosurgery* 1984; **15**: 658–662.

27. Yu C, Petrovich Z, Apuzzo ML, Zelman V, Giannotta SL. Study of magnetic resonance imaging-based arteriovenous malformation delineation without conventional angiography. *Neurosurgery* 2004; **54**: 1104–1110; discussion 1108–1110.

28. Brown RD Jr, Flemming KD, Meyer FB, *et al*. Natural history, evaluation, and management of intracranial vascular malformations. *Mayo Clin Proc* 2005; **80**: 269–281.

29. Jordan JE, Marks MP, Lane B, Steinberg GK. Cost-effectiveness of endovascular therapy in the surgical management of cerebral arteriovenous malformations. *AJNR Am J Neuroradiol* 1996; **17**: 247–254.

30. Soderman M, Rodesch G, Karlsson B, Lax I, Lasjaunias P. Gamma knife outcome models as a reference standard in the embolisation of cerebral arteriovenous malformations. *Acta Neurochir (Wien)* 2001; **143**: 801–810.

147

31. Marks MP, Lane B, Steinberg GK, *et al.* Endovascular treatment of cerebral arteriovenous malformations following radiosurgery. *AJNR Am J Neuroradiol* 1993; **14**: 297–303; discussion 304–305.

32. Martin NA, Khanna R, Doberstein C, Bentson J. Therapeutic embolization of arteriovenous malformations: the case for and against. *Clin Neurosurg* 2000; **46**: 295–318.

33. Meisel HJ, Mansmann U, Alvarez H, *et al.* Cerebral arteriovenous malformations and associated aneurysms: analysis of 305 cases from a series of 662 patients. *Neurosurgery* 2000; **46**(4): 793–800.

Laboratory and other ancillary testing in intracerebral hemorrhage: an algorithmic approach

Michael Chen and Louis R. Caplan

An accurate etiological diagnosis of spontaneous intracerebral hemorrhage (ICH) needs to be determined expeditiously because of the multiple potential causes and corresponding treatments. Possible etiologies range from systemic illnesses such as hypertension, bleeding disorders, and malignancies to specific vascular abnormalities including amyloid angiopathy, vascular malformations, and vasculitides, to exogenous factors such as drugs of abuse and head trauma. Despite the many etiologies, there is some consistency in the relative frequency of these causal factors in patients with ICH, as published in case series (Fig. 12.1).

Important pieces of information to obtain from the medical history that dictate further diagnostic testing include: the presence of an associated headache, a history of hypertension, a history of trauma (physical or psychological), recent cognitive decline, use of anticoagulants or thrombolytics, illicit drugs, heavy alcohol use, and hematological disorders. Particular detail should be elicited about any activities at or before the onset of neurological symptoms. We have seen several patients with ICH associated with new onset hypertension, occurring during a time of increased stress. On examination, findings to look for include the blood pressure, level of consciousness, neurological deficits, evidence of bleeding, signs of drug abuse or head trauma, and a funduscopic examination.

The subsequent diagnostic steps use the information garnered from the history, physical, and neurological examinations with the findings on CT of the head. Computerized tomography clearly differentiates between hemorrhage and ischemic stroke. It also gives valuable information on location. The location, shape, and size of the ICH provide further guidance as to the etiology of the bleed, but the mass of

hemorrhage may obscure clues as to the ICH origin. Any associated intraventricular, subarachnoid, or subdural blood are important details that need to be noted. Hemoglobin appears bright on non-contrast CT but in rare instances of severe anemia may appear isodense. Single hematomas tend to be spontaneous whereas the presence of multiple ICHs without a history of trauma is often due to bleeding diathesis, amyloidosis, venous thrombosis, or hemorrhagic metastases. The presence of perilesional edema within a few hours after the bleed also suggests a secondary cause rather than a spontaneous, primary cause.

In addition to a detailed review of the CT scan, certain initial investigations should be ordered on any patient with ICH, which include: a complete blood count, serum electrolytes, renal function tests, a coagulation profile, an electrocardiogram, and a chest radiograph.

The overriding concern on initial evaluation of a patient with spontaneous ICH is not the underlying etiology but the potential for herniation or mass-related neurological deterioration. Operative intervention may be necessary, particularly with cerebellar hemorrhages, to relieve life-threatening mass effect. Airway protection, normalization of coagulation parameters, and blood pressure control are among the basic management steps that should precede further diagnostic and ancillary testing.

Hematoma volume estimation

An estimate of the hematoma volume on CT or MRI is very useful in not only predicting the clinical course, but also in guiding management decisions. The most reproducible and practical method is known as the (ABC)/2 method described by Kwak [1] (see also

Intracerebral Hemorrhage, ed. J. R. Carhuapoma, S. A. Mayer, and D. F. Hanley. Published by Cambridge University Press.

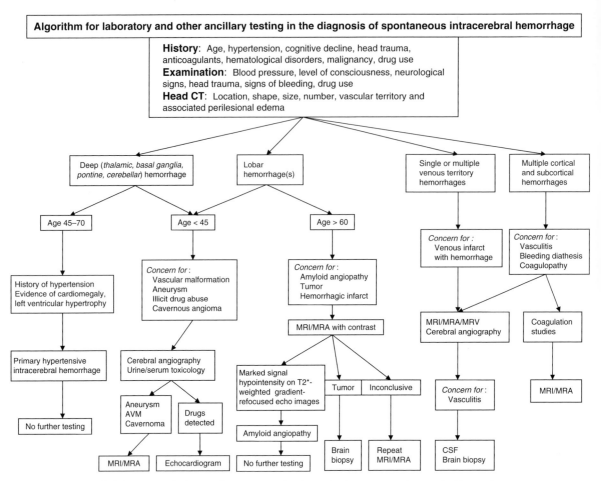

Fig. 12.1 Algorithm for laboratory and other ancillary testing in the diagnosis of spontaneous intracerebral hemorrhage. AVM, arteriovenous malformation; CSF, cerebrospinal fluid.

Chapter 5). This formula assumes an elliptical shape to the hematoma. Because hematoma volume is one of the two most significant predictors of mortality (along with admission level of consciousness), an accurate determination is important not only prognostically, but also in directing how the future evaluation should proceed. Broderick found a Glasgow Coma Scale (GCS) score of 8 or less with ICH hematoma volume $> 60\,cm^3$ predicted a 91% mortality rate at 30 days [2]. Other factors associated with a poor outcome include: intraventricular blood, hematoma expansion, infratentorial vs. supratentorial hemorrhage, presence of midline shift or herniation, and older age [2]. Therapeutic nihilism and acute withdrawal of care, however, was shown by Becker in a retrospective analysis to be the biggest predictor of mortality [3]. He reported a small portion of patients with a hematoma volume $> 60\,cm^3$ and GCS score

< 8 who had treatment maintained and were eventually discharged to rehabilitation.

Limited diagnostic evaluation

Hypertensive hemorrhage

The most common cause of non-traumatic spontaneous ICH is hypertension. The frequency of hypertension underlying spontaneous ICH has been estimated to be between 72% and 81% [4]. Patients aged 45–70 comprise this group and often have hypertension documented in their medical history and a medication list with several antihypertensive medications. There may be evidence of retinal hemorrhages on fundoscopy, cardiomegaly on chest radiograph, or evidence of left ventricular hypertrophy on electrocardiogram.

The characteristic findings on head CT consist of ICH located in the deep portions of the brain such as the basal ganglia, internal capsule, thalamus, pons, or cerebellum. Putaminal hemorrhages, the most common of these, usually originate in the posterior angle of the lentiform nucleus and spread concentrically in an anterior-posterior fashion. The lateral branches of the striate arteries are usually implicated. Thalamic hemorrhages may involve the anterior, lateral, medial, or posterior portions of the thalamus. Medially expanding hematomas may rupture into the third ventricle. The posterior limb of the internal capsule is often involved with lateral thalamic hemorrhages. Pontine hemorrhages are often devastating, and involve the junction between the basis pontis and tegmentum of the mid-pons. Cerebellar hematomas are usually in the region of the dentate nucleus, and usually require emergent surgery when large.

If there is definitive hypertension by history, on initial blood pressure recordings, or by ancillary testing, combined with patient age between 45–70, and a hemorrhage in the deep portions of the cerebral hemisphere, no further diagnostic evaluation is necessary.

Bleeding diathesis

Patients on long-term anticoagulation with warfarin can usually be easily identified on initial history or bloodwork revealing a prolonged prothrombin time. Patients taking warfarin account for approximately 9–11% of all ICH cases [5,6]. It is considered the second most frequent cause of ICH with cerebellar or lobar location [7]. Coagulopathy-related hematomas tend to be larger and more commonly lobar. There is less edema and there are often multiple hemorrhagic lesions [8]. The intensity of anticoagulant treatment, as expected, also raises the risk of ICH. Hylek and Singer reported data from an anticoagulant therapy unit and showed the risk of ICH to double with each 0.5 point increase in the prothrombin time ratio above the recommended limit of 2.0 [9]. Severe and confluent leukoaraiosis was associated with a higher risk of ICH in patients treated with warfarin in the Stroke Prevention in Reversible Ischemia Trial [10]. Characteristic findings on CT scan include blood-fluid levels, which result from "sedimentation" of red blood cells in a hematoma that does not clot because of the anticoagulant effect. Patients who develop ICH while on heparin anticoagulation may have had a preceding cerebral infarction. Other risk factors include excessive prolongation of partial thromboplastin time, large infarct size, and uncontrolled hypertension (> 180/110 mmHg) [11]. Despite the seemingly obvious etiology for hemorrhage on patients taking antithrombotics, an MRI and MRA of the brain are usually performed to exclude structural lesions.

Cerebral ischemia with hemorrhagic transformation

Hemorrhagic transformation of an ischemic infarction is a relatively common occurrence, particularly with cardioembolic strokes and in those treated with thrombolytics. The MR appearance of hemorrhagic transformation of an ischemic infarct is similar to that seen with primary ICH but usually is in the core of the infarct. In patients treated with thrombolytics, hemorrhages tend to occur within the first 24 hours after treatment. In one study, 40% of hemorrhages started during infusion and another 25% occurred within 24 hours [12]. In the National Institute of Neurological Diseases and Stroke rt-PA Stroke Study, the intracranial hemorrhages in the recombinant tissue plasminogen activator (rt-PA) group occurred in both the lobar white matter and the deep gray nuclei and were associated with a high mortality [13].

Extensive diagnostic evaluation

Although pontine, thalamic, basal ganglia, and cerebellar bleeds represent up to 90% of spontaneous ICH and are usually hypertension related, further careful evaluation should proceed when the hemorrhage pattern is not strictly in these locations. These patients are usually young or elderly. Lobar hemorrhages may be spontaneous and hypertensive, but often are secondary to the presence of vascular malformations, tumors, or venous thrombosis. Magnetic resonance imaging effectively and non-invasively detects for these secondary causes and is quite useful in dating previous ICHs and in detecting very small vascular lesions such as cavernous malformations. During the period of the acute bleed, the characteristics of the underlying cause may be obscured by the hematoma. In many patients, it is best to let some time pass and to repeat brain imaging, which usually better differentiates the cause.

Findings on head CT that should prompt consideration of subsequent cerebral angiography include the presence of subarachnoid or intraventricular blood, an abnormal calcification or prominent draining vein, or blood that extends to the perisylvian or interhemispheric fissure. The procedural risk is small, but significant given the often critical condition of patients with ICH. Timing of angiography is important and should be based on the patient's clinical condition. Zhu et al. [14] looked at the clinical variables of age, location of hemorrhage, and history of hypertension, and the correlation with finding an underlying vascular abnormality on cerebral angiography. They showed that age and presence of pre-existing hypertension were both independent negative predictors of angiographic yield. Furthermore, in a hypertensive patient with putaminal, thalamic, and/or posterior fossa hemorrhage, angiographic yield was 0%. Angiographic yield was significantly higher in patients 45 years old or younger who did not have a pre-existing history of hypertension. Lobar hemorrhage had at least a 10% yield in hypertensive older patients and up to 64% yield in younger normotensive patients. Putaminal, thalamic, and posterior fossa ICH grouped together had a yield of 48% in normotensive patients with age less than 45, 7% in normotensive patients older than 45, and 0% in all patients with pre-existing hypertension. They concluded that cerebral angiography has a low yield in identifying an underlying vascular abnormality in patients > 45 years old who have a history of hypertension and a thalamic, putaminal, or posterior fossa ICH. Repeat angiography in patients with subcortical ICH has a high yield and should be considered in younger patients without hypertension. The guidelines of the American Heart Association recommend angiography for all patients with no clear cause of hemorrhage who are candidates for surgery, particularly young patients without hypertension whose condition is stable [15].

Age becomes a useful factor in further focusing the etiological differential diagnosis. With younger patients, the concern is more for vascular abnormalities and drugs of abuse. With older patients, attention should be focused on evaluating for cerebral amyloid angiopathy, and intracranial tumors. There are then other important etiologies with less of an age association.

The younger patient with lobar hemorrhage
Vascular malformations

Spontaneous intracerebral and intraventricular hemorrhages in young people are mainly lobar in location and often result from a vascular malformation [16]. Ruiz-Sandoval et al. collected a series of 200 patients with ICH less than 40 years of age and found mainly lobar hemorrhages caused by vascular malformations. Hypertension remained the cause in most cases of ICH in the basal ganglia [16].

The first etiological possibility that should be thought of is ICH due to aneurysmal rupture. Clues include hematoma location near the Sylvian fissure or frontal parasagittal region and blood in the subarachnoid space. The putative mechanism is that the aneurysm ruptures directly into the brain parenchyma and gives the appearance of a spontaneous ICH. In fact, 28% of cerebral aneurysms may present with intraventricular blood and as many as 40% may present with intraparenchymal hemorrhage [17]. Middle cerebral aneurysms are often associated with temporal lobe hematomas. Vertebrobasilar aneurysms rarely present with ICH. Angiography when the patient is stable is the next logical step.

If there is no suspicion for an aneurysm, a stroke protocol MRI/MRA is often used as the next test to assess for ischemic injury and other vascular malformations. Magnetic resonance angiography has about a 90% sensitivity in detecting structural vascular lesions.

An arteriovenous malformation (AVM) is an abnormal connection between arteries and veins without an intervening capillary bed. In addition to headaches and focal neurological signs, seizures are often part of the medical history. Aneurysms are notoriously associated with AVMs and may be located either in the nidus or on a feeding vessel. Magnetic resonance imaging/MRA and/or CT may suggest the diagnosis, with flow voids in the former and enhancing serpentine structures in the latter. Arteriovenous malformations < 3 cm are associated with statistically larger hematoma volumes [17]. Cerebral angiography is usually necessary to adequately characterize the arterial feeders, venous drainage, and possible associated aneurysms. Seven percent of AVMs have an associated aneurysm, most of them located on the feeding artery [17]. The AVM can then be graded using the Spetzler-Martin system taking into account AVM size, eloquence of adjacent brain, and pattern of venous drainage [18].

Cavernous angiomas tend to have a lower bleeding potential than AVMs. Magnetic resonance imaging most sensitively defines cavernous malformations and has become the diagnostic imaging test of choice [19]. On T2-weighted sequences, cavernous angiomas characteristically appear as irregular lesions with a central core of mixed signal surrounded by a halo of hypodensity corresponding to hemosiderin deposits, which represent previous episodes of bleeding around the malformation. These lesions are generally single, well-demarcated with preference for cortical and subcortical regions of the hemisphere and the pons.

Illicit drug use

Illicit drug use is often suspected in a younger patient with an ICH or subarachnoid hemorrhage (SAH). Cocaine and methamphetamine are the drugs most often implicated in causing both SAH and ICH. Cocaine-related intracranial hemorrhage, especially crack cocaine inhalation, has been associated with a very high frequency of associated aneurysms and vascular malformations while the frequency of amphetamine-hemorrhage-related vascular abnormalities is low. However, several reports have noted the occurrence of ICH and SAH with amphetamine abuse but found no underlying vascular abnormality on detailed pathological examination of cerebral vessels [20]. The hemorrhages were explained by necrotizing angiitis related to amphetamine misuse associated with hypertension [21]. On the other hand, there have been two reports of ruptured AVMs after amphetamine misuse and a single case after ecstasy abuse [22,23]. McEvoy et al. [20] reported 13 patients over seven months who had ICH and a history of drug abuse. Of the ten stable enough for cerebral angiography, all but one had a vascular abnormality. However, it is difficult to link any neurological event with a use of a particular drug. The details of the drug use are not always easy to clarify. Multiple, often adulterated substances may be involved. The patient may not be very forthcoming with details of their drug use.

The mechanisms of amphetamine- and cocaine-related hemorrhages have been variously explained. The first is pharmacologically mediated changes in blood pressure and flow. Amphetamines and cocaine have pressor effects by preventing the reuptake of sympathomimetic neurotransmitters by nerve terminals. An acute sympathetic surge can cause progressive weakening of blood vessels, aneurysm formation, and eventual rupture. More than 90% of cocaine-induced ICH and/or SAH occur during or a few hours after its use [8]. The vascular wall may be further directly compromised by drug contents. Arterial injury can result from embolization of foreign material such as talc and microcrystalline cellulose, or from circulating immune complexes. Another mechanism of ICH from drug abuse, particularly with intravenous drug users, is via endocarditis. Those who inject drugs intravenously are especially likely to develop endocarditis [24]. Embolic material from bacterial vegetations in the heart can involve the cerebral arterial wall and lead to mycotic aneurysms that rupture. Mycotic aneurysms, however, only occur in about 1–3% of cases of endocarditis [25]. A final mechanism includes coagulopathies related to liver damage. Excessive alcohol use is well known to affect platelets and cause a prolongation in the prothrombin time.

The white blood cell count can detect an underlying infection that may suggest endocarditis. Urine screening of drugs of abuse is widely used in the diagnostic evaluation of these patients. Positive results can be confirmed by methods such as gas chromatography and mass spectroscopy. Urine testing only provides qualitative information on recent drug use. As urinary levels depend on time and clearance, they do not correlate with toxic symptoms. A careful search for endocarditis or other source of embolization is warranted, along with an erythrocyte sedimentation rate.

Cerebral angiography is useful if there is a suspicion for vascular malformations, which appear associated with chronic amphetamine or cocaine use, cerebral angiitis, or mycotic aneurysms. All patients with intracranial bleeding after cocaine use should have cerebral angiography because of the high frequency of associated vascular lesions. Hart et al. believe that because of the 1–3% incidence of mycotic aneurysms in patients with endocarditis and the fact that they tend to heal with antibiotics, that angiography is not indicated for evaluation of mycotic aneurysms alone [26]. Brust et al. feel angiography for detection of mycotic aneurysms is justified because surgical options are safe and can prevent the high mortality that comes with rupture of mycotic aneurysms that are treated with antibiotics alone [27]. As for cerebral angiitis, Citron et al. reported 14 cases of necrotizing angiitis related to poly-drug abuse [21]. On angiography, they described a pronounced irregularity and "beading" in the anterior circulation branches. However, these characteristics are non-specific, and may be seen in vasospasm, fibromuscular dysplasia, atherosclerosis, and cerebral emboli. Histological examination for vasculitis may be considered as a confirmatory study but the treatment of this complication is not entirely clear.

The older patient with lobar hemorrhage

Cerebral amyloid angiopathy

Spontaneous ICH due to cerebral amyloid angiopathy (CAA) usually occurs in patients greater than 60 years of age with a preceding history of progressive cognitive decline and head CT findings of single or multiple hemorrhages that extend to the cortical surface. The hemorrhages follow the distribution of the vascular amyloid, located mostly in the corticosubcortical or lobar regions with distinctly less involvement of the cerebellum and brainstem structures [28]. Despite extensive leptomeningeal vessel involvement, SAH from CAA is considered rare [29]. A characteristic finding on MRI which often strongly supports the diagnosis are small corticosubcortical lesions on gradient echo or T2*-weighted images that enhance signal dropout due to hemosiderin deposition [30]. This finding is often helpful in that the first hemorrhage may be indistinguishable from hypertensive ICH on head CT. The presence of multiple lobar chronic hemorrhages suggest a chronicity to the hemorrhages often seen in CAA. Knudsen et al. [31] recently validated the "Boston criteria for diagnosis of CAA-related hemorrhage" (Table 12.1) such that a clinical diagnosis of probable CAA can be reached during life through radiographic demonstration of at least two strictly lobar or corticosubcortical hemorrhagic lesions without other definite hemorrhagic process. APOE ε2 and ε4 have emerged as a strong predictor of risk for sporadic CAA-related ICH. Each of these alleles was overrepresented more than twofold among 182 reviewed pathological cases of CAA-related ICH [32]. A cohort in Greater Cincinnati/Northern Kentucky found the presence of APOE ε2 or ε4 to be associated with an adjusted odds ratio for lobar ICH of 2.3 [33]. Furthermore, these markers seem to increase the risk of a younger age at first hemorrhage and a shorter time until ICH recurrence [34].

Table 12.1. Boston criteria for diagnosis of cerebral amyloid angiopathy-related intracerebral hemorrhage

Definite CAA	Full postmortem examination of brain shows lobar ICH, severe CAA, and no other diagnostic lesion
Probable CAA with supporting pathological evidence	Clinical data and pathological tissue (evacuated hematoma or cortical biopsy specimen) showing some lobar CAA in pathological specimen, and no other diagnostic lesion
Probable CAA	Clinical data and MRI or CT demonstration of two or more hemorrhagic lesions restricted to lobar regions (cerebellar hemorrhage allowed), patient age > 55 years, and no other cause of hemorrhage
Possible CAA	Clinical data and MRI or CT demonstration of single lobar ICH, patient age > 55 years, and no other cause of hemorrhage

Source: [From 31].

When the patient is deemed stable to undergo MRI, gradient echo sequences can suggest the diagnosis. Magnetic resonance imaging also helps to exclude other potential cases of lobar ICH, such as an underlying vascular malformation or tumor. Typically no pathological tissue is available. Despite the association of the Apolipoprotein E genotype with CAA, neither the sensitivity nor specificity has yet been determined with enough accuracy for its routine clinical use. In the future, it may be useful for determining an individual's recurrence risk. Magnetic resonance imaging can then be repeated at 4–6 months to repeat the evaluation for an underlying structural lesion if the diagnosis is still in doubt.

Intracranial neoplasm

Well-recognized but uncommon, an underlying intracranial tumor may account for only about 2–10% of ICH cases in autopsy series and clinical-radiological series [35,36]. However, ICH has been reported to be the first clinical manifestation of a neoplasm in half of reported cases. On CT scan, multiple metastatic lesions make for a relatively easy diagnosis. However, cases of ICH into a single lesion may be more difficult to initially diagnose. Other radiographic findings suggestive of a neoplastic lesion are large areas of low-density edema surrounding the hematoma or an area of ring-shaped contrast enhancement at the periphery of the hematoma [37]. The signal of hematomas secondary to neoplasms is more inhomogeneous and complex than in primary spontaneous hematomas. This is because the hematoma occupies a portion of the tumor. A contrast MRI study may reveal an eccentric enhancing rim or nodular mass. The surrounding edema is characteristically finger-like, consisting of vasogenic edema. A delay in the expected signal evolution of a hematoma is the paramount finding on MRI that suggests tumor [38]. Other findings more suggestive of a brain tumor include ICH in the corpus callosum, a ring-like high-density area corresponding to blood around a low-density center, and/or a low-density indentation of the periphery of an ICH on CT.

Sometimes, the hemorrhage fills the entire tumor cavity, making identification of an underlying tumor impossible. Hence, follow-up MRI examination may unmask a tumor as the hematoma resolves. When the patient is stable, biopsy of the hematoma cavity should be the next step if the preceding investigations are inconclusive. Such an invasive investigation is warranted given the obvious marked differences in therapy and prognosis between a hematoma caused by a tumor or hypertension.

Lobar hemorrhage of any age
Cerebral venous thrombosis

Cerebral venous thrombosis (CVT) manifests with a wide spectrum of symptoms and signs. Headache is the most common symptom, and usually the earliest symptom. Hemorrhagic lesions caused by venous thrombosis are often called hemorrhagic venous infarcts by pathologists. They are typically large, subcortical, often multifocal hematomas with petechial hemorrhages within large hypodensities. Rarely, there may be subarachnoid or subdural hemorrhage associated. They may be unilateral or bilateral, single or multiple. The presence of a hematoma indicates markedly elevated venous pressure which is usually associated with diffuse cerebral swelling and T2-weighted

signal abnormalities in the subcortical white matter [8]. If the superior sagittal sinus is involved, the hematoma may be superficial in the hemispheres and paramedian. If the deep venous system is involved, the hematoma may be in the basal ganglia and thalami [39]. Computerized tomography scanning in CVT is of limited value and is mainly used to exclude other conditions such as arterial stroke, tumor, abscess, and SAH. Magnetic resonance imaging or cerebral angiography is usually required to make the diagnosis.

Cerebral angiography has been the key diagnostic procedure for many years but has now been superseded by MRI. However, for difficult cases, angiography can prove useful and requires visualization of the entire venous phase on at least two projections, with an oblique if possible. Cerebral venous thrombosis manifests as partial or complete lack of filling of veins or sinuses, typically involving the superior sagittal sinus, lateral sinus, or jugular veins. Delayed emptying and the presence of collateral pathways are other important associated angiographic findings. Cerebral angiography is the most sensitive study for cortical veins and cavernous sinus thrombosis.

Magnetic resonance angiography has superseded conventional angiography in the diagnosis of venous thrombosis primarily because of its sensitivity to blood flow, ability to visualize the thrombus itself, and non-invasive nature [7]. Two-dimensional time of flight is the most common sequence used with 1.5 and 3.0 mm-thick slices in the coronal and axial planes. As with conventional arteriography, the diagnostic finding is absent flow. Some difficulty remains in being able to confidently differentiate between thrombus, hypoplastic vessels, or benign anomalous venous anatomy [40].

Cerebrospinal fluid examination is still useful in the diagnosis in that there is often elevated protein content, red cells, and sometimes elevated white cells. Probably more importantly is to exclude a concurrent meningitis, particularly in septic CVT.

After CVT has been established, determining the underlying cause of the thrombosis needs to be pursued, which itself may be difficult because of the multiple causes.

Cerebral vasculitides

Cerebral vasculitides generally lead to arterial occlusion and cerebral infarction rather than ICH. This diagnosis is suggested in cases where there is evidence of multiple cerebral infarcts or hemorrhages in different vascular territories. There are multiple causes of intracranial vasculitis, both autoimmune and infectious. In rare cases, granulomatous angiitis of the nervous system (GANS) may lead to ICH. Clinically, there is an evolving headache, progressive cognitive decline, seizures, and recurrent cerebral infarcts. Because of the primary involvement of the central nervous system, systemic manifestations such as fever, malaise, weight loss, anemia, and elevated sedimentation rates are absent [41]. The diagnosis is strongly suggested with the finding of lymphocytic cerebrospinal fluid pleocytosis with elevated protein. Cerebral angiography may show a beading pattern in multiple medium-sized and small intracranial arteries caused by focal concentric narrowing in the distal vasculature. This appearance may mimic that of vasospasm in SAH.

References

1. Kwak R, Kadoya S, Suzuki T. Factors affecting the prognosis in thalamic hemorrhage. *Stroke* 1983; **14**: 493–500.

2. Broderick JP, Brott TG, Duldner JE, Tomsick T, Huster G. Volume of intracerebral hemorrhage. A powerful and easy-to-use predictor of 30-day mortality. *Stroke* 1993; **24**: 987–993.

3. Becker KJ, Baxter AB, Cohen WA, *et al.* Withdrawal of support in intracerebral hemorrhage may lead to self-fulfilling prophecies. *Neurology* 2001; **56**: 766–772.

4. Mohr JP, Caplan LR, Melski JW, *et al.* The Harvard Cooperative Stroke Registry: a prospective registry. *Neurology* 1978; **28**: 754–762.

5. Kase CS, Robinson RK, Stein RW, *et al.* Anticoagulant-related intracerebral hemorrhage. *Neurology* 1985; **35**: 943–948.

6. Boudouresques G, Hauw JJ, Meininger V, *et al.* Etude neuropathologique des hemorragies intracraniennes de l'adulte. *Rev Neurol (Paris)* 1979; **135**: 197–210.

7. Mohr JP, Choi DW, Grotta JC, Weir B, Wolf PA. *Stroke Pathophysiology, Diagnosis, and Management.* Philadelphia, Churchill Livingstone, 2004.

8. Aygun N, Masaryk TJ. Diagnostic imaging for intracerebral hemorrhage. *Neurosurg Clin N Am* 2002; **13**: 313–334.

9. Hylek EM, Singer DE. Risk factors for intracranial hemorrhage in outpatients taking warfarin. *Ann Intern Med* 1994; **120**: 897–902.

10. A randomized trial of anticoagulants versus aspirin after cerebral ischemia of presumed arterial origin. The Stroke Prevention In Reversible Ischemia Trial (SPIRIT) Study Group. *Neurol* 1997; **42**:857–865.

11. Immediate anticoagulation of embolic stroke: brain hemorrhage and management options. Cerebral Embolism Study Group. *Stroke* 1984; **15**: 779–789.

12. Gore JM, Sloan M, Price TR, *et al.* Intracerebral hemorrhage, cerebral infarction, and subdural hematoma after acute myocardial infarction and thrombolytic therapy in the Thrombolysis in Myocardial Infarction Study. Thrombolysis in Myocardial Infarction, Phase II, pilot and clinical trial. *Circulation* 1991; **83**: 448–459.

13. Tissue plasminogen activator for acute ischemic stroke. The National Institute of Neurological Disorders and Stroke rt-PA Stroke Study Group. *N Engl J Med* 1995; **333**: 1581–1587.

14. Zhu XL, Chan MSY, Poon WS. Spontaneous intracranial hemorrhage: which patients need diagnostic cerebral angiography? *Stroke* 1997; **28**: 1406–1409.

15. Broderick JP, Adams HP Jr, Barsan W, *et al.* Guidelines for the management of spontaneous intracerebral hemorrhage: a statement for healthcare professionals from a special writing group of the Stroke Council, American Heart Association. *Stroke* 1999; **30**: 905–915.

16. Ruiz-Sandoval JL, Cantu C, Barinagarrementeria F. Intracerebral hemorrhage in young people. Analysis of risk factors, location, causes and prognosis. *Stroke* 1999; **30**: 537–541.

17. Barnes B, Cawley CM, Barrow DL. Intracerebral hemorrhage secondary to vascular lesions. *Neurosurg Clin N Am* 2002; **13**: 289–297.

18. Spetzler RF, Martin NA. A proposed grading system for arteriovenous malformations. *J Neurosurg* 1986; **65**: 476–483.

19. Requena I, Arias M, Lopez-Ibor L, *et al.* Cavernomas of the central nervous system: clinical and neuroimaging manifestations in 47 patients. *J Neurol Neurosurg Psychiatry* 1991; **54**: 590–594.

20. McEvoy AW, Kitchen ND, Thomas DG. Intracerebral haemorrhage and drug abuse in young adults. *Br J Neurosurg* 2000; **14**: 449–454.

21. Citron BP, Halpern M, McCarron M, *et al.* Necrotizing angiitis associated with drug abuse. *N Engl J Med* 1970; **283**: 1003–1011.

22. Selmi F, Davies KG, Sharma RR, Neal JW. Intracerebral haemorrhage due to amphetamine abuse: report of two cases with underlying arteriovenous malformations. *Br J Neurosurg* 1995; **9**: 93–96.

23. Lukes SA. Intracerebral hemorrhage from an arteriovenous malformation after amphetamine injection. *Arch Neurol* 1983; **40**: 60–61.

24. Louria DB, Hensle T, Rose J. The major medical complications of heroin addiction. *Ann Intern Med* 1967; **67**: 1–22.

25. Davenport J, Hart RG. Prosthetic valve endocarditis. *Stroke* 1990; **21**: 993–999.

26. Hart RG, Kagan-Hallet K, Joerns SE. Mechanisms of intracranial hemorrhage in infective endocarditis. *Stroke* 1987; **18**: 1048–1056.

27. Brust JC, Dickinson PC, Hughes JE, Holtzman RN. The diagnosis and treatment of cerebral mycotic aneurysms *Ann Neurol* 1990; **27**: 238–246.

28. Itoh Y, Yamada M, Hayakawa M, Otomo E, Miyatake T. Cerebral amyloid angiopathy: a significant cause of cerebellar as well as lobar cerebral hemorrhage in the elderly. *J Neurol Sci* 1993; **116**: 135–141.

29. Yamada M, Itoh Y, Otomo E, Hayakawa M, Miyatake T. Subarachnoid haemorrhage in the elderly: a necropsy study of the association with cerebral amyloid angiopathy. *J Neurol Neurosurg Psychiatry* 1993; **56**: 543–547.

30. Greenberg SM, Finklestein SP, Schaefer PW. Petechial hemorrhages accompanying lobar hemorrhages: detection by gradient-echo MRI. *Neurology* 1996; **46**: 1751–1754.

31. Knudsen K, Rosand J, Karluk D, Greenberg S. Clinical diagnosis of cerebral amyloid angiopathy: validation of the Boston criteria. *Neurology* 2001; **56**: 537–539.

32. McCarron MO, Nicoll JAR. APOE genotype in relation to sporadic and Alzheimer-related CAA. In: Verbeek MM, de Waal MW, Vinters HV, eds. *Cerebral Amyloid Angiopathy in Alzheimer's Disease and Related Disorders*. Dordrecht, Kluwer Academic Publishers. 2000; 81–102.

33. Woo D, Sauerbeck LR, Kissela BM, *et al.* Genetic and environmental risk factors for intracerebral hemorrhage: Preliminary results of a population-based study. *Stroke* 2002; **33**: 1190–1195.

34. O'Donnell HC, Rosand J, Knudsen KA, *et al.* Apolipoprotein E genotype and the risk of recurrent lobar intracerebral hemorrhage. Melbourne Risk Factor Study Group. *N Engl J Med* 2000; **342**: 240–245.

35. Mutlu N, Berry RG, Alpers BJ. Massive cerebral hemorrhage: clinical and pathological correlations. *Arch Neurol* 1963; **8**: 641–661.

36. Little JR, Dial B, Bélanger G, Carpenter S. Brain hemorrhage from intracranial tumor. *Stroke* 1979; **10**: 283–288.

37. Gildersleeve N, Koo AH, McDonald CJ. Metastatic tumor presenting as intracerebral hemorrhage. *Radiology* 1977; **124**: 109–112.

38. Anzalone N, Scotti R, Riva R. Neuroradiologic differential diagnosis of cerebral intraparenchymal hemorrhage. *Neurol Sci* 2004; **24**: S3–5.

39. Ameri A, Bousser MG. Cerebral venous thombosis. *Neurol Clin* 1992; **10**: 87–111.

40. Mas JL, Meder JF, Meary E, Bousser MG. Magnetic resonance imaging in lateral sinus hypoplasia and thrombosis. *Stroke* 1990; **21**: 1350–1356.

41. Moore PM, Cupps TR. Neurological complications of vasculitis. *Ann Neurol* 1983; **14**: 155–167.

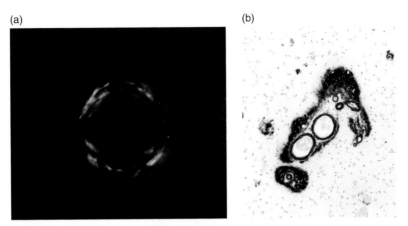

(a)

(b)

Fig. 4.1 Neuropathological appearance of CAA. Congo red stain (a) shows the characteristic green birefringence under polarized light of a vessel with complete replacement of its wall with amyloid. Another brain with advanced CAA (b) demonstrates extensive ß-amyloid immunostaining in vessels and the immediately surrounding brain parenchyma (sometimes referred to as dyshoric CAA) as well as senile plaques. (Images courtesy of Dr. Matthew P. Frosch, Massachusetts General Hospital and Harvard Medical School, Boston, MA.)

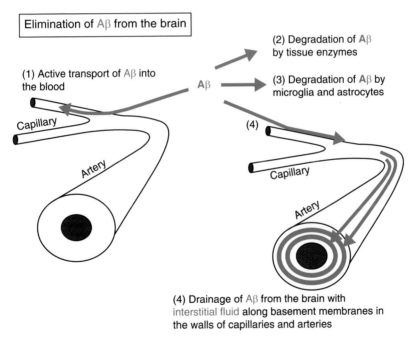

Fig. 4.2 Model for vascular deposition of ß-amyloid. The diagram demonstrates several recognized mechanisms for elimination of Aß from the brain: (1) active transport of Aß into the blood via proteins such as low density lipoprotein receptor-related protein-1 [194,195] and P-glycoprotein [196]; (2) degradation by enzymes in the brain parenchyma [197], (3) microglia [14], and astrocytes [198]; and (4) elimination along the perivascular pathways by which interstitial fluid drains from the brain [17,199]. As mechanisms (1), (2), and (3) fail with age, Aß appears to become increasingly entrapped from the interstitial fluid drainage pathways into the basement membranes of capillaries and small arteries (shown in green) [17,200]. (Figure courtesy of Drs. Roy O. Weller, Roxana Carare-Nnadi, Delphine Boche, and James A. R. Nicoll, University of Southampton School of Medicine, Southampton UK.)

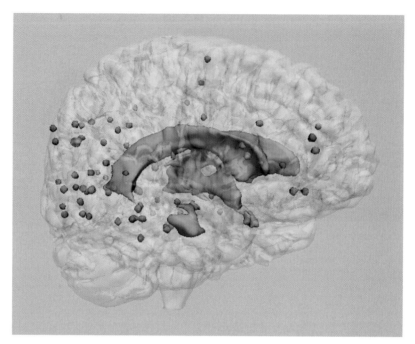

Fig. 4.4 Three-dimensional representation of the distribution of CAA-related hemorrhages. Each dot represents the center of a hemorrhage in a set of 20 patients with probable CAA mapped onto a composite three-dimensional template [135].

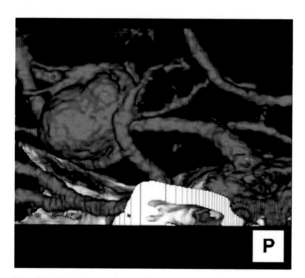

Fig. 9.3 This is bone subtracted 256 slice CTA of the brain in a patient with a large aneurysm. This technique allows dynamic CT to be performed over several cardiac cycles and thus nipples or rupture points can be seen pulsating allowing differentiation of ruptured from unruptured aneurysms. As the whole brain is covered the bone of the skull can be subtracted easily allowing visualization of the skull base region and in particular better visualization of posterior communicating artery aneurysms.

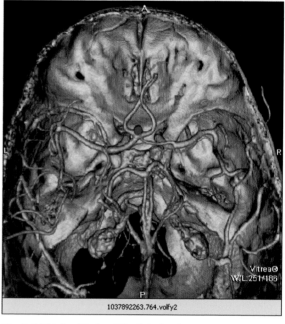

Fig. 9.4 This is a 32 slice CTA of the head reconstructed on a 3-D work station. The beautifully demonstrated anterior communicating artery aneurysm can be seen easily and has been color-coded (red).

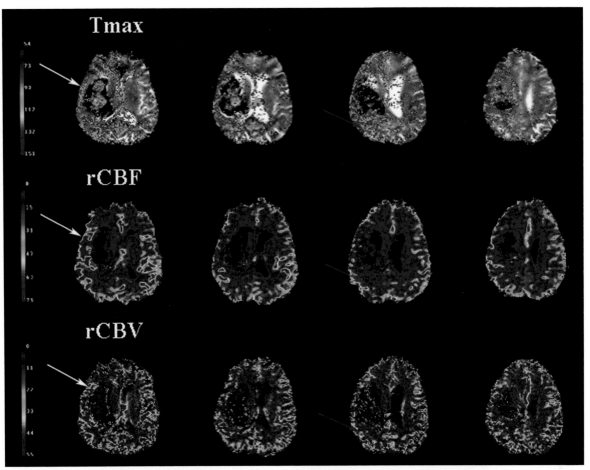

Fig. 10.4 Example of perihematomal blood flow changes in a patient with a putaminal ICH (6 hour after onset). Blood appears black due to the paramagnetic effects of deoxyhemoglobin. Time to peak of the impulse response curve (Tmax) is delayed > 2 seconds (colored voxels) in regions of decreased blood flow (units are 1/10 second). This patient had perihematomal (white arrows) and diffuse ipsilateral hemispheric Tmax delay (red arrows). Relative cerebral blood volume (rCBV; arbitrary units) in the perihematomal region and ipsilateral hemisphere is maintained however, which is inconsistent with ischemia.

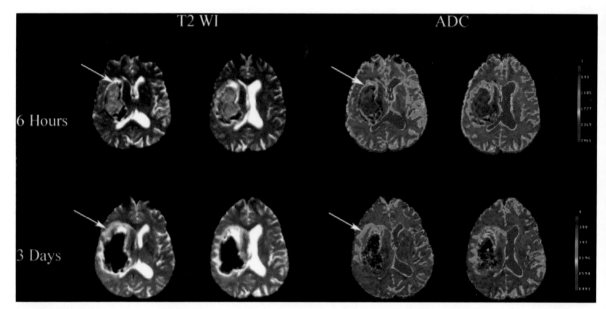

Fig. 10.5 Echoplanar T2-weighted MRI (T2WI; left) demonstrating a large acute putaminal hematoma imaged 6 hours after onset and perihematomal edema (arrows; same patient as Fig. 10.4), which expands over 72 hours. Blood appears hypointense (black) due to the paramagnetic effects of the deoxyhemoglobin, and edema is bright on the acute T2-weighted images. The visibly contracted hematoma contains methemoglobin at 3 days, making it more hypointense. Diffusion-weighted images also demonstrate the hypointense hematoma, as well as perihematomal high signal intensity. This is not diffusion restriction, but an effect known as "shine through" resulting from the heavily T2-weighted edema. The apparent diffusion coefficient (ADC; right) maps indicate elevated rates of water movement in the perihematomal region (arrows; units are $10-6\,mm^2/s$), which are strongly correlated to edema volume both acutely and subacutely. This is consistent with edema of plasma origin and not ischemia.

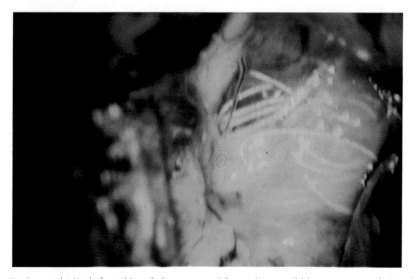

Fig. 11.3 Intra-operative image obtained of a stable coiled aneurysm while another uncoilable aneurysm was being clipped.

13

Medical management of intracerebral hemorrhage

Neeraj S. Naval, Paul A. Nyquist, and J. Ricardo Carhuapoma

Spontaneous intracerebral hemorrhage (ICH) causes 10–15% of first ever strokes and is associated with the highest mortality of all cerebrovascular events, with 30-day mortality after ICH approaching almost 50%. Of note, most survivors never regain functional independence, with only 20% achieving a meaningful level of functional recovery at six months [1,2]. This article discusses the basic principles of management of ICH, including initial stabilization, the prevention of hematoma growth, hemodynamic goal-setting, treatment of potential complications such as cerebral edema, herniation and seizures, and identification of the underlying etiology. Newer treatment options such as minimally invasive surgery (MIS) to reduce clot size are also briefly discussed.

Initial medical stabilization

As in other medical emergencies, initial resuscitative measures should be directed to establishing adequacy of airway, breathing, and circulation (ABCs).

Airway: indications for endotracheal intubation include the lack of adequate airway protection (Glasgow Coma Scale [GCS] Score < 8), herniation syndrome, uncontrolled seizures, and respiratory failure. Airway control might be suboptimal in patients even with GCS > 8 in the absence of a good cough/gag reflex who may be high aspiration risk especially with brainstem hemorrhages.

Breathing: hyperventilation might be necessary in the event of acute herniation, but, extrapolating from brain trauma literature, its prophylactic use is unlikely to be of benefit. Due to the risk of cerebral ischemia with prolonged hyperventilation, cautious slow return to goals of normocarbia ($PaCO_2$ 35–45) after reversal of herniation is recommended.

Circulation (intracranial): if an intracranial pressure (ICP) monitor is available, it seems reasonable to maintain a physiological cerebral perfusion pressure (> 70 mmHg), or in the absence of an ICP monitor, a systolic blood pressure of greater than 90 mmHg to maintain adequate cerebral blood flow [3]. Intracranial pressure monitoring is recommended in patients with GCS < 8. Since > 80% of patients with spontaneous ICH have underlying hypertensive disease in whom the autoregulatory cerebral perfusion pressure/cerebral blood flow (CPP/CBF) curve is shifted to the right (CBF is maintained at a CPP range that is higher than in normotensive patients), the CPP goal > 70 mmHg is more optimal to ensure adequate CBF compared to the CPP goal > 60 mmHg quoted in the Brain Trauma guidelines) (Fig. 13.1).

Control of blood pressure

Because hypertension is the most common cause of spontaneous ICH, its treatment in this setting is of considerable importance, but the therapeutic goals are controversial. The debate on blood pressure control has involved two key points. The first is the possibility that there is a perihematomal "penumbra" of brain tissue that is vulnerable to ischemia if blood pressure is reduced acutely, which results in increased injury in the zone surrounding the hemorrhage. Recent studies using positron emission tomography and MRI do not support the hypothesis of an ischemic perihematomal penumbra; thus, judicious blood pressure control seems to be safe [4].

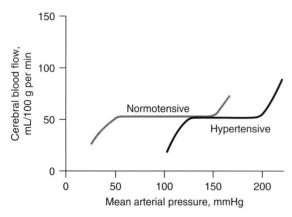

Fig. 13.1 Cerebral autoregulation in hypertension. From [39].

The second issue is the possibility that hematoma growth may be accelerated by hypertension in the setting of acute ICH. The occurrence of ICH is strongly related to premorbid blood pressure; however, the relationship between the growth of hematoma and uncontrolled blood pressure remains to be clarified. Recently, Jauch and colleagues [5] demonstrated that there was no definitive correlation between hemodynamic parameters, such as blood pressure, and hematoma growth.

The recently updated consensus guidelines [3] emphasize aggressive blood pressure control for a systolic blood pressure (SBP) > 200 mmHg or mean arterial blood pressure (MAP) > 150 mmHg [1]. For an SBP > 180 mmHg (or MAP > 130 mmHg), with a suspicion of elevated ICP, ICP monitoring is recommended; on the other hand if ICP elevation is not a concern based on the patient's neurological examination, a goal of SBP < 160 mmHg or MAP < 110 mmHg is recommended (see Tables 13.1 and 13.2).

The question of whether blood pressure control influences survival needs to be evaluated in prospective trials. A multicenter phase I clinical trial is underway to assess the feasibility and safety of antihypertensive treatment (with intravenous nicardipine) for patients who have acute hypertension in the setting of ICH.

Correction of coagulopathy

The presence of coagulopathy, in particular warfarin-related, has been noted to worsen the prognosis of ICH by increasing the rate and time window for hematoma expansion [6]. Mortality exceeds 50% in this patient population with outcomes linked to rate of increase in hematoma size. Early administration of fresh frozen plasma and vitamin K to reverse this

Table 13.1. Recommended guidelines for treating elevated blood pressure in spontaneous ICH

1. If SBP is >200 mmHg or MAP is >150 mmHg, then consider aggressive reduction of blood pressure with continuous intravenous infusion, with frequent blood pressure monitoring every 5 minutes.

2. If SBP is >180 mmHg or MAP is >130 mmHg and there is evidence of or suspicion of elevated ICP, then consider monitoring ICP and reducing blood pressure using intermittent or continuous intravenous medications to keep cerebral perfusion pressure > 60 to 80 mmHg.

3. If SBP is >180 mmHg or MAP is >130 mmHg and there is not evidence of or suspicion of elevated ICP, then consider a modest reduction of blood pressure (e.g., MAP of 110 mmHg or target blood pressure of 160/90 mmHg) using intermittent or continuous intravenous medications to control blood pressure, and clinically re-examine the patient every 15 minutes.

Notes: SBP, systolic blood pressure; MAP, mean arterial pressure.
Source: Adapted from [3].

Table 13.2. Intravenous medications that may be considered for control of elevated blood pressure in patients with ICH

Drug	Intravenous bolus dose	Continuous infusion rate
Labetalol	5 to 20 mg every 15 min	2 mg/min (maximum 300 mg/d)
Nicardipine	NA	5 to 15 mg/h
Esmolol	250 µg/kg IVP loading dose	25 to 300 µg/(kg min)
Enalapril	1.25 to 5 mg IVP every 6 h*	NA
Hydralazine	5 to 20 mg IVP every 30 min	1.5 to 5 µg/(kg min)
Nipride	NA	0.1 to 10 µg/(kg min)
Nitroglycerin	NA	20 to 400 µg/min

Notes: IVP, intravenous push; NA, not applicable.
*Because of the risk of precipitous blood pressure lowering, the enalapril first test dose should be 0.625 mg.
Source: Adapted from [3].

coagulopathy is currently recommended, although recent data suggest that practical issues causing delays in the administration of fresh frozen plasma might lead to continued expansion of hematoma, despite normalization of INR [7]. This argues for alternative or additional treatment options such as prothrombin complex concentrates [8] and perhaps factor VII (in the absence of underlying prothrombotic state) to reverse coagulopathy [9] in the setting of ICH.

New therapeutic approaches

The medical management of acute ICH revolves around the concept of hematoma stabilization. Brott et al. [10] clarified the idea that hematoma size is an important determinant of mortality in the setting of acute ICH, and demonstrated that early hematoma growth does occur. Davis et al. [11] clarified that early hematoma growth is the most strongly predictive variable for poor outcome. Other investigators demonstrated that acute edema formation also is predictive of bad outcome [12]. These observations suggest that reduction in the progression of ICH growth is key to improving survival of these patients in the setting of the ICU.

Activated factor VII

A new therapy offers the promise of reducing hematoma growth. In a recent phase II study, recombinant activated factor VII given within the first four hours of acute ICH improved survival and reduced hematoma expansion. The relative risk for mortality was reduced by 30% for all doses of activated factor VII included in the study [13]. A large randomized controlled study to substantiate these results was recently completed and while the official results have not yet been published, emerging data seem to suggest that this trial failed to demonstrate the effectiveness of recombinant activated factor VII in ICH [14].

Recently published research may help identify patients that are at greater risk of hematoma expansion by the presence of tiny enhancing foci following CT angiography (spot sign) [15] or contrast extravasation [16] and it is to be seen whether the use of hemostatic agents in this patient population might ameliorate outcomes. Alternative hemostatic treatment options include prothrombin complex and factor IX complex concentrates.

Intraventricular thrombolysis

Existing data indicate that in patients who have smaller ICHs ($< 30 \, cm^3$) and intraventricular hemorrhage (IVH) outcomes are related, in large part, to IVH [17].

Therapies that limit the consequences of IVH and reduce the length of stay in the ICU may improve survival significantly. An example of such a therapy is intraventricular thrombolysis of clots in IVH. Several small case series present evidence that supports intraventricular lysis of clot as a safe intervention, yet provide no conclusive evidence about its efficacy. These data were summarized in a Cochrane systematic review [18]. An ongoing clinical trial, Clot Lysis Evaluating Accelerated Resolution of IntraVentricular Hemorrhage, is designed to determine the optimum dose and timing of intraventricular recombinant tissue plasminogen activator (rt-PA) in patients who have IVH.

Minimally invasive surgery (MIS)

The role of MIS in the treatment of ICH has gained importance over the past decade. Surgical therapies have been unable to improve the neurological outcome of these patients, as evidenced by the results of the International Study of the Treatment of Intracranial Hemorrhage, which failed to demonstrate a significant benefit of aggressive surgical treatment over conservative medical treatment for the acute care of ICH [19]. To minimize brain tissue trauma that is induced by surgical manipulation, and in view of the failure of craniotomy/hematoma evacuation to improve survival and neurological outcome after ICH, new modalities (e.g., stereotactic-guided aspiration) have emerged as treatment alternatives that are amenable to testing. If MIS with or without thrombolytic therapy were capable of achieving safe and efficient clot reduction, it might modify patient outcomes positively. The trials looking at clot lysis in the setting of ICH are discussed separately in Chapter 15.

Treatment of complications
Elevated intracranial pressure

Intracranial hypertension has been associated with worse outcomes following ICH, which suggests that ICP monitoring may be of benefit in selected high-risk patients [20]. In the setting of increased ICP or a herniation syndrome, controlled hyperventilation to a $PaCO_2$ of 27–30 mmHg decreases ICP rapidly by causing cerebral vasoconstriction with an almost immediate reduction in cerebral blood flow. Osmotherapy should be instituted using mannitol with a serum osmolality goal of more than 300 mOsm/kg or hypertonic saline with a Na goal of 145–155 mmol/l [20,21]. Use of low-dose mannitol for prophylaxis against development of intracranial hypertension has not been shown to be effective in ameliorating outcomes [22]. For refractory elevations in ICP, additional options include pharmacologically induced coma or decompressive hemicraniectomy [23–25]. Steroids have no role in the management of cerebral edema or increased ICP [26] based on studies that showed either no improvement or worsening outcomes in the group treated with steroids. Whether a more aggressive glycemic control regimen associated with steroid use would show significantly different results remains a mystery.

Recently published retrospective data suggest an association between prior statin use and decreased perihematomal edema as well as decreased 30-day mortality despite correction for other factors that could impact outcomes. These emerging data however need to be prospectively validated before they can be applied to this patient population [27,28].

Seizures

Seizures were believed to occur in 10–15% of patients after ICH [29,30], but more recent data suggest a higher prevalence when these patients are monitored with continuous electroencephalography, especially patients in a comatose state [31,32]. In its guidelines, the Stroke Council of the American Heart Association recommended uniform seizure prophylaxis in the acute period after intracerebral and subarachnoid hemorrhage [3], but it did not define the duration nor classify the patients by location of hemorrhage. Given the possible risk for neuronal damage and elevated ICP secondary to seizures, it seems reasonable to administer phenytoin prophylactically in patients who have lobar hemorrhages, especially in patients with altered mental status. Additionally, in comatose patients with deep hemorrhages, an EEG, preferably continuous, is suggested to rule out non-convulsive status epilepticus. In the absence of seizures, discontinuation of prophylaxis 2–4 weeks after the ICH seems reasonable [33,34].

Supportive treatment

1. Head of bed elevation to > 30 degrees increases jugular venous outflow and decreases ICP.
2. Avoid hypovolemia to maintain CPP goals > 70.
3. Goals of normothermia should be maintained as fever worsens outcome in several experimental models of brain injury [35]. Therapeutic hypothermia may be considered in the setting of refractory ICP elevation for neuroprotection [36].
4. Goals of normoglycemia must be targeted given that high blood glucose on admission independently predicts an increased 28-day case-fatality rate in both non-diabetic and diabetic patients with ICH [37]. The specific ideal blood glucose targeted range is controversial and is being studied in clinical trials.
5. Subcutaneous (SQ) unfractionated heparin, low-molecular-weight heparins/heparinoids, anticoagulants, platelet antiaggregants, and use of mechanical methods such as intermittent pneumatic compression and graduated compression stockings are options with varying strengths of evidence for preventing venous thromboembolism in patients with stroke. Timing of restarting full dose anticoagulation in patients who had an ICH secondary to anticoagulation must be decided on a case-by-case basis based on indication for anticoagulation and etiology of hemorrhage (higher risk of recurrence with amyloid angiopathy).

Identification of underlying etiology

In patients who are older than 45 years with a history of hypertension and an ICH located in the basal ganglia, thalamus, and posterior fossa, further investigations to confirm the etiology of hemorrhage are unnecessary [38]. In younger non-hypertensive individuals, further investigations, such as angiography to rule out aneurysms and arteriovenous malformations, are warranted. Because older patients are at higher risk for tumors and metastasis, MRI might be the first imaging modality used. Amyloid angiopathy is a common etiological factor in older patients, especially those older than 65 years who have multiple lobar hemorrhages. In hemorrhages in patients who are on anticoagulation, a risk–benefit ratio needs to be established before restarting anticoagulation.

References

1. Broderick JP, Brott T, Tomsick T, et al. Intracerebral hemorrhage more than twice as common as subarachnoid hemorrhage. J Neurosurg 1993; 78: 188–191.

2. Qureshi AI, Tuhrim S, Broderick JP, et al. Spontaneous intracerebral hemorrhage. N Engl J Med 2001; 344: 1450–1460.

3. Broderick J, Connolly S, Feldmann E, *et al.* American Heart Association/American Stroke Association Stroke Council; American Heart Association/American Stroke Association High Blood Pressure Research Council; Quality of Care and Outcomes in Research Interdisciplinary Working Group. Guidelines for the management of spontaneous intracerebral hemorrhage in adults: 2007 update: a guideline from the American Heart Association/American Stroke Association Stroke Council, High Blood Pressure Research Council, and the Quality of Care and Outcomes in Research Interdisciplinary Working Group. *Stroke* 2007; **38**(6): 2001–2023. Epub 2007 May 3.

4. Schellinger PD, Fiebach JB, Hoffmann K, *et al.* Stroke MRI in intracerebral hemorrhage: is there a perihemorrhagic penumbra? *Stroke* 2003; **34**: 1674–1679.

5. Jauch EC, Lindsell CJ, Adeoye O, *et al.* Lack of evidence for an association between hemodynamic variables and hematoma growth in spontaneous intracerebral hemorrhage. *Stroke* 2006; **37**(8): 2061–2065.

6. Flibotte JJ, Hagan N, O'Donnell J, *et al.* Warfarin, hematoma expansion, and outcome of intracerebral hemorrhage. *Neurology* 2004; **63**(6): 1059–1064.

7. Lee SB, Manno EM, Layton KF, *et al.* Progression of warfarin-associated intracerebral hemorrhage after INR normalization with FFP. *Neurology* 2006; **67**(7): 1272–1274.

8. Lankiewicz MW, Hays J, Friedman KD, Tinkoff G, Blatt PM. Urgent reversal of warfarin with prothrombin complex concentrate. *J Thromb Haemost* 2006; **4**: 967–970.

9. Baker RI, Coughlin PB, Gallus AS, *et al.* Warfarin reversal: consensus guidelines, on behalf of the Australasian Society of Thrombosis and Haemostasis. *Med J Aust* 2005; **182**: 48. Erratun *Med J Aust* 2004; **181**: 492–497.

10. Brott T, Broderick J, Kothari R, *et al.* Early hemorrhage growth in patients with intracerebral hemorrhage. *Stroke* 1997; **28**(1): 1–5.

11. Davis SM, Broderick J, Hennerici M, *et al.* Recombinant Activated Factor VII Intracerebral Hemorrhage Trial Investigators. Hematoma growth is a determinant of mortality and poor outcome after intracerebral hemorrhage. *Neurology* 2006; **66**(8): 1175–1181.

12. Gebel JM Jr, Jauch EC, Brott TG, *et al.* Relative edema volume is a predictor of outcome in patients with hyperacute spontaneous intracerebral hemorrhage. *Stroke* 2002; **33**(11): 2636–2641.

13. Mayer SA, Brun NC, Begtrup K, *et al.* Recombinant Activated Factor VII Intracerebral Hemorrhage Trial Investigators. Recombinant activated factor VII for acute intracerebral hemorrhage. *N Engl J Med* 2005; **352**(8): 777–785.

14. Fernandez-Concepcion O. [The FAST study fails to demonstrate the effectiveness of recombinant factor VIIa in intracerebral haemorrhage.] *Rev Neurol (Paris)* 2007; **45**(7): 445–446.

15. Wada R, Aviv RI, Fox AJ, *et al.* CT angiography "spot sign" predicts hematoma expansion in acute intracerebral hemorrhage. *Stroke* 2007; **38**(4): 1257–1262.

16. Goldstein JN, Fazen LE, Snider R, *et al.* Contrast extravasation on CT angiography predicts hematoma expansion in intracerebral hemorrhage. *Neurology* 2007; **68**(12): 889–94.

17. Broderick JP, Brott TG, Duldner JE, Tomsick T, Huster G. Volume of intracerebral hemorrhage. A powerful and easy-to-use predictor of 30-day mortality. *Stroke* 1993; **24**: 987–993.

18. Lapointe M, Haines S. Fibrinolytic therapy for intraventricular hemorrhage in adults. *Cochrane Database Syst Rev* 2002; **(3)**: CD003692.

19. Mendelow AD, Gregson BA, Fernandes HM, *et al.* Early surgery versus initial conservative treatment in patients with spontaneous supratentorial intracerebral haematomas in the International Surgical Trial in Intracerebral Haemorrhage (STICH): a randomised trial. *Lancet* 2005; **365**(9457): 387–397.

20. Diringer MN. Intracerebral hemorrhage: pathophysiology and management. *Crit Care Med* 1993; **21**(10): 1591–1603.

21. Bhardwaj A, Ulatowski JA. Hypertonic saline solutions in brain injury. *Curr Opin Crit Care* 2004; **10**(2): 126–131.

22. Misra UK, Kalita J, Ranjan P, *et al.* Mannitol in intracerebral hemorrhage: a randomized controlled study. *J Neurol Sci* 2005; **234**: 41–45.

23. Dereeper E, Berre J, Vandesteene A, *et al.* Barbiturate coma for intracranial hypertension: clinical observations. *J Crit Care* 2002; **17**(1): 58–62.

24. Kang TM. Propofol infusion syndrome in critically ill patients. *Ann Pharmacother* 2002; **36**(9): 1453–1456.

25. Steiner T, Ringleb P, Hacke W. Treatment options for large hemispheric stroke. *Neurology* 2001; **57**(5 Suppl 2): S61–68.

26. Poungvarin N, Bhoopat W, Viriyavejakul A, *et al.* Effects of dexamethasone in primary supratentorial intracerebral hemorrhage. *N Engl J Med* 1987; **316**: 1229–1233.

27. Naval NS, Abdelhak TA, Urrunaga N, *et al.* An association of prior statin use with decreased perihematomal edema. *Neurocrit Care* 2008; **8**(1): 12–18.

28. Naval NS, Abdelhak TA, Zeballos P, *et al.* Prior statin Use reduces mortality in intracerebral hemorrhage. *Neurocrit Care* 2008; **8**(1): 6–12.

29. Bladin C, Alexandrov A, Bellavance A, *et al.* Seizures after stroke: a prospective multicenter study. *Arch Neurol* 2000; **57**: 1617–1622.

30. Kilpatrick C, Davis S, Tress B, *et al.* Epileptic seizures after stroke. *Arch Neurol* 1990; **47**: 157–169.

31. Vespa P. Continuous EEG monitoring for the detection of seizures in traumatic brain injury, infarction, and intracerebral hemorrhage: "to detect and protect". *J Clin Neurophysiol* 2005; **22**(2): 99–106.

32. Vespa PM, O'Phelan K, Shah M, *et al.* Acute seizures after intracerebral hemorrhage: a factor in progressive midline shift and outcome. *Neurology* 2003; **60**(9): 1441–1446.

33. Naidech AM, Kreiter KT, Janjua N, *et al.* Phenytoin exposure is associated with functional and cognitive disability after subarachnoid hemorrhage. *Stroke* 2005; **36**(3): 583–587.

34. Silverman IE, Restrepo L, Mathews GC. Poststroke seizures. *Arch Neurol* 2002; **59**(2): 195–201.

35. Takagi K. Body temperature in acute stroke. *Stroke* 2002; **33**: 2154–2155; author reply 2154–2155.

36. Gupta R, Jovin TG, Krieger DW. Therapeutic hypothermia for stroke: do new outfits change an old friend? *Expert Rev Neurother* 2005; **5**: 235–246.

37. Fogelholm R, Murros K, Rissanen A, Avikainen S. Admission blood glucose and short term survival in primary intracerebral haemorrhage: a population based study. *J Neurol Neurosurg Psychiatry* 2005; **76**: 349–353.

38. Zhu XL, Chan MS, Poon WS. Spontaneous intracranial hemorrhage: which patients need diagnostic cerebral angiography? A prospective study of 206 cases and review of the literature. *Stroke* 1997; **28**: 1406–1409.

39. Kaplan NM. Management of hypertensive emergencies. *Lancet* 1994; **344**(8933): 1335–1338.

Surgical management of intracerebral hemorrhage

A. David Mendelow

Introduction

The clinical problem about whether or not to operate on a patient with an intracerebral hemorrhage (ICH) is a complex one because of the coexistence of three different treatment aims:

1. To stop the bleeding and to avoid rebleeding (seen particularly in patients on anticoagulants and in patients with underlying aneurysms and/or arteriovenous malformations [AVMs]).
2. To remove the mass effect to prevent secondary ischemic brain damage. Such secondary brain damage has been well recognized experimentally [1] and has been confirmed clinically in some studies [2] but not in others [3].
3. To treat secondary complications that include obstructive hydrocephalus with infratentorial (cerebellar) hemorrhage and the hydrocephalus associated with intraventricular hemorrhage (IVH).

It will be obvious to all that open craniotomy aided by modern techniques including image guidance and the operating microscope achieves the first and second of these three aims. However, this usually requires a general anesthetic and, if a clot is deep-seated, access is via normal overlying brain structures. Deep clots may therefore be better treated by minimal interventional techniques that include endoscopic and/or catheter aspiration, aided by the direct use of thrombolytic drugs to avoid catheter obstruction [4,5]. Not unexpectedly the International Surgical Trial in Intracerebral Hemorrhage (STICH) trial [6] suggested that superficial clots treated by open craniotomy resulted in better outcomes than surgery for deep-seated clots or by using less invasive techniques. However, that was

not the primary outcome measure and this suggestion came from prespecified subgroup analysis. In that trial 1033 patients with spontaneous supratentorial ICH were randomized to a policy of early surgery or to a policy of initial conservative treatment. The primary outcome measure was the prognosis-based 8 point Glasgow Coma Scale (GCS) at six months. There was no difference demonstrated between these two policies. The conclusion about superficial lobar hematomas was derived from subgroup analysis. Class 1 evidence needs to be obtained from large prospective randomized controlled trials (PRCTs) that have set clear primary outcomes rather than from such subgroup analyses, which will inevitably be underpowered. The overall result of the STICH trial was therefore neutral.

For this reason, new PRCTs are ongoing to address the question of whether or not there is a role for surgery for supratentorial ICH more specifically. In this chapter, the evidence from PRCTs will be presented and analyzed in the form of meta-analysis. Also, the ongoing PRCTs that address the questions raised will be summarized.

Objective number 3 (the treatment of hydrocephalus) will be addressed separately, but the main method of acute treatment is by external ventricular drainage. The problems created by such operative drainage relate to catheter blockage by blood and exciting new work on the intermittent use of thrombolytic agents will also be summarized [4,7]. The special circumstances of obstructive hydrocephalus with infratentorial (cerebellar) hemorrhage will also be considered because insertion of an external ventricular drain (EVD) is a relatively uncomplicated procedure and sometimes may be substituted with ventriculo-peritoneal shunting or third ventriculostomy [8].

Intracerebral Hemorrhage, ed. J. R. Carhuapoma, S. A. Mayer, and D. F. Hanley. Published by Cambridge University Press.
© J. R. Carhuapoma, S. A. Mayer, and D. F. Hanley 2010.

Surgery for intracerebral hemorrhage

Despite 13 PRCTs that have investigated the role of surgery for spontaneous supratentorial ICH there is no firm conclusion that can be drawn about whether or not to operate on these patients (B. A. Gregson, personal communication, 2008). Ongoing analysis of these trials has helped to identify subgroups of patients that are most likely to benefit from surgery. However, these subgroups need to be evaluated in further trials, which are currently ongoing. This chapter summarizes these trials and sets out the hypotheses for those that are currently underway. There are, as yet, no trials of surgery for infratentorial hemorrhage either of the cerebellum or the brainstem but the limited evidence that is available is summarized at the end.

There is no doubt that early removal of some hematomas is effective: every neurosurgeon knows that. There is thus agreement amongst neurosurgeons that acute traumatic extradural and subdural hematomas, which cause depression of consciousness, need urgent operation [9,10]. However, the role of surgery for traumatic ICH and/or contusion is less clear cut. There is also agreement that postoperative hematomas that cause symptoms should be immediately evacuated. So, the benefit of surgical evacuation of some clots is well recognized by neurosurgeons throughout the world. By contrast, the benefits of surgery for spontaneous intracerebral parenchymal hemorrhage are less clear cut, largely because of the severe disability that is often suffered by the survivors of surgery. Similar problems are created by decompressive craniectomy in stroke patients and following trauma. The HAMLET, Decimal and Destiny trials have shown that surgery saves lives but most survivors remain disabled [11,12].

Nevertheless, it is only through PRCTs that firm conclusions can be drawn because of the heterogeneity of case mix that confounds any non-randomized study. This review therefore gives much greater weight to the 13 trials (B. A. Gregson, personal communication, 2008) than it does to the hundreds of observational studies [13].

Operative techniques

Craniotomy

Standard craniotomy is easily performed either via a scalp flap or through a linear incision. Strategic planning of the bone flap should minimize damage to intact brain overlying the hematoma. Current high-speed drills, craniotomes, ultrasonic aspirators and flap-closure techniques are now so sophisticated that they should not produce further brain damage with superficial hematomas and should allow the entire clot to be removed under direct vision (aided by the magnification and good lighting that is routinely provided by modern operating microscopes). This also allows accurate and complete hemostasis to take place using bipolar diathermy with modern non-stick instruments (e.g., Codman Iso-Cool tips®). Image guidance techniques help ensure accurate flap placement and also improve operative maneuverability with "smart image tracking" and "smart auto focus" (Brain Lab®). Similarly, intra-operative 3D ultrasound (often linked directly to the image guidance equipment) ensures complete clot removal facilitated by real-time re-imaging. Similar real-time intra-operative imaging can be provided by intra-operative MRI or CT but such equipment is very expensive and time consuming to use. By contrast, 3D intra-operative ultrasound is quick and relatively inexpensive.

Rebleeding is also prevented by the use of hemostatic materials such as Surgicel® or Fibrillar®. Topical thrombin products (FloSeal® [Baxter, USA]) can be used on the dura and may also help to ensure that hemostasis is more permanently achieved. These hemostatic techniques all help to minimize the risk of postoperative re-hemorrhage.

Decompressive craniectomy

In some circumstances, when a tight brain is anticipated or encountered, a large bone flap can be planned to provide a decompressive craniotomy. Leaving the dura open allows the brain to swell postoperatively thus maintaining a lower intracranial pressure (ICP) and a better cerebral perfusion pressure (CPP). Another option is to partially open the dura with a series of crisscrossed linear incisions (lattice duroplasty) [14]. Decompressive craniectomy has been shown to reduce mortality in malignant middle cerebral artery (MCA) infarction and three PRCTs have been analyzed to confirm that [11,12]. The problem created by more widespread use of decompressive craniectomy is that it results in a larger number of severely disabled survivors. Nevertheless, in the triple trial meta-analysis [11,12] there were seven Rankin 2 survivors in the decompressive craniectomy group compared with only one in the non-operative group (p = 0.07; Fisher's exact test)

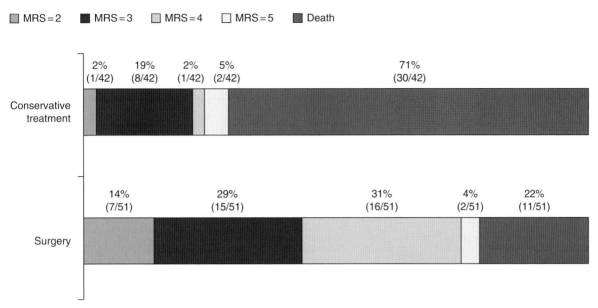

Fig. 14.1 Summary of the outcomes in the Decimal, Destiny and Hamlet trials: note only one single patient with a Rankin 2 outcome with non-operative treatment compared with seven such patients with decompressive craniectomy (Fisher's exact probability = 0.07) [12]. MRS, Modified Rankin Scale.

(Fig. 14.1). So there may be more patients that achieve a better level of independence than if no decompressive craniectomy took place. Full publication of the recent HAMLET trial result [15] presents a less optimistic view than the pooled analysis suggested and indeed meta-analysis of all 134 patients from the three trials does not yield a conclusive result [16]. To date no PRCTs of decompressive craniectomy have been performed in patients with spontaneous ICH. However, if performed in the future, it is likely that reduced mortality will be achieved with an increased number of disabled survivors as has occurred with middle cerebral infarction. A review of decompressive craniectomy for ICH has indicated that its use is not widespread [17]. For these reasons, internal decompression (removal of clot with excellent hemostasis) is likely to remain the treatment of choice when surgery is considered appropriate with supratentorial ICH.

Endoscopy

Realization of the effectiveness of endoscopy began with Auer's trial which showed a significant benefit from endoscopic removal compared with conservative treatment [18]. Several centers perform endoscopy as the main operative method for removal of clot. To date only a few centers have agreed to perform endoscopy as a subsection of the STICH II trial

but no patients have yet been randomized from these centers. Time will tell if there are sufficient numbers of cases with sufficient surgical enthusiasm to conduct an endoscopic subsection of the STICH II trial.

Timing of surgery and clinical trials

It is the appropriateness of craniotomy and internal decompression, and its timing, that has created the controversy in patients with ICH. The first PRCT evaluating surgery in ICH was published in 1961 and showed that surgery had an adverse effect on outcome [19]. That trial was in the pre-CT era and randomization was not concealed by modern standards. Nevertheless, it will be included in the subsequent meta-analysis. It did, however, influence neurosurgical practice in a nihilistic way for a long time until Auer *et al.* published their single center trial of endoscopic removal of supratentorial ICH [18]. They showed a beneficial effect from surgery, thus initiating the controversy that has raged until the present time.

Nobody likes extra work; particularly when it may lead to expensive disability, criticism from colleagues and managers and antagonism from ungrateful relatives. This is a philosophy that pervades the National Health Service (NHS) in the United Kingdom, and many other parts of the world, where most emergency craniotomies are performed by overworked trainee specialist registrars in neurosurgery on fixed salaries. Indeed, many non-neurosurgical emergency operations fall into this category. Recent criticism of delays in the NHS has appeared in the press [20]. Perversely, the incentive of "fee for service" (often thousands of Pounds, Dollars or Euros) may lead to the opposite: unnecessary operations being performed because they generate income for the surgeon and/or institution. Such non-medical factors play a role in influencing the need for and timing of operations for patients with ICH.

Against this background we have to interpret the results of randomized controlled trials in surgical patients. The largest trial of surgery in patients with supratentorial spontaneous ICH was in fact neutral [6]. The prespecified subgroups published in that trial indicated that surgery might have a greater benefit in patients out of coma (GCS Score > 9) with superficial clots (< 1 cm from the cortical surface) (Fig. 14.2). Subsequent analysis of the CT scans in STICH [21] revealed a worse outcome when IVH was present especially if there was associated hydrocephalus (Fig. 14.3). The publication of this trial in the United Kingdom has resulted in fewer patients being referred for surgery and, when they are, trainees may deflect the referral because of unavailability of beds or perhaps just to avoid work in an overstretched service. By contrast, in some countries, the results of subgroup analysis have been used to justify surgery as in both European and American guidelines that have suggested a role for surgery in superficial hematomas [22]. It is premature to adopt such a position and the results of the ongoing STICH II trial should provide class 1 information about the benefit or otherwise of early surgery for superficial lobar ICH where there is no IVH. The justification for STICH II comes from the meta-analysis of the 13 trials about surgery with supratentorial spontaneous ICH that have been published to date (Fig. 14.4). There is a clear benefit from surgery in terms of reducing mortality. Preliminary analysis of both morbidity and mortality, in those seven PRCTs that have provided sufficient data for re-analysis, has also shown a strong trend in favor of reduced morbidity and mortality in lobar hematomas where there is no associated IVH (B. A. Gregson, personal communication, 2008).

The STICH II trial is ongoing and, at this time, has randomized the first 40 of a planned 600 patients. The state of the STICH II trial can be assessed from the website [23].

In additions to STICH II (which focuses on the subgroup of superficial lobar supratentorial spontaneous intracerebral hematomas without ventricular hemorrhage) two other trials are ongoing: the MISTIE trial and CLEAR III:

- MISTIE is a PRCT of minimal interventional surgery (as opposed to craniotomy in STICH II) with insertion of a catheter into the clot and the instillation of regular thrombolytic agents to avoid blockage with clotted blood. The catheter is inserted via a burr hole using image guidance. The state of the MISTIE trial can be evaluated from its website [24].
- In the CLEAR III trial, one or two EVDs are inserted using image guidance to facilitate drainage of blood and cerebrospinal fluid. The Clear trials were initiated following successful drainage with the use of thrombolytic agents such as urokinase [7,25]. The Clear IVH trial used recombinant tissue plasminogen activator (rt-PA) and this phase II study has now been completed. This dose finding safety and feasibility trial has resulted in one milligram (mg) of rt-PA being introduced eight hourly (with drainage over the ensuing seven hours after clamping for one hour to allow the rt-PA to act topically within the ventricle). The CLEAR III trial is soon to be initiated and the status can be examined on their website too [26].

Cerebellar hemorrhage

Patients with cerebellar hemorrhage should be regarded as a special category. No PRCTs have been undertaken and none is likely because of the confounding problem of hydrocephalus. There is no doubt that obstructive hydrocephalus occurs and this produces a secondary reduction in the level of consciousness hours or even days after the primary cerebellar ICH. Patients with cerebellar clots, who are in good condition with preserved level of consciousness, should be carefully monitored. If their level of consciousness deteriorates, then scanning may reveal obstructive hydrocephalus and an emergency EVD should rapidly restore consciousness. However, if there is a large cerebellar clot with obliteration of the basal cisterns, then primary clot removal by craniectomy or craniotomy may be considered usually with an EVD as a preventative measure to avoid postoperative hydrocephalus. This type of obstructive hydrocephalus is quite different from that

Review: STICH
Comparison: 01 Early surgery vs. initial conservative
Outcome: 16 prognosis-based GOS

Study or subcategory	Early surgery n/N	Initial conservative n/N	OR (fixed) 95% CI	OR (fixed) 95% CI
01 age				
< 65	182/262	204/284		0.89 [0.62, 1.29]
>= 65	164/206	174/212		0.85 [0.52, 1.39]
02 GCS				
GCS 5–8	80/88	83/99		1.93 [0.78, 4.75]
GCS 9–12	140/187	158/196		0.72 [0.44, 1.16]
GCS 13–15	126/193	137/201		0.88 [0.58, 1.34]
03 side				
Left hemisphere	186/246	208/265		0.85 [0.56, 1.28]
Right hemisphere	160/222	170/231		0.93 [0.61, 1.40]
04 side				
Lobar	107/181	130/194		0.71 [0.47, 1.08]
Basal ganglia/thalam	236/284	247/300		1.05 [0.69, 1.62]
05 volume				
<= 50 ml	211/302	238/323		0.83 [0.58, 1.17]
> 50 ml	135/166	140/173		1.03 [0.60, 1.77]
06 depth from cortical surface				
<= 1 cm	170/257	192/260		0.69 [0.47, 1.01]
> 1 cm	174/208	184/234		1.39 [0.86, 2.25]
07 intended method of evacuation				
Craniotomy	238/324	267/337		0.73 [0.51, 1.04]
Others	108/144	111/159		1.30 [0.78, 2.15]
08 deficit of affected arm				
Normal/weak	110/182	135/206		0.80 [0.53, 1.21]
Paralyzed	231/279	238/284		0.93 [0.60, 1.45]
09 deficit of affected leg				
Normal/weak	150/229	169/248		0.89 [0.61, 1.30]
Paralyzed	192/232	201/239		0.91 [0.56, 1.48]
10 deficit of speech				
Normal	72/124	92/136		0.66 [0.40, 1.10]
Dysphasic/aphasic	216/276	228/289		0.96 [0.64, 1.44]
Cannot assess	58/68	58/71		1.30 [0.53, 3.20]
11 any antithrombolytic or anticoagulant therapy				
Anticoagulant therapy	24/34	38/46		0.51 [0.17, 1.46]
No anticoagulant therapy	322/434	340/450		0.93 [0.69, 1.26]
12 country				
UK	43/60	49/62		0.67 [0.29, 1.54]
Germany	51/65	66/78		0.66 [0.28, 1.55]
Spain	15/19	15/19		1.00 [0.21, 4.76]
Poland	25/33	33/42		0.85 [0.29, 2.52]
Latvia	20/28	20/29		1.13 [0.36, 3.50]
Lithuania	11/20	16/25		0.69 [0.21, 2.29]
Russia	19/26	15/20		0.90 [0.24, 3.43]
Czech Republic	39/44	33/43		2.36 [0.73, 7.61]
Macedonia	24/36	30/43		0.87 [0.33, 2.24]
South Africa	29/43	27/34		0.54 [0.19, 1.53]
India	26/38	35/43		0.50 [0.18, 1.39]
Others with < 20 patients	44/56	39/58		1.79 [0.77, 4.14]

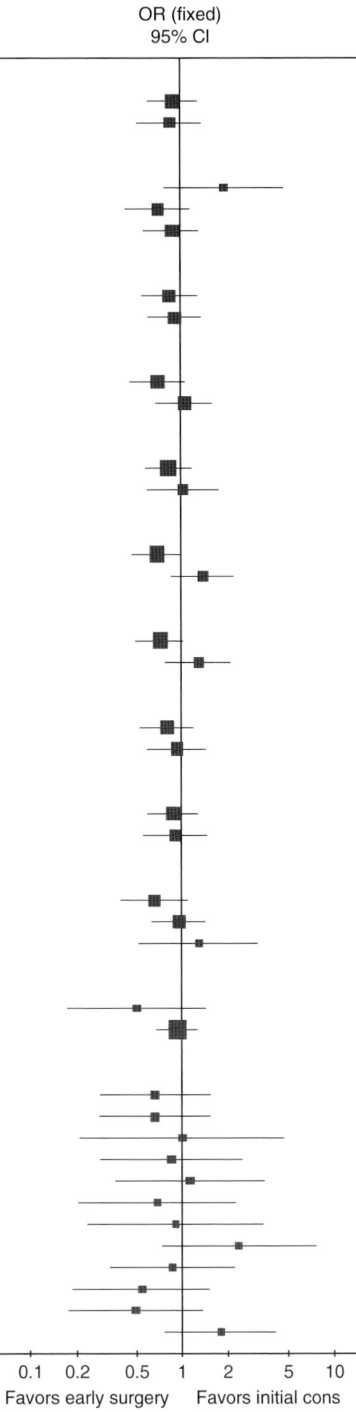

0.1 0.2   0.5   1   2   5   10
Favors early surgery   Favors initial cons

Fig. 14.2 Forrest Plot of subgroups from the STICH trial [6].

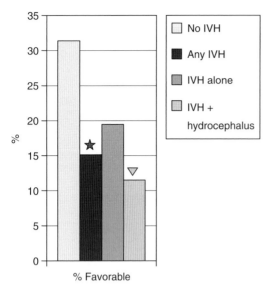

Fig. 14.3 Effect of intraventricular hemorrhage and hydrocephalus on outcome following intracerebral hemorrhage [19]. Star indicates a significant difference (P < 0.00001) between IVH and no IVH. Triangle indicates a significant difference (P < 0.05) between IVH alone and IVH with hydrocephalus.

seen with primary IVH where catheter blockage is a problem and where thrombolytic agents are being evaluated [4,7].

An algorithm for the treatment of cerebellar clots was suggested by Mathew *et al.* [27] and is shown in Fig. 14.5. The surgical results of the removal of the cerebellar clot can be surprisingly good.

Brainstem hemorrhage

Many primary brainstem hemorrhages produce devastating neurological disability. They may be associated with cavernous angiomas and surgery to remove the clot with excision of the cavernous angioma is often considered when the lesion reaches an accessible surface of the brainstem and where removal does not increase the damage done by the bleed itself. Microsurgical approaches to the surfacing hematoma may remove the clot and the cavernous angioma, sometimes with gratifying results [28].

Treatment of the cause of hemorrhage

If an ICH is caused by an AVM or aneurysm, then the risk of rebleeding is a much more major problem. These lesions have been dubbed "ictohemorrhagic" by Mitchell *et al.* [17]. There is evidence from two

PRCTs of surgery for aneurysmal ICH that patients are better treated surgically [29,30]. The trials of spontaneous supratentorial ICH have tended to exclude patients with aneurysmal rupture. For these reasons, surgery is usually recommended when ICH is associated with an aneurysm. Any ICH can be due to an underlying AVM or dural fistula. These lesions should be excluded angiographically at the outset whenever possible. With modern MRA or CT angiography (CTA) it is possible to exclude these lesions non-invasively early in their presentation. If a dural fistula is present, endovascular treatment can often eliminate the lesion and the clot would then be treated on its own merits. Occasionally, when such endovascular treatment is not possible, surgical obliteration of the fistula can be undertaken (Fig. 14.6).

With an AVM, craniotomy may be undertaken at the outset when the clot is identified. However, careful preoperative planning is needed because very vascular AVMs may prove too great a challenge if prior embolization of the inaccessible arterial feeders is not first undertaken. When it is decided not to evacuate a hematoma associated with an AVM, and when subsequent surgery for the AVM is planned to avoid rebleeding (6% in the first year and 3% per year thereafter [31–33]) then such surgery is best undertaken within three months of the ictus. This is because the clot cavity guides the surgeon to the lesion and minimizes new operative dissection with further damage. Careful planning allows the surgeon to identify the AVM in the wall of the clot.

When the initial clot is not planned to be removed and where craniotomy is not being considered or is not feasible, then the best option may be gamma knife stereoradiosurgery [34–36]. Stereoradiosurgery may obliterate the lesion with or without prior angiographic embolization [37].

An important principle is *not* to embark on the treatment of the AVM when it cannot be totally obliterated by either embolization, surgery, or the gamma knife [38]. The details of multimodality treatment of AVMs and the discussions regarding endovascular coiling and clipping of aneurysms are complex and beyond the scope of this chapter. Suffice it to say that unless complete obliteration is envisaged, it is better not to interfere with the circulation with ill-planned embolization or surgery.

The treatment of unruptured AVMs is being evaluated in the ARUBA trial [39] but both incomplete and complete interventions are being lumped

Review: Surgery in intracerebral hemorrhage
Comparison: 01 Surgery vs. Control
Outcome: 02 Death

Study or subcategory	Treatment n/N	Control n/N	Peto OR 95% CI	Peto OR 95% CI
McKissock (1961) [19]	58/89	46/91		1.81 [1.01, 3.27]
Auer (1989) [18]	21/50	35/50		0.32 [0.15, 0.71]
Juvela (1989) [43]	12/26	10/26		1.36 [0.46, 4.05]
Batjer (1990) [44]	4/8	11/13		0.20 [0.03, 1.33]
Chen (1992) [45]	15/64	11/63		1.44 [0.61, 3.40]
Morgenstern (1998) [46]	3/17	5/17		0.53 [0.11, 2.53]
Zuccarello (1999) [47]	2/9	3/11		0.77 [0.11, 5.62]
Cheng (2001) [48]	31/263	43/230		0.58 [0.36, 0.96]
Teernstra (2001) [4]	20/36	20/34		0.88 [0.34, 2.25]
Hosseini (2003) [49]	3/20	9/17		0.19 [0.05, 0.72]
Hattori (2004) [50]	9/121	20/121		0.42 [0.20, 0.92]
Mendelow (2005) [6]	173/477	189/505		0.95 [0.73, 1.23]
Pantazis (2006) [51]	26/54	31/54		0.69 [0.33, 1.47]
Total (95% CI)	1234	1232		0.82 [0.69, 0.98]

Total events: 377 (Treatment), 433 (Control)
Test for heterogeneity: Chi^2 = 27.90, df = 12 (P = 0.006), I^2 = 57.0%
Test for overall effect: Z = 2.16 (P = 0.03)

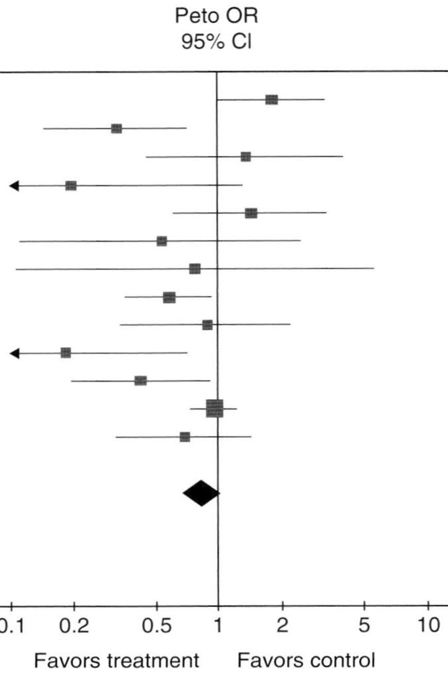

Fig. 14.4 Meta-analysis of mortality in 13 surgical trials of ICH (B.A. Gregson, personal communication, 2008).

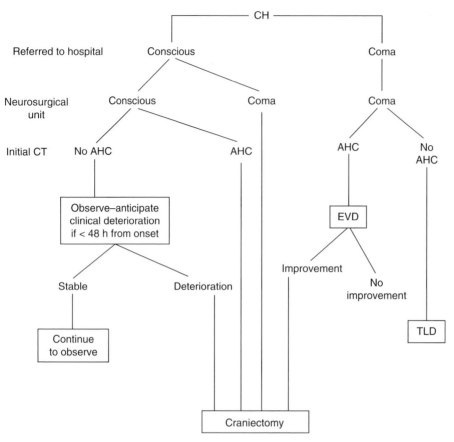

Fig. 14.5 Algorithm for treatment of cerebellar hemorrhage [25] (With permission.) CH = cerebellar hemorrhage; EVD = external ventricular drain; AHC = acute hydrocephalus; TLD = treatment limiting decision.

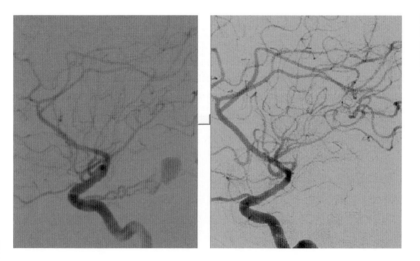

Fig. 14.6 Dural fistula angiogram pre (left) and post (right) craniotomy with division of the tentorium cerebelli and all the arterial feeding vessels within it: the fistula no longer fills (right).

together in that trial. There is therefore likely to be a bias against intervention because it is already known that partial treatment is hazardous. Hopefully the ARUBA investigators will recognize this problem with the trial's design and they will prespecify the subgroups in which complete obliteration is both aimed for at the outset and is achieved in practice at the finish.

Unusual causes of hemorrhage

Sometimes a hemorrhage is found to be associated with a tumor. Under these circumstances the treatment of the tumor itself has to be considered in relation to any planned evacuation of the clot. It is unlikely that the catheter-based approaches (CLEAR III or MISTIE) will become useful in patients with associated tumors or where tumor removal or biopsy are likely to be coordinated. Other causes of ICH that need to be considered are those associated with anti-coagulant usage or bleeding diatheses. In all cases of anti-coagulant or clotting abnormality, the plan should be to rapidly reverse the clotting abnormality with vitamin K, fresh frozen plasma, prothrombin complex concentrate, or recombinant activated factor VII [40].

Conclusions

The best evidence about treatment of ICH to date is summarized in the documents that compare Guidelines and Recommendations from the European Stroke Initiative [41] and the American Heart Association/American Stroke Association [42]. These guidelines and recommendations are compared by Juttler and Steiner [22]. This is a rapidly evolving field and it is likely that the family of trials described here (STICH II, MISTIE and CLEAR III) will shed further light on the best way to manage patients with ICH over the next few years.

References

1. Mendelow AD. Mechanisms of ischaemic brain damage with intracerebral hemorrhage. *Stroke* 1993; **24**(12 Suppl): I 115–117.

2. Siddique MS, Fernandes HM, Wooldridge TD, *et al.* Reversible ischemia around intracerebral hemorrhage: a single-photon emission computerized tomography study. *J Neurosurg* 2002; **96**: 736–741.

3. Qureshi AI, Wilson DA, Hanley DF, Traystman RJ. No evidence for an ischemic penumbra in massive experimental intracerebral hemorrhage. *Neurology* 1999; **52**(2): 266–272.

4. Teernstra O, Evers S, Lodder J, *et al.* Stereotactic treatment of intracerebral hematoma by means of plasminogen activator. A multicentre randomized controlled trial (SICHPA). *Stroke* 2003; **34**: 968–974.

5. Hanley D, Zuccarello M. Minimally Invasive Surgery plus rtPA for Intracerebral Hemorrhage Evacuation. (http://www.strokecenter.org/trials/trialDetail. aspx?tid=690, accessed 2 July 2009).

6. Mendelow AD, Gregson BA, Fernandes HM, *et al.* STICH investigators. Early surgery versus initial conservative treatment in patients with spontaneous supratentorial intracerebral hematomas in the International Surgical Trial in Intracerebral Hemorrhage (STICH): a randomised trial. *Lancet* 2005; **365**(9457): 387–397.

7. Naff NJ, Hanley DF, Keyl PM, *et al.* Intraventricular thrombolysis speeds blood clot resolution: results of a pilot, prospective, randomized, double-blind, controlled trial. *Neurosurgery* 2004; **54**(3): 577–583; discussion 583–584.

8. Dusick JR, McArthur DL, Bergsneider M. Success and complication rates of endoscopic third ventriculostomy for adult hydrocephalus: a series of 108 patients. *Surg Neurol* 2008; **69**(1): 5–15.

9. Mendelow AD, Karmi MZ, Paul KS, Fuller GA, Gillingham FJ. Extradural haematoma: effect of delayed treatment. *Br Med J* 1979; **1**(6173): 1240–1242.

10. Seelig JM, Becker DP, Miller JD, *et al.* Traumatic acute subdural hematoma: major mortality reduction in comatose patients treated within four hours. *N Engl J Med.* 1981; **305**(25): 1511–1518.

11. Vahedi K, Vicaut E, Mateo J, *et al.* DECIMAL Investigators. Sequential-design, multicenter, randomized, controlled trial of early decompressive craniectomy in malignant middle cerebral artery infarction (DECIMAL Trial). *Stroke* 2007; **38**(9): 2506–2517.

12. Vahedi K, Hofmeijer J, Juettler E, *et al.* Early decompressive surgery in malignant infarction of the middle cerebral artery: a pooled analysis of three randomised controlled trials. *Lancet Neurol* 2007; **6**(3): 215–222.

13. Siddique M. Surgery for intracerebral hemorrhage. Unpublished MD thesis, University of Newcastle upon Tyne; 2007.

14. Mitchell P, Tseng M, Mendelow AD. Decompressive craniectomy with lattice duraplasty. *Acta Neurochir (Wien)* 2004; **146**(2): 159–160.

15. Hofmeijer J, Kappelle LJ, Algra A, *et al*. HAMLET investigators. Surgical decompression for space-occupying cerebral infarction (the Hemicraniectomy After Middle Cerebral Artery infarction with Life-threatening Edema Trial [HAMLET]): a multicentre, open, randomised trial. *Lancet Neurol* 2009; **8**(4): 326–333.

16. Mitchell P, Gregson BA, Crossman J, *et al*. Reassessment of the HAMLET Study. *Lancet Neurol* 2009; **8**(7): 602–603.

17. Mitchell P, Gregson BA, Vindlacheruvu RR, Mendelow AD. Surgical options in ICH including decompressive craniectomy. *J Neurol Sci* 2007; **261**(1–2): 89–98.

18. Auer LM, Deinsberger W, Niederkorn K, *et al*. Endoscopic surgery versus medical treatment for spontaneous intracerebral hematoma: a randomized study. *J Neurosurg* 1989; **70**(4): 530–535.

19. McKissock W, Richardson A, Taylor J. Primary intracerebral hemorrhage. A controlled trial of surgical and conservative treatment in 180 unselected cases. *Lancet* 1961; **2**: 221–226.

20. BBC. New Threat to NHS Finances. In: Paulo B, editor. The Politics Show can reveal that the European Union regulation of so-called 'health tourism' could threaten the financial basis of the National Health Service: BBC 1; 2007.

21. Bhattathiri PS, Gregson B, Prasad KS, Mendelow AD. Intraventricular hemorrhage and hydrocephalus after spontaneous intracerebral hemorrhage: results from the STICH trial. *Acta Neurochir Suppl* 2006; **96**: 65–68.

22. Juttler TE, Steiner T. Treatment and prevention of spontaneous intracerebral hemorrhage: comparison of EUSI and AHA/ASA recommendations. *Exp Rev Neurother* 2007; **7**: 401–416.

23. Mendelow AD. STICH II website. In: Chilton L, editor. Newcastle University; 2007. (http://www.ncl.ac.uk/stich).

24. Zuccarello M. MISTIE Trial. 2008. (http://www.mistietrial.com).

25. Naff NJ, Carhuapoma JK, Williams MA, *et al*. Treatment of intraventricular hemorrhage with urokinase: effects on 30-day survival. *Stroke* 2000; **31**: 841–847.

26. Hanley DF. CLEAR III Trial. 2008. (http://www.neuro.jhmi.edu/ivh).

27. Mathew P, Teasdale G, Bannan A, Oluoch-Olunya D. Neurosurgical management of cerebellar haematoma and infarct. *J Neurol Neurosurg Psychiatry* 1995; **59**(3): 287–292.

28. Samii M, Eghbal R, Carvalho GA, Matthies C. Surgical management of brainstem cavernomas. *J Neurosurg* 2001; **95**(5): 825–832.

29. Heiskanen O, Poranen A, Kuurne T, Valtonen S, Kaste M. Acute surgery for intracerebral haemotomas caused by rupture of an intracranial arterial aneurysm. A prospective randomized study. *Acta Neurochir (Wein)* 1988; **90**: 81–83.

30. Tapaninaho A, Hernesniemi J, Vapalahti M. Emergency treatment of cerebral aneurysms with large hematomas. *Acta Neurochir (Wien)* 1988; **91**(1–2): 21–24.

31. Fults D, Kelly DL Jr. Natural history of arteriovenous malformations of the brain: a clinical study. *Neurosurgery* 1984; **15**(5): 658–662.

32. Jane JA, Kassell NF, Torner JC, Winn HR. The natural history of aneurysms and arteriovenous malformations. *J Neurosurg* 1985; **62**(3): 321–323.

33. Wilkins RH. Natural history of intracranial vascular malformations: a review. *Neurosurgery* 1985; **16**(3): 421–430.

34. Steiner L, Lindquist C, Adler JR, *et al*. Clinical outcome of radiosurgery for cerebral arteriovenous malformations. *J Neurosurg* 1992; **77**(1): 1–8.

35. Flickinger JC, Kondziolka D, Pollock BE, Lunsford LD. Radiosurgical management of intracranial vascular malformations. *Neuroimaging Clin N Am*. 1998; **8**(2): 483–492.

36. Pan DH, Guo WY, Chung WY, *et al*. Gamma knife radiosurgery as a single treatment modality for large cerebral arteriovenous malformations. *J Neurosurg* 2000; **93**(Suppl 3): 113–119.

37. Lundqvist C, Wikholm G, Svendsen P. Embolization of cerebral arteriovenous malformations: Part II–Aspects of complications and late outcome. *Neurosurgery* 1996; **39**(3): 460–467; discussion 467–469.

38. Miyamoto S, Hashimoto N, Nagata I, *et al*. Posttreatment sequelae of palliatively treated cerebral arteriovenous malformations. *Neurosurgery* 2000; **46**(3): 589–594; discussion 594–595.

39. Stapf C. The ARUBA Trial. 2008. (http://www.arubastudy.org).

40. Hanley JP. Warfarin reversal. *J Clin Pathol* 2004; **57**: 1132–1139.

41. Steiner T, Kaste M, Forsting M, *et al*. Recommendations for the management of intracranial hemorrhage-part I: spontaneous intracerebral hemorrhage. The European Stroke Initiative Writing Committee and the Writing Committee for the EUSI Executive Committee. *Cerebrovasc Dis* 2006; **22**(4): 294–316. Epub 2006 Jul 28. Erratum in: *Cerebrovasc Dis* 2006; **22** (5–6): 461. Katse Markku [corrected to Kaste Markku].

42. Broderick J, Connolly S, Feldmann E, *et al*. American Heart Association/American Stroke Association Stroke Council; American Heart Association/American

Stroke Association High Blood Pressure Research Council; Quality of Care and Outcomes in Research Interdisciplinary Working Group. Guidelines for the management of spontaneous intracerebral hemorrhage in adults: 2007 update: a guideline from the American Heart Association/American Stroke Association Stroke Council, High Blood Pressure Research Council, and the Quality of Care and Outcomes in Research Interdisciplinary Working Group. *Stroke* 2007; **38**(6): 2001–2023. Epub 2007 May 3.

43. Juvela S, Heiskanen O, Poranen A, *et al.* The treatment of spontaneous intracerebral hemorrhage. A prospective randomized trial of surgical and conservative treatment. *J Neurosurg* 1989; **70**(5): 755–758.

44. Batjer HH, Reisch JS, Allen BC, Plaizier LJ, Su CJ. Failure of surgery to improve outcome in hypertensive putaminal hemorrhage. A prospective randomized trial. *Arch Neurol* 1990; **47**(10): 1103–1106.

45. Chen X, Yang H, Czherig Z. A prospective randomised trial of surgical and conservative treatment of hypertensive intracranial haemorrhage. *Acta Acad Med Shangai* 1992; **19**: 237–240.

46. Morgenstern LB, Frankowski RF, Shedden P, Pasteur W, Grotta JC. Surgical treatment for intracerebral hemorrhage (STICH): a single-center, randomized clinical trial. *Neurology* 1998; **51**(5): 1359–1363.

47. Zuccarello M, Brott T, Derex L, *et al.* Early surgical treatment for supratentorial intracerebral hemorrhage: a randomized feasibility study. *Stroke* 1999; **30**(9): 1833–1839.

48. Cheng XC, Wu JS, Zhao XP, *et al.* The randomised multicentric prospective controlled trial in the standard treatment of hypertensive intracerebral hematomas: the comparison of surgical therapeutic outcomes with conservative therapy. *Chin J Clin Neurosci* 2001; **9**: 365–368.

49. Hosseini H, Leguerinel C, Hariz M, *et al.* Stereotactic aspiration of deep intracerebral hematomas under computed tomographic control. A multicentric prospective randomised trial. In: 12th European Stroke Conference, 2003; Valencia, Spain: Cerebrovascular Diseases. 2003; 57.

50. Hattori N, Katayama Y, Maya Y, Gatherer A. Impact of stereotactic hematoma evacuation on activities of daily living during the chronic period following spontaneous putaminal hemorrhage: a randomized study. *J Neurosurg* 2004; **101**(3): 417–420.

51. Pantazis G, Tsitopoulos P, Constantinos M, *et al.* Early surgical treatment vs. conservative management for spontaneous supratentorial intracerebral hematomas: a prospective randomised controlled trial. *Surg Neurol* 2006; **66**(5): 492–502.

Future therapy in intracerebral hemorrhage and intraventricular hemorrhage: aspiration and thrombolysis

Paul A. Nyquist, Neeraj S. Naval, and J. Ricardo Carhuapoma

Introduction

Thirty-day mortality after intracerebral hemorrhage (ICH) approaches 50%. Within the surviving patients, only 20% achieve a meaningful level of functional recovery at six months [1,2]. Intraventricular hemorrhage (IVH) is the direct hemorrhage of blood into the ventricles of the brain. Mortality estimates for IVH range from 50% to 80% [3–8]. The most common cause of IVH is spontaneous ICH, followed by subarachnoid hemorrhage (SAH). The incidence of IVH in ICH is about twice that in SAH [7]. Approximately 10% of aneurysmal SAH and 40% of primary ICH experience IVH [7,9,10]. Intraventricular hemorrhage in ICH and SAH account for 10% of the 700 000 strokes occurring yearly in the United States [7,9–11]. The total annual incidence of IVH in the United States is estimated to be about 22 000 adults per year [9].

Case-control cohort studies have repeatedly identified hematoma volume and admission Glasgow Coma Scale [GCS] score to be the main prognostic factors affecting survival and neurological outcome in patients with ICH and IVH [12]. Reduction of hematoma volume in both ICH and IVH could lead to improved neurological outcome by several mechanisms. Reduction of clot size will directly reduce local mass effect, thus decreasing the risk of fatal complications such as brainstem compression. In addition, minimizing hematoma volume could also lead to a decreased risk of globally elevated intracranial pressure (ICP) due to obstructive hydrocephalus ("trapped ventricles"). Conceivably, hematoma evacuation could also minimize the process of secondary neuronal injury leading to perihematoma tissue swelling caused by a variety of biochemical mechanisms

triggered by the interaction between blood and viable brain parenchyma (Fig. 15.1) [13].

At present medical management of ICH and IVH revolves around the control of ICP. Despite best medical management mortality remains high with only 38% of patients surviving the first year [14]. Even with best reported medical management mortality is as high as 50% [15]. These studies suggest that measures to control ICP through control of such factors as hydrocephalus have little effect. Diringer *et al.* looked at the independent effect of hydrocephalus on outcome and found that hydrocephalus resulted in increased mortality and greater rates of intubation [16]. Adams *et al.* found that control of hydrocephalus with an external ventricular drain had very little impact on survival in his cohort of 22 patients [17].

Large randomized trials proving the relative benefit of intracranial and intraventricular thrombolytic treatment over conservative medical management or craniotomy alone do not exist yet. However, optimism about this treatment modality is rising in light of the results of small treatment trials summarized in this report (Fig. 15.1). Several methodological issues surrounding this form of treatment remain to be resolved, including comparison of the relative efficacies of various mechanisms of clot aspiration and drainage. A dose-escalation trial showing the fibrinolytic dose that has the optimal risk–benefit ratio is also required. Clinically meaningful study end points should include global outcome measures that emphasize improvement in function in addition to improvement in mortality. Additionally, emphasis should be placed on the timing of the initiation and the cessation of therapy required to establish optimal clinical efficacy. If successful, thrombolytic therapy for IVH and ICH will become an important tool in the growing

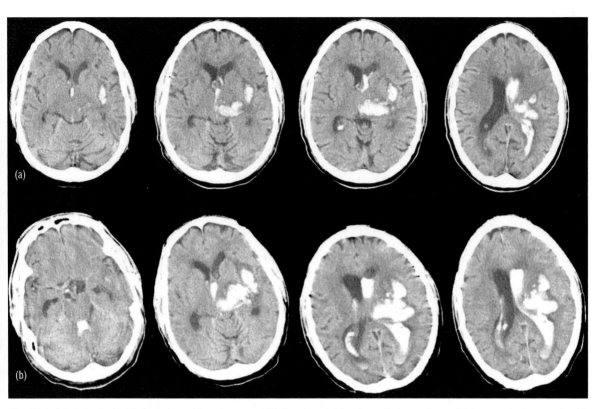

Fig. 15.1 Admission brain CT of a patient with spontaneous ICH showing a left basal ganglia hemorrhage with intraventricular extension (a). Eight hours following admission, the patient developed worsening level of consciousness. Follow-up brain CT demonstrated significant hematoma enlargement as well as worsening intraventricular hemorrhage (b).

treatment armamentarium for IVH and ICH with the potential for a disease modifying impact on these patients.

Minimally invasive surgery (MIS)

The role of minimally invasive surgery (MIS) in the treatment of ICH has gained importance over the past decade. This can be attributed to the lack of validated therapeutic options for this form of stroke as well as to the high associated morbidity and mortality. Traditional medical and surgical approaches, proposed mainly on clinical experience, have been unable to favorably modify the neurological outcome of these patients. Contemporary evidence that corroborates this statement was provided by the results of the International Study of the Treatment of Intracerebral Hemorrhage (STICH), which did not establish significant benefit for aggressive surgical treatment over conservative medical treatment for the acute care of ICH [1].

Prospective research testing novel therapies capable of improving the clinical outcome of ICH victims is lacking. Additionally, fundamental questions clarifying processes involved in the pathophysiology of secondary injury following ICH remain to be investigated. Nevertheless, various clinical studies and case series testing the hypothesis that clot burden plays a significant role in several forms of ICH have become available in the last ten years which seem to suggest that clot reduction plays an important role in limiting brain edema and additional neuronal injury, as well as in reducing the severity of neurological deficits following ICH [2,18–20]. If MIS were capable of achieving safe and efficient clot reduction, it would have a clear potential to positively modify ICH patient outcomes (Fig. 15.2). In this chapter, we attempt to review the available evidence supporting this hypothesis and to delineate the future clinical research needed in the area of thrombolytic therapy in ICH and IVH.

Therapeutic targets

The relationship between blood/blood degradation products and perihematomal edema following ICH

177

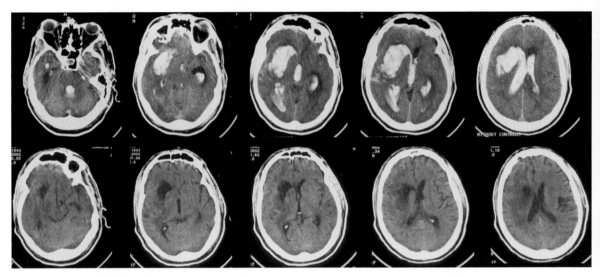

Fig. 15.2 Admission brain CT of a patient with massive spontaneous ICH involving right basal ganglia as well as the ventricular system (Top). Following the stereotactic placement of an intraclot catheter and the administration of 2 mg of rt-PA via this catheter every 12 hours, the follow-up brain CT 5 days later (Bottom) shows near complete resolution of the parenchymal as well as the intraventricular hemorrhage in this patient.

and IVH continues to be unraveled. Hemoglobin and its derivatives (methemoglobin, deoxyhemoglobin, and hemosiderin) have potent molecular and physiological effects on adjacent brain parenchyma. Hemoglobin with its prosthetic iron group is a nitric oxide absorber with long-lasting physiological effects. In addition, thrombin has been shown to induce blood–brain barrier disruption vasogenic cerebral edema [21–24].

In order to minimize brain tissue trauma induced by surgical manipulation and in view of the lack of success that craniotomy/hematoma aspiration has demonstrated in improving survival and neurological outcome after ICH, new modalities such as stereotactic guided aspiration emphasize the role of less invasive methods of clot evacuation as a viable treatment alternative amenable to testing.

Approaches to hematoma evacuation in ICH

Studies testing the safety and efficacy of MIS techniques in the treatment of ICH have taken advantage of mainly two different procedures:

- The use of endoscopic aspiration of the hematoma
- The stereotactic placement of a flexible catheter in the core of the hematoma followed by the administration of thrombolytic agents.

Both approaches are viable treatment alternatives to the surgical stress of craniotomy in clot evacuation that are amenable to testing.

In the late 1980s, Auer and coworkers performed a randomized study comparing hematoma endoscopic aspiration versus medical management in the treatment of ICH patients [25]. Main inclusion criterion in this study was the presence of a supratentorial hematoma with a volume greater than $10\,cm^3$. All hemorrhages that occurred because of identifiable brain lesions such as tumor, arteriovenous malformation (AVM), and aneurysms were excluded. At six months, the mortality rate was 42% in the MIS-treated group, which compared favorably with the mortality in the medically treated group of 70%. Nevertheless, significant differences in the quality of life of patients with large-sized ($> 50\,cm^3$) hematomas between the two cohorts were not observed. In patients with smaller hematomas ($< 50\,cm^3$), quality of life was improved in the MIS-treated group, without a noticeable impact on the mortality. These results generated controversies as many critics suggested that lack of blinding could have led to differences in the medical management of the two treatment groups. Furthermore, benefits of this technique seemed restricted to lobar hemorrhages and patients younger than 60 years old.

A study by Marquardt and coworkers focused on the use of a novel multiple target aspiration technique in 64 patients to aspirate a "sufficient proportion" of the hematoma with minimal risk for the patient. More than 80% of the hematoma volume was successfully aspirated in 73.4% of the patients with only one episode of rebleeding [26].

In recent years, emerging data showing favorable outcomes with the local instillation of fibrinolytic agents into the core of the hematoma has dampened the enthusiasm for endoscopic aspiration without fibrinolysis.

Fibrinolysis with clot aspiration in ICH

Clot evacuation combining the use of fibrinolysis with clot aspiration has emerged as the most promising surgical modality in the acute care of ICH. Clinical trials testing this technique are generating increased interest after the failure of standard craniotomy to achieve outcomes superior to medical management, as proven by the recently published STICH trial [1]. In several ways, stereotactic clot aspiration is similar to endoscopic aspiration. Clot resolution is enhanced by thrombolytic agents such as streptokinase [27], urokinase, recombinant tissue plasminogen activator (or rt-PA) for clot lyses. Several studies using animal models of ICH and IVH have demonstrated the efficacy of thrombolysis in reducing clot volume. Furthermore, the associated increase in perihematomal edema observed when rt-PA is used as therapy for ischemic stroke has not been observed in trials in ICH [2,28–30]. This observation suggests that rt-PA may be used safely to accelerate hematoma volume resolution. The testing of rt-PA in the treatment of ICH has now moved into clinical trials.

The potential role of combining clot lysis with stereotactic aspiration was also studied by Teernstra et al. [18]. This modality was compared with best medical treatment alone in the Stereotactic Treatment of Intracerebral Hematoma by Means of a Plasminogen Activator trial (SICHPA). Thirty-six of the 71 patients enrolled in this multicenter trial were randomized to the surgical group within 72 hours of onset. Inclusion criteria were age > 45, spontaneous supratentorial ICH > 10 cm³, and Glasgow Eye Motor scores between 2 and 10. There was a statistically significant reduction in the volume of the hematoma in the surgically treated group. There was no significant reduction in six-month mortality in the surgical group (56% and 59% in the surgery and medical treatment groups, respectively). Rebleed rate of 22% in the surgical

group, using urokinase as thrombolytic agent, was deemed crucial in negating any benefit of reduced lesion mass. The role of other confounding factors on the study results, such as significantly larger hematoma volumes at baseline in the surgical group, is unclear.

There is reason for optimism based on the findings of smaller studies both in the United States as well as Europe [19,20,31–37]. Montes and coworkers demonstrated that use of clot lysis (using urokinase) combined with stereotactic aspiration is safe and accelerates clot volume reduction. This study was completed in 12 patients. There was a mean reduction in hematoma volume of 57% and an increase in clot size in only one patient [31]. A mean reduction in clot size of 84% was achieved in another small case series by Lippitz et al. [32]. Rohde et al. showed a decrease in clot burden following frameless stereotactically guided catheter placement and clot lysis [33].

The optimal dosing of rt-PA for the treatment of ICH remains unknown. Different groups of investigators have used different regimens, mainly based on empirical reasons. Dose-escalation studies from thrombolytic therapy in the treatment of IVH aimed to clarify this subject further are close to completion. Schaller and coworkers [36] used a novel method to calculate the initial rt-PA dose. The amount of rt-PA was directly proportional to the maximal diameter of the initial hematoma volume. The dose was recalculated daily based on clot diameter as measured by daily CT scans. A recent report by Barrett and coworkers [37] used 2 mg rt-PA every 12 hours for hemorrhages > 35 cm³ in diameter until the hematoma volume was reduced to < 10 cm³, or the catheter fenestrations were no longer in continuity with the clot. This dose was based on safety data obtained from previously published studies in ICH and IVH [33].

Most of the reported clinical experience in the field of stereotactic surgery for ICH comes from studies performed in Japan [38–44]. Matsumoto and Hondo described the use of a 3.5 mm diameter silicone tube which was inserted into the center of the hematoma following three-dimensional CT images or biplane CT images taken to determine the coordinates of the target point in 51 patients (34 basal ganglionic, 11 subcortical, 3 thalamic, and 3 cerebellar hematomas). Following placement of the catheter through a burr hole under local anesthesia, aspiration of the hematoma was attempted with a syringe. Immediately after the first trial of hematoma aspiration, urokinase

(6000 IU/5 ml saline) was administered through this silicone tube and the drain was clipped. Subsequently, aspiration and infusion of urokinase were repeated every 6 or 12 hours until the hematoma was completely evacuated. The silicone tube was removed when repeat CT scanning revealed no residual hematoma [38]. These authors reported over 400 stereotactic aspiration procedures in patients with hypertensive ICH. A favorable outcome at six months was seen in patients with basal ganglionic ICH in comparison to patients who underwent conventional surgery or best medical treatment alone [39,40].

Niizuma and coworkers reported significant rebleeding in only 4 of 97 patients with hypertensive ICH treated with CT-guided stereotactic aspiration. In this study, the authors used urokinase for clot liquefaction, followed by aspiration through a drainage catheter. In 70% of the cases, at least 80% of the clot was evacuated [41].

Studies looking at long-term clinical outcomes in stereotactic clot lysis and removal have been performed in Germany. A retrospective review of outcomes in 85 patients treated at the University of Freiburg Medical School showed favorable long-term clinical outcomes in patients who received local urokinase following stereotactic hematoma evacuation [34]. On the other hand, a retrospective review of 126 patients who had either frame-based or frameless stereotactic hematoma puncture followed by clot irrigation with rt-PA did not have improved clinical outcomes despite the observed decrement in hematoma size. In this study, there was an associated increase in poor outcomes in patients over the age of 65 years [35].

A recently published study by Vespa *et al.* using frameless stereotactic aspiration of deep ICHs followed by local rt-PA instillation reported promising safety results, including improved neurological outcomes that correlated well with the degree of hematoma removal [19]. This study demonstrated not only an improvement in the level of consciousness, but also an improvement in the motor scores on the affected side. Of note, there was no increase in the perihematomal edema in the patients reported by these and other authors [2,19].

Similar beneficial effects have been proposed for the use of thrombolysis in IVH. Based on early data showing a trend towards improved 30-day outcomes in patients who received intraventricular urokinase [45], a randomized double-blinded pilot trial by Naff

and coworkers has showed accelerated clot resolution with intraventricular urokinase [46]. These results seem to enforce the multifactorial nature of the proposed therapeutic effect of rapid clot removal in different paradigms of ICH.

The most recent Cochrane Database Review on this subject [47] concluded that endoscopic evacuation has not yet been shown to significantly decrease the odds of death and dependency among survivors. Sufficient evidence has not yet been obtained to establish this treatment as a standard of care. Reports of treatment benefits from patients treated with endoscopic aspiration of ICH in Japan have led to the routine use of this modality as an alternative to craniotomy in that country. In the United States, this treatment modality has been restricted to research environments in academic stroke centers and is not widely advocated as a preferred method for the treatment of ICH yet.

Intraventricular hemorrhage

Intraventricular hemorrhage contributes to morbidity in many ways. Prolonged presence of IVH clot deep within the brain causes decreased level of consciousness. The greater the volume of blood in the ventricles and the longer the duration of exposure, the greater the length of time of coma [48,49]. One way to combat this is through the placement of external ventricular drains (EVDs). Studies looking at the placement of EVDs suggest that EVDs do not affect the size or damage associated with circulating blood products nor do they change the time required for blood clot resolution [46]. Until now, reducing the size of the intraventricular clot and decreasing the time that deep brain structures are exposed to clot have not been directly addressed by any current IVH treatment. The administration of thrombolytics through the IVH may significantly improve outcomes through the early reduction of clot size and reduction of the cerebrospinal fluid (CSF) blood burden.

Intraventricular hemorrhage forms ventricular blood clots, which block ventricular CSF conduits causing acute obstructive hydrocephalus. If untreated, ICP will increase and as the ICP approaches the arterial perfusion pressure it can cause death. In the setting of IVH, obstructive hydrocephalus is the greatest and most immediate threat to life. External ventricular drains are used to lower ICP quickly and are continued until the ventricular blood clots have dissolved sufficiently to allow normalized CSF circulation. In addition, the mass effect of clots in the IVH may independently increase the risk of cerebral edema and contribute to morbidity and mortality.

Blood degradation products embedded in the subarachnoid granulations by the CSF flow may contribute to morbidity. With prolonged exposure, blood degradation products permanently occlude and scar the subarachnoid granulations and consequently inhibit CSF absorption [50–52]. This may cause communicating hydrocephalus, which impairs cognition, gait and balance, and urinary continence. This syndrome of normal pressure or elevated pressure hydrocephalus may require the placement of a permanent ventricular shunt to facilitate treatment. Early clearance of IVH blood through the use of thrombolytics may significantly improve outcomes in this setting [5,45,46].

Two animal studies have looked at the effects of injected blood in the ventricles of dogs and porcine. Pang et al. utilized a dog model to show that thrombolysis of intraventricularly injected blood improved mortality, resulted in earlier decreased clot size, and improved level of consciousness in treated animals [48,53]. Mayfrank showed similar results in a porcine model of IVH using rt-PA as a lytic agent [54]. Ventricular dilatation with blood affected outcomes in a manner independent of the effects related to clot volume or mass effect supporting the hypothesis that there is an independent biochemical effect of ventricular blood on outcomes. There was a significant decline in mass effect in pigs treated with rt-PA. In both porcine and dog models there were no detectable signs of inflammation in the meninges of sacrificed experimental animals. The volume of injected blood was directly proportional to mortality [53,54].

In the Pang dog model three important observations were made: that intraventricular urokinase significantly hastened the resolution of intraventricular blood, urokinase promoted rapid return of consciousness, and improved neurological outcome. These observations support the conclusion that the existence of blood and heme products in the ventricles affected outcome separately from the influence of the mechanical effect of the clot and its effects on hydrodynamics.

In the last 15 years the concept that lysis of intraventricular blood will improve outcome has gained acceptance. A number of small case series present evidence that supports intraventricular lysis of clot as a safe intervention, yet provide no conclusive evidence about its efficacy. However, the investigation of techniques used to lyse clot in this disease have been plagued by a number of false starts. The thrombolytic first used for the lysis of intraventricular clot in the setting of IVH was urokinase. Until recently the vast majority of published studies used urokinase. Todo et al. first published a case series demonstrating the safe and efficacious use of urokinase for the lysis of IVH clot in the 1990s. In this study six patients received intraventricular urokinase. There were no observed secondary hemorrhages, supporting the idea that urokinase could be used safely for intraventricular lysis in the setting of IVH [55]. Coplin et al. published a case series with 20 IVH patients treated with intraventricular urokinase and compared their outcomes with historic controls. Clot life span was reduced and no complications associated with EVD placement where observed [56]. Naff et al. completed a case series in which 20 patients were treated with urokinase, with doses ranging from 5000 IU to 25 000 IU. Urokinase was given every 12 hours until resolution of clot [45]. Earlier resolution of clot with minimal complications were reported. Recently Naff et al. completed a prospective randomized controlled trial using urokinase. Patients were randomized into a treatment group in which 25 000 IU of urokinase were administered every 12 hours until prespecified clinical criteria were obtained [46]. Twelve patients were enrolled, seven treatment, and five placebo. Earlier resolution of clot was observed in the treated group [46]. However urokinase was withdrawn from use by the FDA for concerns about drug safety. There were issues concerning the safe manufacture of the drug. The unavailability of urokinase ended a successful line of inquiry emphasizing urokinase as the lytic of choice in IVH. At present rt-PA has become the predominant investigational agent for intraventricular thrombolysis in IVH. Studies are ongoing to examine the safety of rt-PA in IVH, and a large randomized control study has been funded.

The safety of thrombolysis for IVH is a question of great concern. Recently a comprehensive Cochrane review completed by Lapointe and Haines, reviewed the safety and efficacy of thrombolysis in the Cochrane collaboration format [57]. There are a number of case series and some prospective randomized trials. In seven independent studies, the use of intraventricular thrombolytic agents has been reported in 74 patients with ICH or SAH. Seventeen patients were treated with urokinase and 57 with rt-PA. The dose of rt-PA ranged from 4 to 20 mg daily. Good neurological outcome was reported in 50 of the 74 patients as measured by each group's criteria. Complications potentially attributable to treatment or EVD use associated with treatment included: five cases of bacterial meningitis, one patient had an increase in hematoma volume, and two extradural hematomas were noted. Based on the conclusions of this review, insufficient evidence exists to support clinical efficacy. The preliminary analysis does suggest rt-PA can be administered safely in IVH. At present there is concensus in the clinical community that a large randomized prospective study of rt-PA in IVH is needed [57].

Some safety concerns about the indirect systemic effects of rt-PA have arisen. In a rat model Wang et al. reported a number of findings. They observed that there was a dose-dependent effect on the rate of clot resolution. They also observed that the flow of CSF did not occur in concordance with a reduction in clot size. There also appeared to be an independent toxic effect of rt-PA administration. These included inflammatory changes in the choroid plexus and leukocyte infiltration in the periventricular white matter of the brains of treated rodents [58]. No human clinical data report the observation of these toxic effects of rt-PA in the ventricles of humans. Whether or not these findings are clinically relevant remains to be seen. These concerns over safety often arise from a series of clinical observations seen in the use of rt-PA for ischemic stroke. In that setting there is concern about the effect of rt-PA as an independent risk factor for cerebral edema and ICH.

Thrombolysis is a potential therapy for the treatment of IVH in the setting of SAH. Thrombolytics have been used extensively in small clinical trials aimed at reducing the burden of blood associated with SAH. The goal of such therapy is to reduce the risk of occurrence and the intensity of vasospasm observed in the setting of aneurysmal SAH. This has led to studies looking at intracisternal thrombolysis in the setting of SAH. The most recent study used a single intra-operative dose of rt-PA in comparison to a placebo. This was associated with a trend in the reduction of angiographic vasospasm [59].

In the setting of IVH, thrombolytics could also reduce the amount of blood in the ventricular system and help to reduce the risk of vasospasm as well as treat the side effects of IVH. The possibility that thrombolytics may facilitate rebleeding in this setting is of great concern. Intraventricular rt-PA in the

setting of acute IVH has also been used and examined retrospectively in a large number of case series and a few small prospective trials. One of the first case series to be completed was by Findlay et al. in 1993. In this series they had patients with IVH and SAH, IVH and ruptured AVM, as well as a case of IVH from a surgical catheter placement. They were treated with individual doses of rt-PA in the range of 2–12 mg. Treatment was initiated within 24 hours of surgery. No hemorrhagic strokes secondary to the rt-PA were reported. The drug was dosed one time every 24 hours with most patients receiving only one dose [59]. In this series with a large number of patients with ruptured aneurysms, no cases of rebleeding were associated with the use of this drug. This suggests that this treatment may be safe and effective in the setting of IVH and SAH [59]. Recently, Varelas et al. reported their experience with rt-PA for IVH in a prospective study in IVH in the setting of SAH. Ten patients received the drug and their outcomes were compared with ten age-matched controls. They found that the rt-PA group had a statistically shorter length of stay, more rapidly improving GCS score, and a decreased need for shunt placement. The average dose was 3.5 mg of rt-PA administered on admission to the hospital. The rt-PA was only administered after the aneurysm had been secured [60].

Mayfrank et al. reported a case series of 12 patients with IVH who were treated within 24 hours of onset of symptoms with 2–5 mg of rt-PA [61]. The dose was given at 6–14 hours until a substantial reduction in IVH volume was achieved, as recognized on CT scan. The average time for marked reduction to normalization of the CT scan was 24–48 hours from the beginning of thrombolytic therapy. Improved ICP control was observed in this study and only one complication, a case of meningitis, was observed. Goh and Poon reported a case series of ten patients, seven with negative angiograms and three with AVMs. Follow-up at three months identified no rebleeding, and no cases of meningitis. Total doses of 6–12 mg of rt-PA were used in this study with a 24-hour dosing interval [62]. These studies support the idea that rt-PA can be safely administered in the setting of AVMs.

The most recently published study on the use of rt-PA in IVH was completed at Mercer in Georgia. Fountas et al. reported the results of a prospective trial of rt-PA in IVH in 21 patients. These patients were exclusively ICH patients without aneurysms or AVMs. Thrombolytics were administered on a

24-hour schedule with a dose of 3 mg. There was an observed hemorrhage rate of 19%, and an infection rate of 14.3%. A CSF pleocytosis was observed in all 21 patients [63].

Intraventricular hemorrhage is also commonly seen in premature infants. The estimates of the incidence of IVH in this population range as high as 24.6% of all premature infants [64]. In this population bleeding occurs at the site of the immature germinal matrix. Hypoxia secondary to respiratory distress results in an increase stress on the highly vascular germinal matrix. This causes hemorrhage from the germinal matrix directly into the ventricles. Protocols incorporating streptokinase in the setting of neonatal hydrocephalus and IVH have shown no benefit at this time [65]. Whitelaw completed a Cochrane meta-analysis suggesting that intraventricular lysis of clot with streptokinase did not reduce the frequency of shunt dependency in infants with IVH and hydrocephalus [65]. Whitelaw *et al.* have completed a phase I trial examining the use of rt-PA in IVH in infants and have reported the safe use of low doses of rt-PA in infants. The doses used were 1.0 mg or 0.5 mg with dosing intervals of 1–7 days. The half-life of rt-PA in CSF in this setting was determined to be 24 hours. Further study is needed to determine the efficacy of this treatment at reducing dependency on shunts and avoidance of hydrocephalus [66]. These studies have provided valuable data for further study of IVH in the adult setting. They have shown that smaller doses of rt-PA given at more frequent intervals may be efficacious; they have also aided in the establishment of rt-PA's half-life in the ventricular system. Further testing of this technique in adults will undoubtedly help to clarify concerns over safety and efficacy in neonates.

Conclusion

There is evidence suggesting that thrombolytics used for the lysis of blood in the setting of IVH and ICH in humans may improve outcomes. The potential clinical benefits include: faster reduction of IVH and ICH clot size, faster removal of blood from the ventricular systems, reduction in the incidence of hydrocephalus, reduced time in coma, and reduced mortality. This may result in improved patient survival, reductions in the number of patients requiring long-term shunting, reduced length of stay in the ICU, and improved neurological outcomes. At this time there appears to be a clinical consensus that rt-PA is the most commonly used thrombolytic and studies are testing rt-PA in this setting. Future clinical trials using this drug are under way and rt-PA appears to be the drug for which the most accurate information about safety and efficacy will exist. There are number of issues that must be resolved about the use of rt-PA in the setting of IVH. These include what dose is safest, what period of dosing is safest, when to stop treatment, and which ventricles to place catheters in for maximum clot reduction. Many of these questions will be answered by ongoing clinical trials. With the completion of these trials it is the hope of physicians that we will at last have a treatment for lyses of IVH that is safe and effective. The use of thrombolysis in the setting of IVH may be one of many clinical tools that will improve outcomes associated with ICH and IVH. Hopefully this new tool may help to change the attitude of many physicians in the setting of IVH from therapeutic nihilism to dogmatic optimism.

There is a current FDA sponsored randomized prospective trial on the efficacy and safety of rt-PA in IVH. This study is the Clot Lysis: Evaluating Accelerated Resolution of IntraVentricular Hemorrhage (CLEAR IVH). This study is designed to determine the optimum dose and timing of rt-PA in IVH. It will help to establish standard procedures about the use of rt-PA in the setting of IVH and resolve many of the issues discussed above.

Similarly in ICH the use of intra clot thrombolysis and aspiration in MIS has advanced to the point where clinical trials are now under way to test stereotactically guided clot lysis and aspiration. The MISTIE (Minimally Invasive Surgery plus rt-PA for ICH Evacuation) trial, a National Institutes of Health (NIH) funded exploratory trial using rt-PA as a thrombolytic, is presently under way. The data to answer the key questions of lytic dose, optimum timing, and optimal treatment candidates are yet to be determined. The use of endoscopically based MIS is alive and well in countries other than the United States. Its application here will depend on the interest of clinicians and the availability of technology.

References

1. Mendelow AD, Gregson BA, Fernandes HM, *et al.* STICH investigators. Early surgery versus initial conservative treatment in patients with spontaneous supratentorial intracerebral haematomas in the International Surgical Trial in Intracerebral Haemorrhage (STICH): a randomised trial. *Lancet* 2005; **365**(9457): 387–397.

2. Wagner KR, Xi G, Hua Y, *et al.* Ultra-early clot aspiration after lysis with tissue plasminogen activator in a porcine model of intracerebral hemorrhage: edema reduction and blood-brain barrier protection. *J Neurosurg* 1999; **90**(3): 491–498.

3. Adams RE, Diringer MN. Response to external ventricular drainage in spontaneous intracerebral hemorrhage with hydrocephalus. *Neurology* 1998; **50**: 519–523.

4. Daverat P, Castel JP, Dartigues JF, Orgogozo JM. Death and functional outcome after spontaneous intracerebral hemorrhage. A prospective study of 166 cases using multivariate analysis. *Stroke* 1991; **22**(1): 1–6.

5. Tuhrim S, Dambrosia JM, Price TR, *et al.* Intracerebral hemorrhage: external validation and extension of a model for prediction of 30-day survival. *Ann Neurol* 1991; **29**(6): 658–663.

6. Young WB, Lee KP, Passin MS. Prognostic significance of ventricular blood in supratentorial hemorrhage: a volumetric study. *Neurology* 1990; **40**: 616–619.

7. Adams HP, Torner JC, Kassell NF. Intraventricular hemorrhage among patients with recently ruptured aneurysms: a report of the Cooperative Aneurysm Study. *Stroke* 1992; **23**: 140.

8. Tuhrim S, Horowitz DR, Sacher M, *et al.* Validation and comparison of models predicting survival following intracerebral hemorrhage. *Crit Care Med* 1995; **23**: 950–954.

9. Naff NJ. Intraventricular hemorrhage in adults. *Curr Treat Options Neurol* 1999; **1**(3): 173–178.

10. Broderick JP, Brott T, Tomsick T, Miller R, Huster G. Intracerebral hemorrhage more than twice as common as subarachnoid hemorrhage. *J Neurosurg* 1993; **78**(2): 188–191.

11. Mohr G, Ferguson G, Khan M. Intraventricular hemorrhage from ruptured aneurysm. *J Neurosurg* 1983; **58**: 482–487.

12. Broderick JP, Brott TG, Duldner JE, Tomsick T, Huster G. Volume of intracerebral hemorrhage. A powerful and easy-to-use predictor of 30-day mortality. *Stroke* 1993; **24**: 987–993.

13. Gebel JM Jr, Jauch EC, Brott TG, *et al.* Natural history of perihematomal edema in patients with hyperacute spontaneous intracerebral hemorrhage. *Stroke* 2002; **33**: 2631–2635.

14. Qureshi AI, Tuhrim S, Broderick JP, *et al.* Spontaneous intracerebral hemorrhage. *N Engl J Med* 2001; **344**: 1450–1460.

15. Zurasky JA, Aiyagari V, Zazulia AR, Shackelford A, Diringer MN. Early mortality following spontaneous intracerebral hemorrhage. *Neurology* 2005; **64**(4): 725–727.

16. Diringer MN, Edwards DF, Zazulia AR. Hydrocephalus: a previously unrecognized predictor of poor outcome from supratentorial intracerebral hemorrhage. *Stroke* 1998; **29**: 1352–1357.

17. Adams RE, Diringer MN. Response to external ventricular drainage in spontaneous intracerebral hemorrhage with hydrocephalus. *Neurology* 1998; **50**(2): 519–523.

18. Teernstra OP, Evers SM, Lodder J, *et al.* Stereotactic treatment of intracerebral hematoma by means of plasminogen activator: a multicenter randomized controlled trial (SICHPA). *Stroke* 2003; **34**: 968–974.

19. Vespa P, Miller C, McArthur D, *et al.* Frameless stereotactic aspiration and thrombolysis of deep intracerebral hemorrhage is associated with reduction of hemorrhage volume and neurological improvement. *Neurocrit Care* 2005; **2**(3): 274–281.

20. Miller DW, Barnett GH, Kormos DW, Steiner CP. Stereotactically guided thrombolysis of deep cerebral hemorrhage: preliminary results. *Cleve Clin J Med* 1993; **60**: 321–324.

21. Azarov I, Huang KT, Basu S, *et al.* Nitric oxide scavenging by red blood cells as a function of hematocrit and oxygenation. *J Biol Chem* 2005; **280**(47): 39024–39032.

22. Lee KR, Colon GP, Betz AL, *et al.* Edema from intracerebral hemorrhage: the role of thrombin. *J Neurosurg* 1996; **84**: 91–96.

23. Lee KR, Betz AL, Keep RF, *et al.* Intracerebral infusion of thrombin as a cause of brain edema. *J Neurosurg* 1995; **83**: 1045–1050.

24. Yang GY, Betz AL, Hoff JT. The effects of blood or plasma clot on brain edema in the rat with intracerebral hemorrhage. *Acta Neurochir Suppl (Wien)* 1994; **60**: 555–557.

25. Auer LM, Deinsberger W, Niederkorn K, *et al.* Endoscopic surgery versus medical treatment for spontaneous intracerebral hematoma: a randomized study. *J Neurosurg* 1989; **70**: 530–535.

26. Marquardt G, Wolff R, Seifert V. Multiple target aspiration technique for subacute stereotactic aspiration of hematomas within the basal ganglia. *Surg Neurol* 2003; **60**(1): 8–13.

27. Tzaan WC, Lee ST, Lui TN. Combined use of stereotactic aspiration and intracerebral streptokinase infusion in the surgical treatment of hypertensive intracerebral hemorrhage. *J Formos Med Assoc* 1997; **96**(12): 962–967.

28. Rohde V, Rohde I, Thiex R, *et al.* Fibrinolysis therapy achieved with tissue plasminogen activator and aspiration of the liquefied clot after experimental intracerebral hemorrhage: rapid reduction in hematoma volume but intensification of delayed edema formation. *J Neurosurg* 2002; **97**(4): 954–962.

29. Narayan RK, Narayan TM, Katz DA, Kornblith PL, Murano G. Lysis of intracranial hematomas with urokinase in a rabbit model. *J Neurosurg* 1985; **62**(4): 580–586.

30. Kaufman HH, Schochet S, Koss W, Herschberger J, Bernstein D. Efficacy and safety of tissue plasminogen activator. *Neurosurgery* 1987; **20**(3): 403–407.

31. Montes JM, Wong JH, Fayad PB, Awad IA. Stereotactic computed tomographic-guided aspiration and thrombolysis of intracerebral hematoma: protocol and preliminary experience. *Stroke* 2000; **31**: 834–840.

32. Lippitz BE, Mayfrank L, Spetzger U, *et al.* Lysis of basal ganglia haematoma with recombinant tissue plasminogen activator (rtPA) after stereotactic aspiration: initial results. *Acta Neurochir (Wien)* 1994; **127**: 157–160.

33. Rohde V, Rohde I, Reinges MH, Mayfrank L, Gilsbach JM. Frameless stereotactically guided catheter placement and fibrinolytic therapy for spontaneous intracerebral hematomas: technical aspects and initial clinical results. *Minim Invasive Neurosurg* 2000; **43**: 9–17.

34. Mohadjer M, Braus DF, Myers A, Scheremet R, Krauss JK. CT-stereotactic fibrinolysis of spontaneous intracerebral hematomas. *Neurosurg Rev* 1992; **15**: 105–110.

35. Thiex R, Rohde V, Rohde I, *et al.* Frame-based and frameless stereotactic hematoma puncture and subsequent fibrinolytic therapy for the treatment of spontaneous intracerebral hemorrhage. *J Neurol* 2004; **251**(12): 1443–1450.

36. Schaller C, Rohde V, Meyer B, Hassler W. Stereotactic puncture and lysis of spontaneous intracerebral hemorrhage using recombinant tissue-plasminogen activator. *Neurosurgery* 1995; **36**: 328–333; discussion 333–335.

37. Barrett RJ, Hussain R, Coplin WM, *et al.* Frameless stereotactic aspiration and thrombolysis of spontaneous intracerebral hemorrhage. *Neurocrit Care* 2005; **3**(3): 237–245.

38. Matsumoto K, Hondo H. CT-guided stereotactic evacuation of hypertensive intracerebral hematomas. *J Neurosurg* 1984; **61**: 440–448.

39. Hondo H, Uno M, Sasaki K, *et al.* Computed tomography controlled aspiration surgery for hypertensive intracerebral hemorrhage. Experience of more than 400 cases. *Stereotact Funct Neurosurg* 1990; **54–55**: 432–437.

40. Hondo H, Matsumoto K, Tomida K, Shichijo F. CT-controlled stereotactic aspiration in hypertensive brain hemorrhage. Six-month postoperative outcome. *Appl Neurophysiol* 1987; **50**: 233–236.

41. Niizuma H, Otsuki T, Johkura H, Nakazato N, Suzuki J. CT-guided stereotactic aspiration of intracerebral hematoma–result of a hematoma-lysis method using urokinase. *Appl Neurophysiol* 1985; **48**: 427–430.

42. Horimoto C, Yamaga S, Toba T, Tsujimura M. Stereotactic evacuation of massive hypertensive intracerebral hemorrhage. *No Shinkei Geka* 1993; **21**(6): 509–512.

43. Amano K, Kawamura H, Tanikawa T, *et al.* Surgical treatment of hypertensive intracerebral haematoma by CT-guided stereotactic surgery. *Acta Neurochir Suppl (Wien)* 1987; **39**: 41–44.

44. Tanikawa T, Amano K, Kawamura H, *et al.* CT-guided stereotactic surgery for evacuation of hypertensive intracerebral hematoma. *Appl Neurophysiol* 1985; **48**(1–6): 431–439.

45. Naff NJ, Carhuapoma JR, Williams MA, *et al.* Treatment of intraventricular hemorrhage with urokinase: effects on 30-day survival. *Stroke* 2000; **31**: 841–847.

46. Naff NJ, Hanley DF, Keyl PM, *et al.* Intraventricular thrombolysis speeds blood clot resolution: results of a pilot, prospective, randomized, double-blind, controlled trial. *Neurosurgery* 2004; **54**: 577–583; discussion 583–584.

47. Prasad K, Shrivastava A. Surgery for primary supratentorial intracerebral haemorrhage. *Cochrane Database Syst Rev* 2000; **(2)**: CD000200. Review.

48. Pang D, Sclabassi RJ, Horton JA. Lysis of intraventricular blood clot with urokinase in a canine model: part 1: canine intraventricular blood cast model. *Neurosurgery* 1986; **19**: 540–546.

49. Steinke W, Sacco RL, Mohr JP. Thalamic stroke. Presentation and prognosis of infarcts and hemorrhages. *Arch Neurol* 1992; **49**: 703–710.

50. Bagley C. Blood in cerebrospinal fluid. Resultant functional and organic alterations in the central nervous system. *Arch Surg* 1928; **17**: 39–81.

51. Ellington E, Margolis G. Block of arachnoid villus by subarachnoid hemorrhage. *J Neurosurg* 1969; **30**: 651–657.

52. Kibler RF, Couch RSC, Crompton MR. Hydrocephalus in the adult following spontaneous hemorrhage. *Brain* 1961; **84**: 45–61.

53. Pang D, Sclabassi RJ, Horton JA. Lysis of intraventricular blood clot with urokinase in a canine model: part 2: in vivo safety study of intraventricular urokinase. *Neurosurgery* 1986; **19**: 547–552.

54. Mayfrank L, Kissler J, Raoofi R. Ventricular dilatation in experimental intraventricular hemorrhage in pigs. Characterization of cerebrospinal fluid dynamics and the effects of fibrinolytic treatment. *Stroke* 1997; **28**: 141–148.

55. Todo T, Usui M, Takakura K. Treatment of severe intraventricular hemorrhage by infusion of urokinase. *J Neurosurg* 1991; **74**(1): 81–86.

56. Coplin WM, Vinas FC, Agris JM, *et al.* A cohort study of the safety and feasibility of intraventricular urokinase for nonaneurysmal spontaneous intraventricular hemorrhage. *Stroke* 1998; **29**(8): 1573–1579.

57. Lapointe M, Haines S. Fibrinolytic therapy for intraventricular hemorrhage in adults. *Cochrane Database Syst Rev* 2002; **(3)**: CD003692. Review.

58. Wang YV, Lin CW, Shen CC, Lai SC, Kuo JS. Tissue plasminogen activator for the treatment of intraventricular hematoma: the dose effect relationship. *J Neurol Sci* 2002; **202**(1–2): 35–41.

59. Findlay JM, Kassell NF, Weir BK. A randomized trial of intraoperative, intracisternal tissue plasminogen activator for the prevention of vasospasm. *Neurosurgery* 1995; **37**: 168–176.

60. Varelas PN, Rickert KL, Cusick J, *et al.* Intraventricular hemorrhage after aneurysmal subarachnoid hemorrhage: pilot study of treatment with intraventricular tissue plasminogen activator. *Neurosurgery* 2005; **56**(2): 205–213.

61. Mayfrank L, Lippitz B, Groth M, Bertalanffy H, Gilsbach JM. Effect of recombinant tissue plasminogen activator on clot lysis and ventricular dilatation in the treatment of severe intraventricular haemorrhage. *Acta Neurochir (Wien)* 1994; **122**(1–2): 32–38.

62. Goh KY, Poon WS. Recombinant tissue plasminogen activator for the treatment of spontaneous adult intraventricular hemorrhage. *Surg Neurol* 1998; **50**(6): 526–531.

63. Fountas KN, Kapasalaki EZ, Parish DC, *et al.* Intraventricular administration of rt-PA in patients with intraventricular hemorrhage. *South Med J* 2005; **98**(8): 767–773.

64. Paneth N, Pinto-Martin J, Gardiner J, *et al.* Incidence and timing of germinal matrix/intraventricular hemorrhage in low birth weight infants. *Am J Epidemiol* 1993; **137**(11): 1167–1176.

65. Whitelaw A. Intraventricular streptokinase after intraventricular hemorrhage in newborn infants. *Cochrane Database Syst Rev* 2007; **(4)** CD000498.

66. Whitelaw A, Saliba E, Fellman V, *et al.* Phase I study of intraventricular recombinant tissue plasminogen activator for treatment of posthaemorrhagic hydrocephalus. *Arch Dis Child Fetal Neonatal Ed* 1996; **75**(1): F20–26.

16

Mathematical models of intracerebral hemorrhage and intraventricular hemorrhage outcomes prediction: their comparison, advantages, and limitations

Stanley Tuhrim

Clinical outcomes prediction in rudimentary form began as clinical observations of associations between single characteristics and pertinent outcomes. The advent of computerized statistical analysis made feasible multivariate modeling in which the contributions of several factors to a particular outcome could be considered simultaneously and their colinearity and interactions could be analyzed. As a result, the roles of characteristics that were interdependent could be more clearly elucidated. Broadly speaking, multivariate modeling in intracerebral hemorrhage (ICH) has focused on two types of applications: determining outcomes, such as short-term survival or long-term recovery, and examining the independent effects of specific characteristics (e.g., intraventricular hemorrhage [IVH]) that could help explicate pathophysiological mechanisms and identify potential targets for intervention. Modeling also provides a mathematical means for adjusting for variables that may affect outcomes and complicate the assessment of the effect of another variable, in the context of either an observational study or a clinical trial.

Published nearly 20 years ago, the initial multivariate models addressing outcome in ICH focused on 30-day mortality [1,2] and identified Glasgow Coma Scale (GCS) score, ICH size, and IVH as important predictors of short-term outcome. Since then over 25 similar analyses have confirmed the importance of these variables and suggested a number of others (listed in Table 16.1) about which there is less consensus [3–27]. In general, these models are accurate and easily applied in a clinical setting. There are several limitations however. First, with a few exceptions, these models have not been confirmed by testing

in independent data sets distinct from those from which they were derived. This would be a more significant concern were it not for the consistency of the results of most of these models. Second, it has been suggested that these models have become "self-fulfilling prophecies" [28] because they could be used as tools for triaging patients with little chance of survival to less aggressive forms of care, thereby depriving them of life-sustaining interventions. While this assertion is difficult to confirm or disprove, there is actually little evidence that any of these models are used for triage [17]. The consistency of the factors appearing in the earliest models, developed using data collected in clinical settings naïve to predictive instruments, and those appearing in subsequently derived models, suggests that the impact of these factors predates any triage effect that could lead to a self-fulfilling prophecy. In addition, the similarity of the factors predicting short-term mortality and long-term disability indicates that it is likely that if more aggressive care could prevent some short-term mortality, the longer-term outcome in these survivors would remain poor.

Perhaps the greatest limitation of these models as predictive instruments is their inability to provide relative certitude regarding outcome in the majority of cases. Typically the accuracy of these models is assessed by comparing the predicted likelihood of an outcome (e.g., 30-day mortality) in a particular category of patient with the observed outcomes in a specified population. While the performance assessed in this way has generally been quite good, most patients fall in categories associated with intermediate likelihoods of stated outcomes, limiting the model's practical value. For example, a model may indicate

Intracerebral Hemorrhage, ed. J. R. Carhuapoma, S. A. Mayer, and D. F. Hanley. Published by Cambridge University Press.
© J. R. Carhuapoma, S. A. Mayer, and D. F. Hanley 2010.

Table 16.1. ICH outcome models

	Age	ICH size	IVH +/−	IVH vol	GCS	Location	Hydro	BP	Glu	4th vent
Portenoy [1]	N	+	+	N	+	−	N	−	N	N
Tuhrim [2]	N	+	+	N	+	N	N	+	−	N
Dixon [3]	−	+	+	N	+	+	N	−	N	N
Senant [4]	+	+	+	N	+	−	N	−	−	N
Daverat [5]	+	+	+	N	+	−	N	N	N	N
Broderick [6]	−	+	N	+	+	−	N	−	N	N
Lisk [7]	+	+	+	+	+	−	−	−	N	N
Shapiro [8]	−	+	+	N	+	N	N	N	N	+
Masè [9]	−	+	+	N	+	−	N	−	−	N
Qureshi [10]	−	+	+	N	+	−	N	−	N	N
Fogelholm [11]	−	−	−	N	+	N	−	+	+	N
Diringer [12]	−	−	−	−	+	−	+	−	N	N
Fujii [13]	+	+	−	N	+	N	N	−	N	N
Razzaq [14]	−	+	+	N	+	−	+	+	N	N
Tuhrim [15]	N	+	−	+	+	N	+	+	N	−
Phan [16]	−	+	+	N	+	−	+	−	−	N
Hemphill [17]	+	+	+	N	+	+	N	−	−	N
Hallevy [18]	+	+	+	N	+	−	N	−	N	+
Cheung [19]	−	−	+	+	+	−	−	+	−	N
Fang [20]	+	+	+	N	+	+	N	−	+	N
Leira [21]	+	+	+	N	+	−	N	−	N	N
Roquer [22]	+	+	+	N	+	−	N	−	+	N
Toyoda [23]	−	+	+	N	+	N	N	+	+	N
Franke [24]	−	+	−	N	+	N	N	−	+	N
Schwarz [25]	+	+	+	N	+	−	N	+	+	N
Berwaerts [26]	−	+	−	N	+	−	N	N	N	N
Nilsson [27]	+	+	−	N	+	+	N	N	N	N

Notes: GCS, Glasgow coma scale; Hydro, hydrocephalus; BP, blood pressure; Glu, glucose; N, not determined.

that in a group of patients with a GCS score ≤ 8 and intraventricular extension of a small ICH the expected 30-day mortality would be 55% and, indeed, six of ten patients with those characteristics were observed to die [29]. While this may indicate the accuracy of the model it provides little of practical value for the patients in this category beyond that of a two-sided coin. Put another way, if the predicted probability of an outcome does not differ much from the natural history of the group as a whole for many patients, then that model provides little added value beyond knowing that the patient has had an ICH.

Having established the importance of factors such as ICH size and GCS score in predicting outcome, multivariate modeling can be used to determine if other factors present in a subset of ICH patients are independent contributors to morbidity or mortality, thereby establishing their importance as potential targets for intervention. A primary example of this application is the confirmation of the volume of IVH as an important contributor to short-term morbidity. In contradistinction to primary IVH, which generally results in a good short-term outcome [29], IVH was initially identified by clinical observation as carrying a poor prognosis in ICH. Because intraventricular extension generally occurred in the setting of large parenchymal hemorrhages, confirmation of the independent contribution of IVH to poor outcome required multivariate modeling. The significance of the presence of IVH was initially demonstrated by Portenoy *et al.* [1] and has subsequently been confirmed and expanded upon, so that the volume and location of IVH are now recognized as important contributors to morbidity [15,30]. In conjunction with animal studies demonstrating both the noxious effect of IVH and the amelioration of this effect by its rapid lysis and removal, this has lead to the development and assessment of an intervention (thrombolysis via injection of a thrombolytic agent through an intraventricular catheter).

Prognostic models have also fostered the development of prognosis-based clinical trial methodology in which prognostic models are used to stratify patients. The recently completed International Surgical Trial in Intracerebral Hemorrhage (STICH) divided patients into good and poor prognosis groups on the basis of their prognosis as estimated from an equation based on prior observational studies. For subjects in the poor prognosis group, those with a prognosis score below the median, a favorable outcome included the good recovery, moderate disability, and upper severe disability categories in the Glasgow Outcome Scale, while for the good prognosis group a favorable outcome included only good recovery and moderate disability [31]. While this study, as most others of surgical intervention in ICH, failed to show a benefit of evacuation over conservative management, the use of prognosis-based outcome measures has been advocated as an important advance in avoiding missing clinically significant treatment effects [32].

Another area that has garnered much recent attention is the early growth of ICH. The frequency and clinical significance of early expansion of ICH was recognized as a consequence of the early investigations into the use of intravenous tissue plasminogen activator (t-PA) for acute ischemic stroke [33] but, more recently, modeling of outcomes has lead to the recognition of the importance of early hematoma growth in early neurological deterioration (END)

and the significance of both of these interrelated phenomena on ultimate outcome [21]. In these studies END serves as both an outcome measure (dependent variable) and a predictive factor (independent variable) associated with an eightfold increase in a poor ultimate outcome. Factors recorded during the first 48 hours after admission that were identified as independently associated with END were age, male sex, time from onset, severity as measured by Canadian Stroke Scale score, IVH, and systolic blood pressure. Each of these factors was also associated with poor functional outcome, although systolic blood pressure was of borderline statistical significance. Factors present on admission that were independent predictors of END included elevated body temperature, neutrophil count, and plasma fibrinogen levels, but no CT scan findings, such as ICH volume or location or presence of IVH.

Utilizing modeling in this way provided evidence for a scenario in which inflammation (as evidenced by the association with inflammatory markers) leads to early hematoma growth and through that (and perhaps other mechanisms) to END, which in turn is associated with a poor functional outcome. As a result of this mathematical modeling of outcomes a pathophysiological model can be created that suggests several possible avenues for intervention: reduction of blood pressure and possibly other approaches to the elimination of early hematoma growth such as enhancement of clotting mechanisms. Other studies have confirmed the associations between elevation of inflammatory markers [34] and blood pressure levels [35] and ICH enlargement, further substantiating the potential importance of these hypotheses. Indeed, a prospective feasibility study suggests modest blood pressure lowering may be a safe and effective means of reducing early hematoma growth [36].

Recently, a similar approach has been used by multiple investigators to investigate the contribution of prior antiplatelet use to early deterioration in ICH. Using mortality, early hematoma enlargement, and need for surgical evaluation as outcome measures and adding antiplatelet use to conventional variables associated with these outcomes in ICH, three separate groups of investigators recently demonstrated a significant, intuitively plausible and clinically important relationship between recent antiplatelet use, early hematoma growth, and outcome [22,23,37]. Again, this suggests a possible therapeutic strategy applicable to as much as one-third of all ICH patients [38].

Conclusion

Mathematical models of outcomes in ICH have proved useful in several ways. They have identified consensus clinical and imaging characteristics of ICH that are strongly associated with short- and long-term outcome, including GCS score or level of alertness on admission, intraparenchymal hematoma size, and presence and quantity of IVH. They have fostered the development of predictive instruments that are sufficiently accurate that they could be used to counsel patients and families regarding the likelihood of survival and recovery. These models could also be used to differentiate between those who may benefit from intensive care and those whose prognosis is so poor that they would be very unlikely to benefit from any intervention, although there is little evidence that this is done in practice.

Models can be used to provide a sophisticated historical comparison for data collection in observational studies. Models are also used to define patient groups suitable for specific clinical trials and help to define relevant endpoints that can be prespecified for a particular group according to their expected outcome. Finally, mathematical outcome models have been used to identify specific findings (e.g., IVH, hydrocephalus) or other characteristics (e.g., aspirin use) that may affect outcome and be targets for intervention.

References

1. Portenoy RK, Lipton RB, Berger AR, Lesser ML, Lantos G. Intracerebral haemorrhage: a model for the prediction of outcome. *J Neurol Neurosurg Psychiatry* 1987; **50**: 976–979.

2. Tuhrim S, Dambrosia JM, Price TR, *et al.* Prediction of intracerebral hemorrhage survival. *Ann Neurol* 1998; **24**: 258–263.

3. Dixon AA, Holness RO, Howes WJ, Garner J. Spontaneous intracerebral haemorrhage: an analysis of factors affecting prognosis. *Can J Neurol Sci* 1985; **12**: 267–271.

4. Senant J, Samson M, Proust B, Szeibert J, Onnient Y. [A multi-factorial approach in the vital prognosis of spontaneous intracerebral hematoma]. *Rev Neurol (Paris)* 1988; **144**: 279–283.

5. Daverat P, Castel JP, Dartigues JF, Orgogozo JM. Death and functional outcome after spontaneous intracerebral hemorrhage. A prospective study of 166 cases using multivariate analysis. *Stroke* 1991; **22**: 1–6.

6. Broderick JP, Brott TG, Duldner JE, Tomsick T, Huster G. Volume of intracerebral hemorrhage. A powerful and easy-to-use predictor of 30-day mortality. *Stroke* 1993; **24**: 987–993.

7. Lisk DR, Pasteur W, Rhoades H, Putnam RD, Grotta JC. Early presentation of hemispheric intracerebral hemorrhage: prediction of outcome and guidelines for treatment allocation. *Neurology*, 1994; **44**: 133–139.

8. Shapiro SA, Campbell RL, Scully T. Hemorrhagic dilation of the fourth ventricle: an ominous predictor. *J Neurosurg* 1994; **80**: 805–809.

9. Masè G, Zorzon M, Biasutti E, Tasca G, Vitrani B. Immediate prognosis of primary intracerebral hemorrhage using an easy model for the prediction of survival. *Acta Neurol Scand* 1995; **91**: 306–309.

10. Qureshi AI, Safdar K, Weil J, *et al.* Predictors of early deterioration and mortality in black Americans with spontaneous intracerebral hemorrhage. *Stroke* 1995; **26**: 1764–1767.

11. Fogelholm R, Avikainen S, Murros K. Prognostic value and determinants of first-day mean arterial pressure in spontaneous supratentorial intracerebral hemorrhage. *Stroke* 1997; **28**: 1396–1400.

12. Diringer MN, Edwards DF, Zazulia AR. Hydrocephalus: a previously unrecognized predictor of poor outcome from supratentorial intracerebral hemorrhage. *Stroke* 1998; **29**: 1352–1357.

13. Fujii Y, Takeuchi S, Sasaki O, Minakawa T, Tanaka R. Multivariate analysis of predictors of hematoma enlargement in spontaneous intracerebral hemorrhage. *Stroke* 1998; **29**: 1160–1166.

14. Razzaq AA, Hussain R. Determinants of 30-day mortality of spontaneous intracerebral hemorrhage in Pakistan. *Surg Neurol* 1998; **50**: 336–342; discussion 342–343.

15. Tuhrim S, Horowitz DR, Sacher M, Godbold JH. Volume of ventricular blood is an important determinant of outcome in supratentorial intracerebral hemorrhage. *Crit Care Med* 1999; **27**: 617–621.

16. Phan TG, Koh M, Vierkant RA, Wijdicks EF. Hydrocephalus is a determinant of early mortality in putaminal hemorrhage. *Stroke* 2000; **31**: 2157–2162.

17. Hemphill JC 3rd, Bonovich DC, Besmertis L, Manley GT, Johnston SC. The ICH score: a simple, reliable grading scale for intracerebral hemorrhage. *Stroke* 2001; **32**: 891–897

18. Hallevy C, Ifergane G, Kordysh E, Herishanu Y. Spontaneous supratentorial intracerebral hemorrhage. Criteria for short-term functional outcome prediction. *J Neurol* 2002; **249**(12): 1704–1709.

19. Cheung RT, Zou LY. Use of the original, modified, or new intracerebral hemorrhage score to predict

mortality and morbidity after intracerebral hemorrhage. *Stroke* 2003; **34**: 1717–1722.

20. Fang HY, Lin CY, Ko WJ. Hematology and coagulation parameters predict outcome in Taiwanese patients with spontaneous intracerebral hemorrhage. *Eur J Neurol* 2005; **12**: 226–232.

21. Leira R, Davalos A, Silva Y, *et al*. Early neurologic deterioration in intracerebral hemorrhage: predictors and associated factors. *Neurology* 2004; **63**: 461–467.

22. Roquer J, Campello A. Rodriguez M, *et al*. Previous antiplatelet therapy is an independent predictor of 30-day mortality after spontaneous supratentorial intracerebral hemorrhage. *J Neurol* 2005; **252**: 412–416.

23. Toyoda K, Okada Y, Minematsu K, *et al*. Antiplatelet therapy contributes to acute deterioration of intracerebral hemorrhage. *Neurology* 2005; **65**: 1000–1004.

24. Franke CL, van Swieten JC, Algra A, van Gijn J. Prognostic factors in patients with intracerebral haematoma. *J Neurol Neurosurg Psychiatry* 1992; **55**: 653–657.

25. Schwarz S, Hafner K, Aschoff A, Schwab S. Incidence and prognostic significance of fever following intracerebral hemorrhage. *Neurology* 2000; **54**: 354–361.

26. Berwaerts J, Dijkhuizen RS, Robb OJ, Webster J. Prediction of functional outcome and in-hospital mortality after admission with oral anticoagulant-related intracerebral hemorrhage. *Stroke* 2000; **31**: 2558–2562.

27. Nilsson OG, Lindgren A, Brandt L, Saveland H. Prediction of death in patients with primary intracerebral hemorrhage: a prospective study of a defined population. *J Neurosurg* 2002; **97**: 531–536.

28. Becker KJ, Baxter AB, Cohen WA, *et al*. Withdrawal of support in intracerebral hemorrhage may lead to self-fulfilling prophecies. *Neurology* 2001; **56**: 766–772.

29. de Weerd AW. The prognosis of intraventricular hemorrhage. *J Neurol* 1979; **222**: 46–51.

30. Coplin WM, Vinas FC, Agris JM, *et al*. A cohort study of the safety and feasibility of intraventricular urokinase for nonaneurysmal spontaneous intraventricular hemorrhage. *Stroke* 1998; **29**: 1573–1579.

31. Mendelow AD, Gregson BA, Fernandes HM, *et al*. STICH Investigators. Early surgery versus initial conservative treatment in patients with spontaneous supratentorial intracerebral haematomas in the International Surgical Trial in Intracerebral Haemorrhage (STICH): a randomised trial. *Lancet* 2005; **365**: 387–397.

32. Berge E, Barer D. Could stroke trials be missing important treatment effects? *Cerebrovasc Dis* 2002; **13**: 73–75.

33. Broderick JP, Brott TG, Tomsick T, Barsan W, Spilker J. Ultra-early evaluation of intracerebral hemorrhage. *J Neurosurg* 1990; **72** 195–199.

34. Silva Y, Leira R, Tejada J, *et al*. Molecular signatures of vascular injury are associated with early growth of intracerebral hemorrhage. *Stroke* 2005; **36**: 86–91.

35. Chen ST, Chen SD, Hsu CY, Hogan EL. Progression of hypertensive intracerebral hemorrhage. *Neurology* 1989; **39**: 1509–1514.

36. Qureshi AI, Mohammad YM, Yahia AM, *et al*. A prospective multicenter study to evaluate the feasibility and safety of aggressive antihypertensive treatment in patients with acute intracerebral hemorrhage. *J Intensive Care Med* 2005; **20**: 34–42.

37. Saloheimo P, Ahonen M, Juvela S, *et al*. Regular aspirin use preceding the onset of primary intracerebral hemorrhage is an independent predictor for death. *Stroke* 2006; **37**: 4–5.

38. Rosand J, Eckman MH, Knudsen KA, Singer DE, Greenberg SM. The effect of warfarin and intensity of anticoagulation on outcome of intracerebral hemorrhage. *Arch Intern Med* 2004; **164**: 880–884.

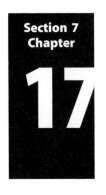

17 Animal models and experimental treatments of intracerebral hemorrhage

Kenneth R. Wagner and Mario Zuccarello

Introduction

Considerable interest has developed over the past decade in experimental studies of intracerebral hemorrhage (ICH) in animal models. This interest has focused not only on the pathophysiological, biochemical, and molecular mechanisms underlying brain tissue injury following ICH, but also on new pharmacological, surgical, and rehabilitative therapies in experimental ICH models. Our goal in this chapter is to focus on the details of producing ICH in animals. We will discuss the two standard methods to induce ICH, i.e. intracerebral blood infusion and bacterial collagenase infusion, and review their pros and cons. We will also review the animal species that have been employed in ICH research. We will describe the advantages and disadvantages of these models and will suggest the "best" models and methods based on the goals of the study, the experimental plan, the desired hematoma volumes, and the expense. Lastly, we will discuss specific mechanistic and therapeutic findings that have been reported during the past several years in these models.

Comprehensive reviews of experimental ICH models have been published by Kaufman and Schochet in 1992 [1] and by ourselves in 2002 [2]. Recently, we updated the subject in a broad overview and evaluation of animal models used in ICH research [3]. For more information about mechanisms of ICH-induced injury, the reader is referred to several recent comprehensive reviews [4–10].

Overview of ICH models and species

Classically, intracerebral hematomas have been induced in experimental animals by directly infusing autologous blood into the brain parenchyma. Using this method, experimental ICH has been studied in several animal species, including rat, rabbit, cat, dog, pig, primate (reviewed in [1] and [2]). The brain region of choice for ICH production has been the basal ganglia, especially in rodents. In pigs, infusions into the frontal white matter enable larger blood volumes to be studied. Recently, several laboratories have employed this method to induce ICH in the mouse [11,12]. In our laboratory, we have developed a large animal (porcine) lobar ICH model in which we infuse up to 3.0 ml of arterial blood into the frontal hemispheric white matter [13]. We have used this model to examine ICH pathophysiology, pathochemistry, and surgical clot evacuation [13–15] (reviewed in [6,7,16]).

A second commonly used model that was developed by Rosenberg and colleagues employs a local injection of bacterial collagenase usually into the basal ganglia [17,18]. Collagenase dissolves the extracellular matrix, which ultimately leads to blood vessel rupture causing ICH. This model, which was originally developed in rats, has been extended recently to include mice. It is discussed in more detail below.

These models have contributed significantly to our knowledge of ICH-induced injury to gray and white matter and to the development of brain atrophy. Specifically, they have provided information on the roles of mass effect and elevated intracranial pressure (ICP), alterations in blood flow and metabolism, and the impact of specific blood components on brain edema formation and blood–brain barrier (BBB) disruption. Currently, these models are providing details of ICH-induced biochemical and molecular events as well as enabling the testing of potential pharmacological and surgical therapies.

Intracerebral Hemorrhage, ed. J. R. Carhuapoma, S. A. Mayer, and D. F. Hanley. Published by Cambridge University Press.
© J. R. Carhuapoma, S. A. Mayer, and D. F. Hanley 2010.

In this chapter we first describe the classical blood infusion ICH models. We then review the collagenase model. In each section we first detail the findings from individual species. We then discuss the brain neuropathological responses to ICH in these models and compare them to observations in human ICH. Lastly, we address the limitations of animal models and discuss their ability to fully capture the complexities of ICH development in humans.

Intracerebral blood infusion ICH models

Intraparenchymal infusion (or injection) of autologous arterial blood has been the traditional technique to generate an intracerebral hematoma. This method clearly does not reproduce the arterial vessel rupture that occurs in spontaneous ICH in humans. However, it does permit the infused blood volume to be controlled, thereby enabling the generation of reasonably reproducible hematoma sizes and mass effects. As described below, blood infusion models have been very useful for studying the pathophysiological and biochemical consequences of the presence of blood within the brain tissue. Some disadvantages of blood infusion models are the possibility of the blood causing ventricular rupture during the infusion and for the infused blood to back flow along the needle track [19,20]. These problems can lead to intraventricular and/or subarachnoid leakage of blood.

To avoid these problems, Deinsberger and colleagues [19] have introduced a double hemorrhage method. In their model, a small volume of blood is initially infused into the brain tissue at a slow rate. A seven-minute wait then follows which allows the infused blood to clot along the needle track. The remaining blood is then infused to produce the hematoma. This method, by enabling blood to clot around the needle shaft, helps to prevent the backflow of blood into the subarachnoid space during the subsequent blood infusion to generate the hematoma. Several other groups have reported studies successfully employing this double infusion approach in rats [21] and in mice [11].

Rats

Rats have been the most frequently used species for experimental ICH studies with the basal ganglia being the most commonly injected site. Among the earliest comprehensive ICH studies were those conducted by Mendelow and colleagues in the mid-to-late 1980s in which they examined relationships between mass effect, perihematomal blood flow, and ICP [22–26]. In addition, to examine the relationships between mass volumes, elevations of ICP, and local perfusion this group also conducted studies using inflatable microballoons [27]. Based on their findings in the rat model that ICH markedly reduced perihematomal blood flow, they concluded that ischemia was responsible for secondary damage after ICH ([28,29], reviews).

It should be noted, however, not all studies support the conclusion that severe ischemia is responsible for perihematomal tissue injury after ICH. Ropper et al. [30] observed a significant but small degree of ischemia (20–30% below baseline) initially. This was followed by flow recovery and even hyperemia in the hours following ICH. More recently, Yang and colleagues [20] using [14C]-iodoantipyrine to measure local cerebral blood flow (CBF), found 50% reductions in CBF at 1 hour after ICH with a return to control values by 4 hours. These workers concluded that although ischemia does occur during the early hours after blood infusion in the rat, the reduction in flow is not severe nor is it the basis for perihematomal edema development [20]. Similarly in ICH patients, Powers and colleagues [31,32] concluded from positron emission studies, that while ICH reduced local blood flow ipsilateral to the hematoma, it was coupled with reduced perihematomal tissue metabolism which is indicative of the absence of ischemia.

It is noteworthy that in addition to these observations that ischemia may be insufficient to cause damage, and that reduced flow appears to be coupled to reduced metabolism, other workers have reported perihematomal hyperemia after ICH [26]. Furthermore, we recently reported increased glucose metabolism in rat perihematomal brain due to glutamate receptor activation [33]. This finding may explain the hyperemia and also the marked increases in perihematomal lactate that we previously reported in our porcine ICH model [14] [16,34].

Mechanisms underlying edema formation following ICH have been long debated. This issue has been resolved by studies in rats (and in pigs) in recent years [10]. These findings have established that coagulation cascade activation and specific plasma proteins are required for perihematomal edema development. Studies by the University of Michigan

ICH group directly demonstrated that thrombin produces edema that is comparable to that generated by infusions of whole blood [35]. Support for this conclusion has come from additional studies both in rat and in porcine ICH models in which infusions of heparinized (versus unheparinized) blood generated very little edema [36].

Additional studies in the rat ICH model related to edema formation have demonstrated that the contribution of the hematoma's red blood cells is delayed. Thus, infused red cells do not produce edema in the basal ganglia until after the first 24 hours postinfusion [10]. This is due to the time required for red cell membrane breakdown and hemoglobin leakage, since infusions of lysed autologous erythrocytes into the rat brain produce marked edema within the first 24 hours after infusion.

The important role of iron and hemoglobin in ICH-related neuronal death [37–39] are supported by a recently developed new hippocampal infusion model. Song and colleagues [40] found that hemoglobin or iron injection versus saline caused marked hippocampal neuronal death. Importantly, systemic treatment with deferoxamine reduced hemoglobin-induced DNA damage, hippocampal neuronal death, and atrophy.

Complement activation and membrane attack complex formation also appear to contribute to perihematomal edema formation since N-acetylheparin, which inhibits complement activation, diminished this edema [41]. Importantly, these results in an animal ICH model suggest that the complement system could be a target for future ICH treatment.

Lastly, studies in a rat cortical ICH model demonstrate the additional toxicity of hemorrhage as compared to cerebral ischemic insults [42]. These investigators showed that extravasated whole blood causes a greater degree of cell death and inflammation than ischemic lesions of similar size [43].

Cats

Experimental ICH in cats has been produced by autologous blood infusions. A report in the late 1970s demonstrated important relationships between hematoma size and location, functional deficits, and ICP elevations [44]. Relationships between neurological deficits and hematoma volume were also observed by Dujovny et al. [45] and by Kobari et al. [46] who demonstrated that increased ICP was the main cause of blood volume/flow reductions shortly after basal ganglia ICH. Dujovny et al. [45] also reported that urokinase treatment resolved internal capsule hematomas and also improved neurological outcomes. Interestingly, these important findings in a cat ICH model support the findings in human ICH where a strong relationship between hematoma size and clinical outcome has been reported [47].

Rabbits

Kaufman and colleagues [48] stereotactically injected autologous blood into the thalamus of rabbits to study the effect of hematoma volumes on survival. Rabbits only tolerated clots that were 3%–5% of their brain volume, a clot volume that approximates a $50 \, cm^3$ hematoma in humans.

A rabbit ICH model was employed in an early study of hematoma removal with thrombolytics by Narayan et al. [49]. Hematomas were effectively lysed with urokinase in 86% of animals. In contrast, only 23% of saline controls showed evidence of hematoma resolution. Urokinase treatment did not increase damage or inflammation. The authors concluded that urokinase was safe and effective even if treatment was delayed for 24 hours. Recently, Zuccarello and colleagues [50] demonstrated the efficacy of stereotactic urokinase administration for human ICH treatment.

Koeppen and colleagues [51] have conducted detailed studies of the perihematomal cellular response in a rabbit thalamic ICH model. Their findings also demonstrated that hematoma resolution after whole blood infusion occurred more slowly than after red blood cell infusions indicating that plasma proteins themselves are important contributors to ICH injury processes.

Other studies in rabbit ICH models have been reported. Gustafsson et al. [52] demonstrated that susceptibility-weighted gradient echo imaging at 1.5 Tesla is highly sensitive in detecting hyperacute parenchymal as well as subarachnoid and intraventricular hemorrhages. Qureshi et al. [53] developed a new model in which autologous blood was infused into the frontal white matter under arterial pressure. This model was used to investigate the degree of injury at 24 hours within and outside the hematoma.

Dogs

Canine models were among the first animals used to study ICH pathophysiology. Steiner et al. [54], in their examination of the brain's tolerance to the presence of a hematoma, found different lethal volumes for specific ICH sites. They concluded that lethal hematoma volumes were due to marked elevations of ICP.

Enzmann and colleagues [55] used high-resolution sonography, CT and neuropathology in a canine parietal lobe hematoma model to examine the evolution of brain tissue injury following ICH. They reported that the sequence of imaging changes in their ICH model showed good correlation with their findings in ICH patients. Early MRI studies of ICH were conducted by Weingarten et al. [56] in a canine model. Based on their studies of venous and arterial blood infusions and intraventricular locations of blood, they recommended that gradient echo sequences would be highly useful in detecting and delineating hemorrhages in ICH patients.

Computerized tomography imaging and histological studies were conducted by Takasugi et al. [57] in an internal capsule ICH model in dogs. These workers identified three distinct stages:

- During the acute stage (< 5 days), homogeneous high density was present on CT at the hematoma's periphery, while histologically, a necrotic layer of perihematomal tissue was present.
- In the subacute stage (5–14 days), perihematomal CT density was decreased with ring enhancement after contrast injection. This corresponded histologically to the presence of immature connective tissue with argentophilic fibers.
- In the chronic stage (> 15 days), contraction of the enhancing ring was noted and corresponded to mature connective tissue with collagen fibers.

Quereshi et al. [58] conducted an important study of the effect of massive ICH on regional CBF (rCBF) and metabolism in a canine ICH model. In testing the hypothesis that perihematomal ischemia develops after ICH and is responsible for secondary injury (discussed above), these investigators failed to find an ischemic penumbra within the first 5 hours after hemorrhage. Ischemia was absent despite prominent ICH-induced increases in ICP and mean arterial pressure (MAP).

In their studies of ICH treatment in their canine model, Qureshi et al. [59] reported that hypertonic saline (3% and 23.4%) was as effective as mannitol in controlling intracranial hypertension with the 3% concentration having a longer effect. These agents did not affect rCBF or cerebral metabolism. This group also demonstrated, in this canine model, that pharmacological reduction of MAP with intravenous labetalol, within the normal cerebral perfusion pressure autoregulatory curve, had no adverse effects on ICP and perihematomal or distant rCBF [53]. Thus, acute MAP reduction within autoregulation limits after ICH is safe.

Monkeys

A few experimental ICH studies have been conducted in monkeys. Pathophysiological studies in vervet monkeys were conducted by Bullock and colleagues [60]. These workers generated hematomas in the caudate nucleus by connecting a femoral arterial catheter to a stereotactically implanted needle. Intracranial pressure peaked at 51 ± 8 mmHg at three minutes after blood infusion and remained elevated through three hours. At one hour, rCBF was significantly reduced in all brain regions. Perihematomal rCBF values were the lowest and were below the ischemic threshold for 90 minutes after the hemorrhage. Segal et al. [61] reported an early ICH treatment study in Macaque monkeys using the thrombolytic, urokinase, which promoted basal ganglia hematoma resorption that correlated with improved clinical examinations.

Pigs

During the past decade, our laboratory developed a porcine white matter (lobar ICH) model and extensively studied ICH pathophysiology, pathochemistry, and treatment [13] ([6,7,16], reviews). The pig has distinct advantages as an ICH model including its large gyrated brain, large amounts of hemispheric white matter, its relatively low cost, and its non-companion animal status. Hematoma volumes up to about 3 cm^3 (equivalent to a 50 cm^3 clot in humans) can be generated in the frontal white matter by slowly (10–15 minutes) infusing autologous arterial blood through an implanted plastic catheter. Furthermore, this porcine lobar ICH model has clinical relevance since:

- White matter bleeds are common in human ICH and occur with almost the same frequency as basal ganglia hemorrhages [62]
- Lobar ICH is the most frequent hemorrhage site in the young [63]
- White matter damage is an important contributor to long-term morbidity following ICH [64,65].

Lastly, white matter has been shown to be more vulnerable to vasogenic edema development than gray matter [66], so this model is especially useful for studying edema-associated injury.

Our previous studies in this model have investigated ICP, blood flow, edema development, the role of blood components, metabolism, transcription factor activation, and inflammatory gene expression [14,16,67] ([6,7,68], reviews). We have also used the large hematoma volumes that can be generated in this model to study neurosurgical clot evacuation [15,69]. We have also used this model to study focal hypothermia treatment [70,71].

Previous studies in our laboratory demonstrated the important role of clot formation, retraction, and plasma protein accumulation in perihematomal edema development [13,16]. While the red cell component of the blood is responsible for much of the hematoma's mass effect, experimental studies with packed red cell infusions demonstrate that it is not responsible for early perihematomal edema [10]. As described above, blood that does not clot also fails to produce significant perihematomal edema in both rat and porcine models [36]. Thus, the early and substantial perihematomal edema that develops following ICH does not result from the mass effect and potentially reduced perfusion induced by the hematoma. Rather, these findings indicate that this very early edema results primarily from the coagulation cascade activation and clot retraction. Clot retraction results in the concentration of the red cells at the core of the clot and extrusion of the fluid/serum components to the perimeter [7,9,16,36,72]. In this regard, confirmation that perihematomal edema development in human ICH is also plasma derived has recently been reported by Butcher et al. [73] based on measurements of increased rates of water diffusion by MRI in ICH patients. Lastly, the importance of coagulation cascade activation in ICH-induced edema development is also translatable to human patients. Specifically, Gebel et al. reported that patients who developed ICH after anticoagulant or thrombolytic treatment failed to develop significant edema despite large intracerebral masses [74].

Recently, Yin and colleagues [75] examined the time course of perihematomal neuronal injury in the pig lobar ICH model to determine the optimal time for surgical intervention. Metabolic changes were examined by MRS, Bax gene expression by in situ hybridization, apoptosis by TUNEL staining, and neuropathology by electron microscopy in the first day following ICH. Both the number of Bax positive and apoptotic cells increased over time and reached peak at 24 hours. Neuropathologically, neuronal damage surrounding the hematoma increased from early hours to 24–48 hours. The authors concluded that since secondary indicators of injury, including apoptosis, perihematomal neuronal damage, and metabolic disturbance, increased from the acute state (3–6 hours) to 24–48 hours, targeting surgical intervention during the early hours after ICH could be effective in reducing the development of secondary damage. Interestingly, we previously observed a rapid and marked increase in lactate in perihematomal white matter after ICH using standard metabolite measurement methods [14]. Hypermetabolism induced by excess glutamate may drive this increased lactate production following ICH [5,33].

We have conducted several treatment studies in the porcine lobar ICH model. We demonstrated that early (3.5 hours) tissue plasminogen activator (t-PA)-induced clot lysis followed by aspiration markedly reduced (by > 70%) both clot volume and perihematomal edema and protected the BBB at 24 hours following ICH [15]. Tissue plasminogen activator liquification of the clot followed by aspiration enabled a significantly greater reduction in clot volume than the 37% reduction obtained by mechanical aspiration without t-PA. In another clot removal study we tested the Possis AngioJet rheolytic thrombectomy catheter [76]. This mechanical clot aspiration device rapidly removed intracerebral hematomas producing an average 61% decrease in clot volumes in approximately 30 seconds. Other treatments studied in this model include inhibiting heme oxygenase by a metalloporphyrin [77].

Bacterial collagenase ICH model

The bacterial collagenase ICH model was developed by Rosenberg and colleagues in 1990 [18] and it has been used by this group (e.g. [78]) and others in numerous ICH studies. In this model, collagenase is locally infused into a specific brain region (generally the basal ganglia) to induce an intracerebral bleed. In this regard, the model mimics spontaneous ICH in humans. The spontaneous, reproducible hemorrhages are straightforward to produce and have volumes that correlate with the amount of collagenase injected. Significant blood leakage does not develop along the needle track. A disadvantage of the model for studying the inflammatory response to ICH is that bacterial collagenase introduces a significant inflammatory reaction that is more intense than that observed in blood infusion ICH models [43,79,80] or following human ICH [81]. Since collagenase dissolves the extracellular matrix around capillaries to produce hemorrhage, this model also differs from the punctate arterial rupture that produces human ICH.

The collagenase ICH model, which has been commonly used in the rat and more recently in the mouse, has shed light on various pathochemical events following ICH. Furthermore, several new experimental treatments for ICH have been tested in this model. Rosenberg and coworkers demonstrated that matrix metalloproteinases (MMPs) contribute to BBB opening and edema development following collagenase-induced ICH and that administration of MMP inhibitors is an effective treatment [82,83]. Furthermore, studies by Power et al. [84] demonstrated that increased expression of specific MMPs develops after ICH and that minocycline is neuroprotective by suppressing monocytoid cell activation and downregulating MMP-12 expression. Tsirka and colleagues [8,85,86] reported that the tripeptide macrophage/microglial inhibitory factor (MIF), when given before as well as after the onset of collagenase-induced ICH, inhibits microglial activation and results in functional improvement. Other reports using this model have described detailed studies of the collagenase dose effect [87], the imaging features and histopathology [79,88], neurobehavioral results and therapy [89–91], and the influence of hyperglycemia [92]. Several drug treatments aimed at different molecular mechanisms of injury have also been studied including: free radical scavengers/spin traps [93,94], neurotransmitter receptor agonists [95,96] and antagonists [97], cytokines and inflammation [80,98–101], and neuroprotectives [102].

In addition to rodents, the collagenase model has also been applied to larger animals, i.e. pigs, by Mun-Bryce et al. [103–105]. In these studies the investigators infused collagenase into the primary sensory cortex in the pig. They have reported on alterations in somatosensory-evoked potentials elicited by electrical stimulation of the contralateral snout as well as changes in DC-coupled potential monitored in the somatosensory region following ICH.

Ischemia-reperfusion hemorrhage model

An interesting and potentially clinically relevant ICH model was described in the rhesus monkey by Laurent et al. [106] in 1976. However, although there have been several citations of this model in clinical reports, there has not been any further work. In this model, hematomas were induced during the vasoproliferative stages of a maturing ischemic infarct. The investigators elevated mean arterial blood pressure at five days after permanent middle cerebral artery (MCA) occlusion causing hemorrhagic infarct conversion. In other interesting studies, previous MCA-occluded animals that were made hypercarbic with 5% carbon dioxide/air at five days post-ischemia, had slowly progressive elevation in ICP and MAP and developed ICH involving the putamen, external capsule, and claustrum, occasionally dissecting through to the ipsilateral ventricle.

Brain pathological response to ICH in animal models

In general, the brain pathological responses to ICH in experimental animal models are consistent with those seen in human ICH [16,55,57,81,107–109]. In animal models, the three stages of perihematomal tissue injury defined by Spatz in 1939 (reference in [108]), i.e., initial deformation, edema and necrosis, and clot absorption and scar or cavity formation, also occur, although at a faster rate. Jenkins et al. [109] have reported an excellent description of the temporal course of these pathological changes in the rat. They observed that regions of pallor and spongiform change due to edema formation develop adjacent to clots within 2 hours. By 6–15 hours, disrupted myelinated nerve fibers and degeneration bulbs were present along with increasing swelling of the corona radiata as edema fluid continued to accumulate. At 24 hours, white matter edema is more marked and extensive. By 48 hours, hematomas in rat and dog ICH models were surrounded by edema, vacuolation, and acellular plasma accumulations, with astrocytic swelling present adjacent to and distant from the hematoma.

Similarly, in our porcine ICH model, we observed that marked, rapidly developing edema with a very high water content was already present in perihematomal white matter by 1 hour after ICH

[13]. This prominent edema can be seen as perihematomal hyperintensity on T2-weighted MRI [16,34] and is comparable to that in ICH patients [110]. In the porcine model, we also observe 50% increases in edema volumes during the first 24 hrs due to delayed BBB opening as evidence by Evans blue leakage [13,16,111,112]. Similarly, in the collagenase ICH model, hyperintensities on T2-weighted imaging are observed surrounding hematomas and extending along posterior white matter fiber tracts [88]. Histologically, by three days, we observe decreased Luxol fast blue staining in edematous white matter suggestive of myelin injury and markedly increased glial fibrillary acidic protein (GFAP) immunoreactivity, indicative of reactive astrocytosis [16]. By seven days, neovascularization is present. After two weeks, continued hematoma resolution and glial scar and cyst formation are consistent in the porcine model to both rodent and human ICH pathologies. A similar brain pathological response occurs in porcine white matter in which only plasma is infused, thereby demonstrating the significance of the blood's plasma protein component in ICH-induced brain injury [16,113].

The time course of inflammation and cell death following infusions of whole blood into the rat striatum have been carefully examined by several workers [43,114]. These workers have also characterized the cellular perihematomal inflammatory response, including the immune cell infiltration and microglial activation. Several workers, including ourselves, examined DNA fragmentation using TUNEL staining [113,115–117]. In addition, molecular analyses of the pro-inflammatory transcription factor, nuclear factor-kappaB (NF-κB), and cytokine responses to ICH have been carried out in other laboratories and by ourselves [6,21,68,71,118–120].

An interesting report that addresses the mechanisms of cell death after ICH has been published by Felberg et al. [121]. In this study, these investigators showed that histological damage from ICH is very prominent in the immediate perihematomal region in the rat. Except for substantia nigra pars reticulata, they found no evidence of neuronal loss in distal regions. They proposed the term "black hole" for this pattern of hemorrhagic damage since it refers to the localized and continued destruction of neurons, which occurs over the first three days as the neurons come into proximity to the hematoma.

Limitations of animal models

It should be noted that despite the strengths and the importance of animal models to study ICH that are described in this chapter, several characteristics of the spontaneous disease in humans are not well-mimicked. Human ICH is linked to advancing age. The incidence of spontaneous ICH is about 25 times higher for those age 75 and above versus those age 45 or below [122]. Thus, current ICH models in young animals do not reproduce the pre-existing degenerative changes in small arteries, arterioles, the neurovascular unit, or the surrounding brain tissue. Additionally, the genetic response capacity to brain injury in humans is now known to change with advancing age [123]. Recently, in an effort to address this problem, Gong et al. [124] compared the ICH response in young (3 months) versus aged rats (18 months old). These investigators reported that brain tissue injury was more severe and the neurological deficits persisted for a longer time in the aged rats after ICH [124]. Additionally, older rats showed greater microglial activation and a greater induction of perihematomal heat shock proteins, HSP-27 and HSP-32. An important goal for future ICH research is to further determine the comparability between the brain tissue responses to ICH in young versus older animals and with ICH in aged human patients.

Another issue that is not generally addressed in animal ICH models is that human ICH often occurs in the setting of longstanding co-morbidities, such as tobacco use, diabetes, and/or hypertension. In addition, ICH patients are commonly being treated with various medicines including antiplatelet, anticoagulant, and statin drugs. These conditions cannot be easily reproduced in animal models. For example, even spontaneously hypertensive rats are not likely to reproduce the often decades-long effects of elevated arterial pressure in patients. Human ICH also varies by race, in incidence overall, and in incidence by age epoch, suggesting important and as yet-to-be discovered variations in genetic susceptibility. Inferences regarding treatment must also be drawn with caution. Our findings and those of others that have demonstrated significant benefits from mechanical and pharmacological interventions have not yet been reproduced in human trials, whether small and focused [50,125] or large and inclusive [126]. There are several potential explanations for these discrepancies with delays in the time to treatment in ICH patients being a likely possibility [127]. However, it is important that future studies in animal models consider their limitations in translating the findings to human ICH treatment. An understanding of the limitations should help to improve the design of future ICH models.

Summary of animal species and ICH induction methods

In this review we have described the various animal species and models that have been employed in ICH research. In addition, we have discussed the several methodologies that have been employed to produce intracerebral hematomas, presenting the pros and cons of the individual species and the ICH induction techniques. In this present section, we have summarized these advantages and disadvantages and have suggested the "best" models and methods based on the goals of the study, the experimental plan, the desired hematoma volumes, and the expense.

Rodents have the advantage of being the most commonly used species in ICH research. The literature on neurobehavioral testing is well developed and the reagents for immunocytochemistry and molecular biology have been extensively studied. The recent development of mouse ICH models enables the study of transgenic and knockout animals, which is a clear advantage for uncovering the detailed molecular pathophysiological events underlying the development of tissue injury following ICH.

Large animals (pigs, dogs, primates) have certain advantages over rodents in ICH research. These include their large gyrated brains with a significant amount of white matter. Large animals enable the induction of greater hematoma volumes to test the efficacy of surgical evacuation techniques or combined surgery and drug treatments. The well-developed frontal white matter in the pig has been especially useful for pathophysiological studies of ICH-induced white matter injury as well as surgical clot evacuation studies. In addition, pigs have the advantage as compared to dogs and cats that they are less expensive to purchase and are considered non-companion animals. Primates are exceedingly expensive to purchase and house and require special facilities and veterinary care.

Regarding the methods for inducing an intracerebral hematoma, as described above, the two commonly used methods are the classical blood infusion method and the collagenase injection method. Neither method exactly models the human event, i.e., sudden arterial rupture with a rapid intraparenchymal accumulation of blood. Currently, there is no model of intracerebral blood vessel rupture to induce ICH. Although both the direct blood infusion model and the collagenase model have their artificialities, the arterial blood infusion through an indwelling catheter described throughout the review is generally considered to be the method of choice by many workers for inducing experimental ICH. The use of the bacterial collagenase enzyme to "dissolve" the extracellular matrix has been considered to be more artificial due to its severe inflammatory response and secondary pathophysiology that occurs in the setting of an already damaged brain parenchyma.

Overall summary

As described in this review, experimental animal ICH models reproduce important pathophysiological events that develop in human ICH including perihematomal edema and alterations in metabolism as well as comparable brain tissue pathological responses. Overall, these animal ICH models are highly important tools to explore new mechanisms underlying brain injury after an intracerebral bleed. The recent publications from several laboratories describing ICH models in the mouse will enable new investigations into secondary inflammatory responses, intracellular signaling, and molecular events that are expected to provide future therapeutic targets for treating ICH. The continued use of a large non-companion animal such as the pig enables studies of ICH-induced white matter injury, an important contributor to patient morbidity. Large animal models also permit studies of surgical treatments that could be combined with pharmacological approaches. There is a continued need for an animal model that would mimic a spontaneous and enlarging hematoma with continued bleeding, a clinical finding that is observed in about 30% of human ICH patients [128].

Acknowledgements

The studies described herein from the authors' laboratory were supported by funding from the National Institute of Neurological Diseases and Stroke (R01NS-30652) and the Department of Veterans Affairs Medical Research Service.

References

1. Kaufman HH, Schochet SS. Pathology, pathophysiology and modeling, In: Kaufman HH, ed. *Intracerebral Hematomas: Etiology, Pathophysiology, Clinical Presentation and Treatment*. New York, Raven Press. 1992; 13–20.

2. Andaluz N, Zuccarello M, Wagner KR. Experimental animal models of intracerebral hemorrhage. *Neurosurg Clin N Am* 2002; **13**: 385–393.

3. Wagner KR, Brott TG. Animal models of intracerebral hemorrhage. In: Bhardwaj A, Alkayed N, Kirsch J, Traystman R, eds. *Acute Stroke: Bench to Bedside*. New York, Informa Healthcare USA. 2007; 112–122.

4. Hua Y, Keep RF, Hoff JT, Xi G. Brain injury after intracerebral hemorrhage: the role of thrombin and iron. *Stroke* 2007; **38**: 759–762.

5. Thiex R, Tsirka SE. Brain edema after intracerebral hemorrhage: mechanisms, treatment options, management strategies, and operative indications. *Neurosurg Focus* 2007; **22**: E6.

6. Wagner KR. Modeling intracerebral hemorrhage: glutamate, nuclear factor-kappaB signaling and cytokines. *Stroke* 2007; **38**: 753–758.

7. Wagner KR, Sharp FR, Ardizzone TD, Lu A, Clark JF. Heme and iron metabolism: role in cerebral hemorrhage. *J Cereb Blood Flow Metab* 2003; **23**: 629–652.

8. Wang J, Dore S. Inflammation after intracerebral hemorrhage. *J Cereb Blood Flow Metab* 2007; **27**(5): 894–908.

9. Xi G, Keep RF, Hoff JT. Pathophysiology of brain edema formation. *Neurosurg Clin N Am* 2002; **13**: 371–383.

10. Xi G, Keep RF, Hoff JT. Mechanisms of brain injury after intracerebral haemorrhage. *Lancet Neurol* 2006; **5**: 53–63.

11. Belayev L, Saul I, Curbelo K, *et al.* Experimental intracerebral hemorrhage in the mouse: histological, behavioral, and hemodynamic characterization of a double-injection model. *Stroke* 2003; **34**: 2221–2227.

12. Nakamura T, Xi G, Hua Y, *et al.* Intracerebral hemorrhage in mice: model characterization and application for genetically modified mice. *J Cereb Blood Flow Metab* 2004; **24**: 487–494.

13. Wagner KR, Xi G, Hua Y, *et al.* Lobar intracerebral hemorrhage model in pigs: rapid edema development in perihematomal white matter. *Stroke* 1996; **27**: 490–497.

14. Wagner KR, Xi G, Hua Y, *et al.* Early metabolic alterations in edematous perihematomal brain regions following experimental intracerebral hemorrhage. *J Neurosurg* 1998; **88**: 1058–1065.

15. Wagner KR, Xi G, Hua Y, *et al.* Ultra-early clot aspiration after lysis with tissue plasminogen activator in a porcine model of intracerebral hemorrhage: edema reduction and blood-brain barrier protection. *J Neurosurg* 1999; **90**: 491–498.

16. Wagner KR, Broderick JP. Hemorrhagic stroke: pathophysiological mechanisms and neuroprotective treatments. In: Lo EH, Marwah J, eds. *Neuroprotection*. Scottsdale, Prominent Press. 2001; 471–508.

17. Rosenberg GA, Estrada E, Kelley RO, Kornfeld M. Bacterial collagenase disrupts extracellular matrix and opens blood-brain barrier in rat. *Neurosci Lett* 1993; **160**: 117–119.

18. Rosenberg GA, Mun-Bryce S, Wesley M, Kornfeld M. Collagenase-induced intracerebral hemorrhage in rats. *Stroke* 1990; **21**: 801–807.

19. Deinsberger W, Vogel J, Kuschinsky W, Auer LM, Boker DK. Experimental intracerebral hemorrhage: description of a double injection model in rats. *Neurol Res* 1996; **18**: 475–477.

20. Yang GY, Betz AL, Chenevert TL, Brunberg JA, Hoff JT. Experimental intracerebral hemorrhage: relationship between brain edema, blood flow, and blood-brain barrier permeability in rats. *J Neurosurg* 1994; **81**: 93–102.

21. Hickenbottom SL, Grotta JC, Strong R, Denner LA, Aronowski J. Nuclear factor-kappaB and cell death after experimental intracerebral hemorrhage in rats. *Stroke* 1999; **30**: 2472–2477; discussion 2477–2478.

22. Bullock R, Mendelow AD, Teasdale GM, Graham DI. Intracranial haemorrhage induced at arterial pressure in the rat. Part 1: Description of technique, ICP changes and neuropathological findings. *Neurol Res* 1984; **6**: 184–188.

23. Kingman TA, Mendelow AD, Graham DI, Teasdale GM. Experimental intracerebral mass: description of model, intracranial pressure changes and neuropathology. *J Neuropathol Exp Neurol* 1988; **47**: 128–137.

24. Mendelow AD, Bullock R, Teasdale GM, Graham DI, McCulloch J. Intracranial haemorrhage induced at arterial pressure in the rat. Part 2: Short term changes in local cerebral blood flow measured by autoradiography. *Neurol Res* 1984; **6**: 189–193.

25. Nath FP, Jenkins A, Mendelow AD, Graham DI, Teasdale GM. Early hemodynamic changes in experimental intracerebral hemorrhage. *J Neurosurg* 1986; **65**: 697–703.

26. Nath FP, Kelly PT, Jenkins A, *et al.* Effects of experimental intracerebral hemorrhage on blood flow,

capillary permeability, and histochemistry. *J Neurosurg* 1987; **66**: 555–562.

27. Kingman TA, Mendelow AD, Graham DI, Teasdale GM. Experimental intracerebral mass: time-related effects on local cerebral blood flow. *J Neurosurg* 1987; **67**: 732–738.

28. Mendelow AD. Spontaneous intracerebral haemorrhage. *J Neurol Neurosurg Psychiatry* 1991; **54**: 193–195.

29. Mendelow AD. Mechanisms of ischemic brain damage with intracerebral hemorrhage. *Stroke* 1993; **24**: I115–117.

30. Ropper AH, Zervas NT. Cerebral blood flow after experimental basal ganglia hemorrhage. *Ann Neurol* 1982; **11**: 266–271.

31. Powers WJ, Zazulia AR, Videen TO, *et al.* Autoregulation of cerebral blood flow surrounding acute (6 to 22 hours) intracerebral hemorrhage. *Neurology* 2001; **57**: 18–24.

32. Zazulia AR, Diringer MN, Videen TO, *et al.* Hypoperfusion without ischemia surrounding acute intracerebral hemorrhage. *J Cereb Blood Flow Metab* 2001; **21**: 804–810.

33. Ardizzone TD, Lu A, Wagner KR, *et al.* Glutamate receptor blockade attenuates glucose hypermetabolism in perihematomal brain after experimental intracerebral hemorrhage in rat. *Stroke* 2004; **35**: 2587–2591.

34. Wagner KR, Hua Y, Xi G, *et al.* Pathophysiologic mechanisms underlying edema development in experimental intracerebral hemorrhage: magnetic resonance studies. *Stroke* 1997; **28**: 264.

35. Lee KR, Kawai N, Kim S, Sagher O, Hoff JT. Mechanisms of edema formation after intracerebral hemorrhage: effects of thrombin on cerebral blood flow, blood-brain barrier permeability, and cell survival in a rat model. *J Neurosurg* 1997; **86**: 272–278.

36. Xi G, Wagner KR, Keep RF, *et al.* Role of blood clot formation on early edema development after experimental intracerebral hemorrhage. *Stroke* 1998; **29**: 2580–2586.

37. Hua Y, Nakamura T, Keep RF, *et al.* Long-term effects of experimental intracerebral hemorrhage: the role of iron. *J Neurosurg* 2006; **104**: 305–312.

38. Nakamura T, Keep RF, Hua Y, *et al.* Deferoxamine-induced attenuation of brain edema and neurological deficits in a rat model of intracerebral hemorrhage. *J Neurosurg* 2004; **100**: 672–678.

39. Wan S, Hua Y, Keep RF, Hoff JT, Xi G. Deferoxamine reduces CSF free iron levels following intracerebral hemorrhage. *Acta Neurochir Suppl* 2006; **96**: 199–202.

40. Song S, Hua Y, Keep RF, Hoff JT, Xi G. A new hippocampal model for examining intracerebral hemorrhage-related neuronal death: effects of deferoxamine on hemoglobin-induced neuronal death. *Stroke* 2007; **38**: 2861–2863.

41. Hua Y, Xi G, Keep RF, Hoff JT. Complement activation in the brain after experimental intracerebral hemorrhage. *J Neurosurg* 2000; **92**: 1016–1022.

42. Xue M, Del Bigio MR. Intracortical hemorrhage injury in rats : relationship between blood fractions and brain cell death. *Stroke* 2000; **31**: 1721–1727.

43. Xue M, Del Bigio MR. Intracerebral injection of autologous whole blood in rats: time course of inflammation and cell death. *Neurosci Lett* 2000; **283**: 230–232.

44. Mohr CP, Lorenz R. The effect of experimentally produced intracerebral hematoma upon ICP. *Neurosurgery* 1979; **4**: 468.

45. Dujovny M, Yokoh ACP. Experimental intracranial hemorrhage: urokinase treatment. *Stroke* 1987; **18**: 280.

46. Kobari M, Gotoh F, Tomita M, *et al.* Bilateral hemispheric reduction of cerebral blood volume and blood flow immediately after experimental cerebral hemorrhage in cats. *Stroke* 1988; **19**: 991–996.

47. Broderick JP, Brott TG, Duldner JE, Tomsick T, Huster G. Volume of intracerebral hemorrhage. A powerful and easy-to-use predictor of 30-day mortality. *Stroke* 1993; **24**: 987–993.

48. Kaufman HH, Pruessner JL, Bernstein DP, *et al.* A rabbit model of intracerebral hematoma. *Acta Neuropathol* 1985; **65**: 318–321.

49. Narayan RK, Narayan TM, Katz DA, Kornblith PL, Murano G. Lysis of intracranial hematomas with urokinase in a rabbit model. *J Neurosurg* 1985; **62**: 580–586.

50. Zuccarello M, Brott T, Derex L, *et al.* Early surgical treatment for supratentorial intracerebral hemorrhage: a randomized feasibility study. *Stroke* 1999; **30**: 1833–1839.

51. Koeppen AH, Dickson AC, McEvoy JA. The cellular reactions to experimental intracerebral hemorrhage. *J Neurol Sci* 1995; **134** Suppl: 102–112.

52. Gustafsson O, Rossitti S, Ericsson A, Raininko R. MR imaging of experimentally induced intracranial hemorrhage in rabbits during the first 6 hours. *Acta Radiol* 1999; **40**: 360–368.

53. Qureshi AI, Wilson DA, Hanley DF, Traystman RJ. Pharmacologic reduction of mean arterial pressure does not adversely affect regional cerebral blood flow and intracranial pressure in experimental intracerebral hemorrhage. *Crit Care Med* 1999; **27**: 965–971.

54. Steiner L, Lofgren J, Zwetnow NN. Lethal mechanism in repeated subarachnoid hemorrhage in dogs. *Acta Neurol Scand* 1975; **52**: 268–293.

55. Enzmann DR, Britt RH, Lyons BE, Buxton JL, Wilson DA. Natural history of experimental intracerebral hemorrhage: sonography, computed tomography and neuropathology. *AJNR Am J Neuroradiol* 1981; **2**: 517–526.

56. Weingarten K, Zimmerman RD, Deo-Narine V, *et al.* MR imaging of acute intracranial hemorrhage: findings on sequential spin-echo and gradient-echo images in a dog model. *AJNR Am J Neuroradiol* 1991; **12**: 457–467.

57. Takasugi S, Ueda S, Matsumoto K. Chronological changes in spontaneous intracerebral hematoma–an experimental and clinical study. *Stroke* 1985; **16**: 651–658.

58. Qureshi AI, Wilson DA, Hanley DF, Traystman RJ. No evidence for an ischemic penumbra in massive experimental intracerebral hemorrhage. *Neurology* 1999; **52**: 266–272.

59. Qureshi AI, Wilson DA, Traystman RJ. Treatment of elevated intracranial pressure in experimental intracerebral hemorrhage: comparison between mannitol and hypertonic saline. *Neurosurgery* 1999; **44**: 1055–1063.

60. Bullock R, Brock-Utne J, van Dellen J, Blake G. Intracerebral hemorrhage in a primate model: effect on regional cerebral blood flow. *Surg Neurol* 1988; **29**: 101–107.

61. Segal R, Dujovny M, Nelson D. Local urokinase treatment for spontaneous intracerebral hematoma. *Clin Res* 1982; **30**: 412A.

62. Kase CS, Caplan LR. *Intracerebral Hemorrhage.* Newton, MA, Butterworth-Heinemann, 1994.

63. Toffol GJ, Biller J, Adams HP Jr. Nontraumatic intracerebral hemorrhage in young adults. *Arch Neurol* 1987; **44**: 483–485.

64. Fukui K, Iguchi I, Kito A, Watanabe Y, Sugita K. Extent of pontine pyramidal tract Wallerian degeneration and outcome after supratentorial hemorrhagic stroke. *Stroke* 1994; **25**: 1207–1210.

65. Kazui S, Kuriyama Y, Sawada T, Imakita S. Very early demonstration of secondary pyramidal tract degeneration by computed tomography. *Stroke* 1994; **25**: 2287–2289.

66. Kimelberg HK. Current concepts of brain edema. Review of laboratory investigations. *J Neurosurg* 1995; **83**: 1051–1059.

67. Wagner KR, Packard BA, Hall CL, *et al.* Protein oxidation and heme oxygenase-1 induction in porcine white matter following intracerebral infusions of whole blood or plasma. *Dev Neurosci* 2002; **24**: 154–160.

68. Wagner KR, Beiler S, Dean C, *et al.* NFκB activation and pro-inflammatory cytokine gene upregulation in white matter following porcine intracerebral hemorrhage. In: Krieglstein J, Klumpp S, eds. *Pharmacology of Cerebral Ischemia 2004.* Stuttgart, Medpharm Scientific Publishers. 2004; 185–194.

69. Zuccarello M, Andaluz N, Wagner KR. Minimally invasive therapy for intracerebral hematomas. *Neurosurg Clin N Am* 2002; **13**: 349–354.

70. Wagner KR, Zuccarello M. Focal brain hypothermia for neuroprotection in stroke treatment and aneurysm repair. *Neurol Res* 2005; **27**: 238–245.

71. Wagner KR, Beiler S, Beiler C, *et al.* Delayed profound local brain hypothermia markedly reduces interleukin-1 beta gene expression and vasogenic edema development in a porcine model of intracerebral hemorrhage. *Acta Neurochir Suppl* 2006; **96**: 177–182.

72. Wagner KR, Xi G, Hua Y, de Courten-Myers GM, Broderick JP. Blood components and acute white matter edema development following intracerebral hemorrhage: are hemolysates edemogenic? *Stroke* 2000; **31**: 345.

73. Butcher KS, Baird T, MacGregor L, *et al.* Perihematomal edema in primary intracerebral hemorrhage is plasma derived. *Stroke* 2004; **35**: 1879–1885.

74. Gebel JM, Brott TG, Sila CA, *et al.* Decreased perihematomal edema in thrombolysis-related intracerebral hemorrhage compared with spontaneous intracerebral hemorrhage. *Stroke* 2000; **31**: 596–600.

75. Yin X, Zhang X, Wang W, *et al.* Perihematoma damage at different time points in experimental intracerebral hemorrhage. *J Huazhong Univ Sci Technolog Med Sci* 2006; **26**: 59–62.

76. Zuccarello M, Dean C, Packard BA, *et al. Minimally invasive removal of intracerebral hematomas: Experience with the Possis AngioJet Catheter in a porcine model.* Presented at the 51st Annual Meeting of the Congress of Neurological Surgeons, San Diego, CA. 2001.

77. Wagner KR, Hua Y, de Courten-Myers GM, *et al.* Tin-mesoporphyrin, a potent heme oxygenase inhibitor, for treatment of intracerebral hemorrhage: in vivo and in vitro studies. *Cell Mol Biol (Noisy-le-grand)* 2000; **46**: 597–608.

78. Mun-Bryce S, Kroh FO, White J, Rosenberg GA. Brain lactate and pH dissociation in edema: 1H- and 31P-NMR in collagenase-induced hemorrhage in rats. *Am J Physiol* 1993; **265**: R697–R702.

79. Del Bigio MR, Yan HJ, Buist R, Peeling J. Experimental intracerebral hemorrhage in rats. Magnetic resonance imaging and histopathological correlates. *Stroke* 1996; **27**: 2312–2319.

203

80. Del Bigio MR, Yan HJ, Campbell TM, Peeling J. Effect of fucoidan treatment on collagenase-induced intracerebral hemorrhage in rats. *Neurol Res* 1999; **21**: 415–419.

81. Weller RO. Spontaneous intracranial hemorrhage. In: Adams JHDL, ed. *Greenfield's Neuropathology*. New York, Oxford University Press. 1992; 269–301.

82. Rosenberg GA. Matrix metalloproteinases in neuroinflammation. *Glia* 2002; **39**: 279–291.

83. Rosenberg GA, Navratil M. Metalloproteinase inhibition blocks edema in intracerebral hemorrhage in the rat. *Neurology* 1997; **48**: 921–926.

84. Power C, Henry S, Del Bigio MR, *et al*. Intracerebral hemorrhage induces macrophage activation and matrix metalloproteinases. *Ann Neurol* 2003; **53**: 731–742.

85. Wang J, Rogove AD, Tsirka AE, Tsirka SE. Protective role of tuftsin fragment 1–3 in an animal model of intracerebral hemorrhage. *Ann Neurol* 2003; **54**: 655–664.

86. Wang J, Tsirka SE. Tuftsin fragment 1–3 is beneficial when delivered after the induction of intracerebral hemorrhage. *Stroke* 2005; **36**: 613–618.

87. Terai K, Suzuki M, Sasamata M, Miyata K. Amount of bleeding and hematoma size in the collagenase-induced intracerebral hemorrhage rat model. *Neurochem Res* 2003; **28**: 779–785.

88. Brown MS, Kornfeld M, Mun-Bryce S, Sibbitt RR, Rosenberg GA. Comparison of magnetic resonance imaging and histology in collagenase-induced hemorrhage in the rat. *J Neuroimaging* 1995; **5**: 23–33.

89. Chesney JA, Kondoh T, Conrad JA, Low WC. Collagenase-induced intrastriatal hemorrhage in rats results in long-term locomotor deficits. *Stroke* 1995; **26**: 312–316.

90. DeBow SB, Davies ML, Clarke HL, Colbourne F. Constraint-induced movement therapy and rehabilitation exercises lessen motor deficits and volume of brain injury after striatal hemorrhagic stroke in rats. *Stroke* 2003; **34**: 1021–1026.

91. Lee HH, Kim H, Lee MH, *et al*. Treadmill exercise decreases intrastriatal hemorrhage-induced neuronal cell death via suppression on caspase-3 expression in rats. *Neurosci Lett* 2003; **352**: 33–36.

92. Song EC, Chu K, Jeong SW. Hyperglycemia exacerbates brain edema and perihematomal cell death after intracerebral hemorrhage. *Stroke* 2003; **34**: 2215–2220.

93. Peeling J, Del Bigio MR, Corbett D, Green AR, Jackson DM. Efficacy of disodium 4-[(tert-butylimino) methyl]benzene-1,3-disulfonate N-oxide (NXY-059), a free radical trapping agent, in a rat model of hemorrhagic stroke. *Neuropharmacology* 2001; **40**: 433–439.

94. Peeling J, Yan HJ, Chen SG, Campbell M, Del Bigio MR. Protective effects of free radical inhibitors in intracerebral hemorrhage in rat. *Brain Res* 1998; **795**: 63–70.

95. Lyden P, Shin C, Jackson-Friedman C, *et al*. Effect of ganaxolone in a rodent model of cerebral hematoma. *Stroke* 2000; **31**: 169–175.

96. Lyden PD, Jackson-Friedman C, Lonzo-Doktor L. Medical therapy for intracerebral hematoma with the gamma-aminobutyric acid-A agonist muscimol. *Stroke* 1997; **28**: 387–391.

97. Terai K, Suzuki M, Sasamata M, *et al*. Effect of AMPA receptor antagonist YM872 on cerebral hematoma size and neurological recovery in the intracerebral hemorrhage rat model. *Eur J Pharmacol* 2003; **467**: 95–101.

98. Del Bigio MR, Yan HJ, Xue M. Intracerebral infusion of a second-generation ciliary neurotrophic factor reduces neuronal loss in rat striatum following experimental intracerebral hemorrhage. *J Neurol Sci* 2001; **192**: 53–59.

99. Mayne M, Fotheringham J, Yan HJ, *et al*. Adenosine A2A receptor activation reduces proinflammatory events and decreases cell death following intracerebral hemorrhage. *Ann Neurol* 2001; **49**: 727–735.

100. Mayne M, Ni W, Yan HJ, *et al*. Antisense oligodeoxynucleotide inhibition of tumor necrosis factor-alpha expression is neuroprotective after intracerebral hemorrhage. *Stroke* 2001; **32**: 240–248.

101. Rodrigues CM, Sola S, Nan Z, *et al*. Tauroursodeoxycholic acid reduces apoptosis and protects against neurological injury after acute hemorrhagic stroke in rats. *Proc Natl Acad Sci U S A* 2003; **100**: 6087–6092.

102. Clark W, Gunion-Rinker L, Lessov N, Hazel K. Citicoline treatment for experimental intracerebral hemorrhage in mice. *Stroke* 1998; **29**: 2136–2140.

103. Mun-Bryce S, Roberts L, Bartolo A, Okada Y. Transhemispheric depolarizations persist in the intracerebral hemorrhage swine brain following corpus callosal transection. *Brain Res* 2006; **1073–1074**: 481–490.

104. Mun-Bryce S, Roberts LJ, Hunt WC, Bartolo A, Okada Y. Acute changes in cortical excitability in the cortex contralateral to focal intracerebral hemorrhage in the swine. *Brain Res* 2004; **1026**: 218–226.

105. Mun-Bryce S, Wilkerson AC, Papuashvili N, Okada YC. Recurring episodes of spreading depression are spontaneously elicited by an intracerebral hemorrhage in the swine. *Brain Res* 2001; **888**: 248–255.

106. Laurent JP, Molinari GF, Oakley JC. Primate model of cerebral hematoma. *J Neuropathol Exp Neurol* 1976; **35**: 560–568.

107. Courville CB. Intracerebral hematoma; its pathology and pathogenesis. *AMA Arch Neurol Psychiatry* 1957; **77**: 464–472.

108. Garcia JH, Ho K-L, Caccamo DV. Intracerebral hemorrhage: pathology of selected topics. In: Kase CS, Caplan LR, eds. *Intracerebral Hemorrhage*. Boston, MA, Butterworth-Heinemann. 1994; 45–72.

109. Jenkins A, Maxwell WL, Graham DI. Experimental intracerebral haematoma in the rat: sequential light microscopical changes. *Neuropathol Appl Neurobiol* 1989; **15**: 477–486.

110. Dul K, Drayer BP. CT and MR imaging of intracerebral hemorrhage. In: Kase CS, Caplan LR, eds. *Intracerebral Hemorrhage*. Boston, MA, Butterworth-Heinemann. 1994; 73–98.

111. Loftspring MC, Beiler S, Beiler C, Wagner KR. Plasma proteins in edematous white matter after intracerebral hemorrhage confound immunoblots: an ELISA to quantify contamination. *J Neurotrauma* 2006; **23**: 1904–1911.

112. Loftspring MC, Clark JF, Wagner KR. A novel duplex ELISA method for quantitation of plasma proteins in areas of brain edema. *Brain Res* 2007; **1162**: 130–132.

113. Wagner KR, Dean C, Beiler S, *et al*. Plasma infusions into porcine cerebral white matter induce early edema, oxidative stress, pro-inflammatory cytokine gene expression and DNA fragmentation: implications for white matter injury with increased blood-brain barrier permeability. *Curr Neurovasc Res* 2005; **2**: 149–155.

114. Gong C, Hoff JT, Keep RF. Acute inflammatory reaction following experimental intracerebral hemorrhage in rat. *Brain Res* 2000; **871**: 57–65.

115. Matsushita K, Meng W, Wang X, *et al*. Evidence for apoptosis after intercerebral hemorrhage in rat striatum. *J Cereb Blood Flow Metab* 2000; **20**: 396–404.

116. Wagner KR, Bryan DW, Hall CL, de Courten-Myers GM, Broderick JP. White matter injury after intracerebral hemorrhage: infused plasma but not red blood cells induces early DNA fragmentation. *J Cereb Blood Flow Metab* 1999; **19**(Suppl 1): S55.

117. Wu J, Hua Y, Keep RF, *et al*. Oxidative brain injury from extravasated erythrocytes after intracerebral hemorrhage. *Brain Res* 2002; **953**: 45–52.

118. Qureshi AI, Suri MF, Ling GS, *et al*. Absence of early proinflammatory cytokine expression in experimental intracerebral hemorrhage. *Neurosurgery* 2001; **49**: 416–420.

119. Wagner KR, Dean C, Beiler S, *et al*. Rapid activation of pro-inflammatory signaling cascades in perihematomal brain regions in a porcine white matter intracerebral hemorrhage model. *J Cereb Blood Flow Metab* 2003; **23**(Suppl 1): 277.

120. Wagner KR, Knight J, Packard BA, *et al*. Rapid nuclear factor kappaB activation and cytokine and heme oxygenase-1 gene expression in edematous white matter after porcine intracerebral hemorrhage. *Stroke* 2001; **32**: 327.

121. Felberg RA, Grotta JC, Shirzadi AL, *et al*. Cell death in experimental intracerebral hemorrhage: the "black hole" model of hemorrhagic damage. *Ann Neurol* 2002; **51**: 517–524.

122. Broderick JP, Brott T, Tomsick T, Huster G, Miller R. The risk of subarachnoid and intracerebral hemorrhages in blacks as compared with whites. *N Engl J Med* 1992; **326**: 733–736.

123. Lu T, Pan Y, Kao SY, *et al*. Gene regulation and DNA damage in the ageing human brain. *Nature* 2004; **429**: 883–891.

124. Gong Y, Hua Y, Keep RF, Hoff JT, Xi G. Intracerebral hemorrhage: effects of aging on brain edema and neurological deficits. *Stroke* 2004; **35**: 2571–2575.

125. Morgenstern LB, Demchuk AM, Kim DH, Frankowski RF, Grotta JC. Rebleeding leads to poor outcome in ultra-early craniotomy for intracerebral hemorrhage. *Neurology* 2001; **56**: 1294–1299.

126. Mendelow AD, Gregson BA, Fernandes HM, *et al*. STICH investigators. Early surgery versus initial conservative treatment in patients with spontaneous supratentorial intracerebral haematomas in the International Surgical Trial in Intracerebral Haemorrhage (STICH): a randomised trial. *Lancet* 2005; **365**: 387–397.

127. Broderick JP. The STICH trial: what does it tell us and where do we go from here? *Stroke* 2005; **36**: 1619–1620.

128. Brott T, Broderick J, Kothari R, *et al*. Early hemorrhage growth in patients with intracerebral hemorrhage. *Stroke* 1997; **28**: 1–5.

Thrombin and secondary brain damage following intracerebral hemorrhage

Guohua Xi, Richard F. Keep, and Julian T. Hoff

Introduction

Thrombin is an essential component of the coagulation cascade and forms immediately in the brain after an intracerebral hemorrhage (ICH). Thrombin may also be formed as a result of prothrombin entry into the brain because of ICH-induced blood–brain barrier (BBB) breakdown [1]. Experiments have demonstrated that thrombin at high concentrations within the brain parenchyma is harmful [2–6]. Thrombin contributes to ICH-induced BBB disruption and acute perihematomal edema formation [2–6]. Hirudin and argatroban, two thrombin inhibitors, reduce hemorrhagic brain injury in a rat ICH model [7–9]. However, thrombin at low concentrations is neuroprotective [10–14]. A better understanding of the two faces of thrombin may lead to potentially novel therapies for ICH. In this chapter, the evidence concerning the role of thrombin in secondary brain injury following ICH is described and discussed.

Brain thrombin, thrombin receptors, and thrombin inhibitors

Brain thrombin

Thrombin, a serine protease, is an essential component in the coagulation cascade. Prothrombin, which is synthesized primarily in the liver, is present in plasma at micromolar levels. Activation of the intrinsic or extrinsic coagulation pathway (or normally a combination of the two) results in the production of factor Xa which cleaves prothrombin to thrombin. Thrombin, in turn, cleaves fibrinogen to fibrin and clot formation.

Prothrombin is present in normal human cerebrospinal fluid (CSF) [15,16]. However, the concentrations are much lower than in plasma. Thus,

Lewczuk et al. [15] reported CSF concentrations of 0.55 mg/l compared to 122 mg/l in plasma. This CSF: plasma ratio is similar to that found for albumin suggesting that CSF prothrombin in normal patients is derived from blood [15]. There is, though, evidence that the brain can be a site of prothrombin production. Prothrombin mRNA is expressed in the neurons and glial cells [17]. It has been reported that prothrombin mRNA is upregulated after spinal cord injury [18]. There is an increase of prothrombin expression in the brain after cerebral ischemia [19] and we have also detected prothrombin mRNA in the perihematomal zone after rat ICH ([20], Xi et al. unpublished data). Such data suggest that thrombin may be formed and contribute to brain injury even if the BBB is intact, particularly since the mRNA for factor X is present in brain [21].

Reports indicate that thrombin may regulate a variety of activities in the brain. Thrombin enhances the synthesis and secretion of nerve growth factor in glial cells [22], modulates neurite outgrowth [23], reverses process-bearing stellate astrocytes to epithelial-like astrocytes [24], stimulates astrocyte proliferation [24–26], and modulates the cytoskeleton of endothelial cells.

Thrombin receptors in the brain

The primary role of thrombin in hemostasis is through cleaving fibrinogen to fibrin, but other important cellular activities of thrombin may be related to thrombin receptor activation. Carney and Cunningham identified thrombin receptors on cell surfaces in 1978 [27]. The thrombin receptor cDNA was cloned in 1991 [28,29]. Since then, three protease-activated receptors (PARs), PAR-1, PAR-3 and PAR-4, have been identified as thrombin receptors [30–32].

Intracerebral Hemorrhage, ed. J. R. Carhuapoma, S. A. Mayer, and D. F. Hanley. Published by Cambridge University Press.
© J. R. Carhuapoma, S. A. Mayer, and D. F. Hanley 2010.

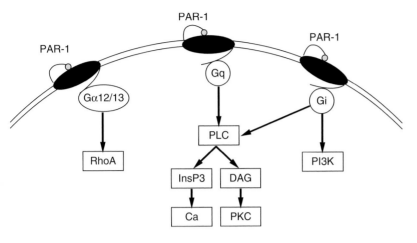

Fig. 18.1 Upstream signaling cascades that result from PAR-1 activation in neural cells. The activation of such cascades can result in a wide range of effects dependent on cell type and dose of thrombin. Effects include inducing apoptosis, neuroprotection, astrocyte/microglial proliferation, neurite retraction, growth factor secretion, and cytoskeletal changes. The mitogen activated protein (MAP) kinase pathway appears to play a key role in several of these events and it can be activated by multiple signaling cascades. See Wang and Reiser [35], Noorbakhsh et al. [42] and Ossovskaya and Bunnet [44] for details. G_i, G_q and $G_{12/13}$ are G proteins that are coupled to PAR-1. PLC, phospholipase C; InsP$_3$, inositol triphosphate; DAG, diacylglycerol; PKC, protein kinase; 3 phosphatidylinositol 3-kinase.

Thrombin receptor mRNA expression is found in neurons and astrocytes [33,34], with both cells types expressing PAR-1, -3 and -4 [35]. Microglia express PAR-1 and PAR-4 [36,37] and there is evidence that oligodendrocytes express PAR-1 [38]. Protease-activated receptor 1 immunoreactivity has been found in human brain tissue [39]. Thrombin receptors are activated by proteolytic cleavage rather than by ligand binding and thrombin receptor-activated peptides are able to mimic many cellular activities of thrombin [40,41]. Recent studies indicate that PARs mediate some of the pathological effects of thrombin and PARs are involved in the pathophysiology of the nervous system [1,42]. For example, PAR-1 mediates thrombin-induced pulmonary microvascular permeability [43]. In addition, Junge et al. reported that brain infarction is reduced in PAR-1 knockout mice and intracerebroventricular injection of the PAR-1 antagonist BMS-200261 reduces infarct volume in a transient mouse focal cerebral ischemia model [39].

Protease-activated receptors can activate a wide range of signaling molecules within cells [42,44]. For example, in neural cells, PAR-1 can be linked to different G proteins ($G_{o/i}$, G_q $G_{12/13}$) that in turn modulate phosphatidylinositol 3-kinase (PI3K), phospholipase C and Rho GTPases, and further downstream signaling moieties [42] (Fig. 18.1). These pathways may regulate many processes, including neurite retraction and other cytoskeletal changes, astrocyte proliferation, apoptosis, and nerve growth factor production [42].

Thrombin inhibitors in the brain

The effects of thrombin in the brain are modulated by endogenous serine protease inhibitors (serpins) and other thrombin inhibitors such as thrombomodulin (TM). Serpins are a superfamily of proteins including antithrombin III. Of the serpins that inhibit thrombin, only protease nexin-1 (PN-1) and plasminogen activator inhibitor-1 (PAI-1) appear to be present in normal brain although another serpin, colligin, can be induced [13].

Protease nexin-1, also known as glia-derived nexin, is found in high concentrations in brain. It is localized around blood vessels and it appears to be the main brain thrombin inhibitor [45,46]. Its expression is not limited to glia since PN-1 mRNA has also been detected in neurons using in situ hybridization. Protease nexin-1 can modulate the mitogenic effects of thrombin, and promote stellation of astrocytes [24]. Delayed PN-1 upregulation in the brain has been observed after cerebral ischemia and peripheral nerve lesion. Plasminogen activator inhibitor-1 is an inhibitor of plasminogen activators, but it can also inhibit thrombin in the presence of vitronectin, which acts as a cofactor [47]. Colligin (also known as heat shock protein 47) is induced in microglia and astrocytes after cerebral ischemia, subarachnoid hemorrhage and an intracerebral infusion of thrombin [13]. The effects of colligin against thrombin may occur through restructuring the extracellular matrix rather than direct protease inhibition.

Thombomodulin, an important thrombin-binding protein, is detected in endothelial cells and astrocytes [48]. It inhibits thrombin by forming a TM–thrombin complex that then induces the activation of protein C, an anticoagulant. Thrombomodulin gene expression is increased in astrocytes after injury and this upregulation might be mediated by thrombin via PAR-1 [48]. Sarker et al. reported that either a recombinant TM or a minimum functional domain of TM reduces thrombin-induced neuronal cell death [49].

Intracerebral hemorrhage-induced injury: the role of thrombin

Thrombin after intracerebral hemorrhage

Normally, after an ICH there is immediate thrombin production that leads to a cessation in bleeding soon after ictus. However, in about one-third of patients [20,50], thrombin production and the coagulation cascade is not adequate to stop bleeding and the hematoma expands for a period. Thus, for example, Brott et al. [50] examined 103 patients with ICH and found that 38% of patients had hematoma expansion within 20 hours. A clinical trial focused on early treatment with activated factor VIIa. It aimed at increasing thrombin production and, thus, preventing hematoma enlargement and ICH-induced brain injury [51]. In phase III, however, this treatment failed to significantly improve patient outcome, although there was some evidence of reduced hematoma expansion.

Thus, after ICH, thrombin has a crucial role in limiting hematoma size and preventing brain injury. However, there is also evidence (outlined below) that thrombin can cause secondary brain injury following ICH and that thrombin inhibitors can reduce ICH-induced injury [2,8]. Therapeutically, it may be possible to separate these beneficial and adverse effects of thrombin because they may occur in different compartments, occur over different time frames, or involve different mechanisms. Thus, in terms of stopping bleeding, the beneficial effects of thrombin are primarily vascular, they involve thrombin-mediated cleavage of fibrinogen (although PAR activation on platelets also plays a role), and they occur relatively soon after the hemorrhage. In contrast, adverse effects of thrombin may be parenchymal (e.g., activation of microglia), they may be PAR-mediated, and thrombin-induced injury may occur hours after ictus (e.g., there is evidence that the thrombin inhibitor,

argatroban, can reduce injury when given several hours after ICH [8]). Although thrombin is produced immediately after a hemorrhage, thrombin remains associated with the clot [52] and may be only slowly released into the surrounding parenchyma. In addition, ICH-induced BBB disruption, which begins to occur several hours after ICH [53,54], will result in an influx of prothrombin and delayed thrombin generation.

Thrombin, blood–brain barrier disruption and perihematomal edema

The primary type of edema after ICH is vasogenic although the cellular form is also present. Vasogenic edema follows an increase in permeability of the BBB and, apart from an open BBB, it is characterized by an accumulation of plasma protein-rich fluid within the extracellular space.

After an ICH, the BBB remains intact to large molecules such as albumin for several hours [53]. Eight to twelve hours later, however, BBB permeability in the perihematomal region increases markedly and continues to rise for 48 hours [54]. Early BBB disruption following ICH is related to thrombin formation since thrombin, in amounts produced by the hematoma, causes significant increases in BBB leakage [4].

Activation of the coagulation cascade plays a key role in early edema formation following ICH [6,55,56]. In an experimental model, non-clotting heparinized autologous whole blood fails to produce perihematomal edema within 24 hours in pigs [6]. The same phenomenon happens in humans too. In the Global Utilization of Streptokinase and Tissue Plasminogen Activator for Occluded Coronary Arteries (GUSTO-1) trial, investigators found that brain edema around the clot is diminished in thrombolysis-related ICH compared to spontaneous ICH in patients with normal clotting [55,57]. In patients with significant anticoagulation, the hematoma appears multilayered on CT scan because of a separation of plasma and erythrocytes. Intracerebral hemorrhage in anticoagulated patients is associated with little perihematomal edema (Fig. 18.2). Reasons for less brain edema around an unclotted hematoma include no clot retraction and less thrombin production stemming from interrupted coagulation.

Thrombin is responsible for early brain edema development after ICH [2,6,56,58]. Intracerebral injection of thrombin induces brain edema (Fig. 18.3). It is known that 1 ml of whole blood can produce about 260 to 360 units of thrombin and intracerebral infusion of five units of thrombin causes marked edema in the rat [2]. Hirudin, a specific thrombin inhibitor found in leeches, inhibits edema formation in a rat ICH model [2]. In addition,

perihematomal edema is attenuated by another thrombin inhibitor, N-α-(2-Naphthalenesulfonylglycyl)-4-amidino-DL-phenylalaninepiperidide (α-NAPAP) [56]. Thrombin-induced brain edema is partly due to breakdown of the BBB [4].

It is still not clear whether or not thrombin-induced BBB disruption is matrix metalloproteinases (MMPs)-mediated. The MMPs are members of a family of zinc-dependent proteases that can degrade extracellular matrix and cause BBB disruption. Thrombin can activate MMP-2 inendothelial cells [59]. Inhibition of MMP reduces thrombolytic-induced hemorrhage after thromboembolic stroke in rabbits [60].

Thrombin, complement activation, and inflammation after intracerebral hemorrhage

Thrombin can activate the complement cascade in the brain. Intracerebral infusion of thrombin results in a sevenfold increase of complement C9 and a deposition of complement C9 on neuronal membranes. Clusterin, an inhibitor of membrane attack complex (MAC) formation, is upregulated and found in neurons after intracerebral thrombin infusion [61]. In addition, the increase of lung vascular permeability after thrombin-induced pulmonary microembolism is mediated by the complement system [62,63].

The effects of coagulation cascade on complement activation are not well studied. However, studies

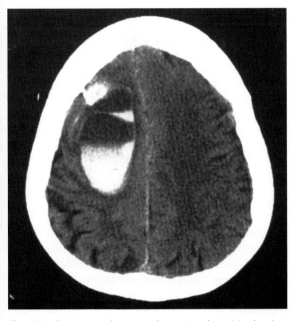

Fig. 18.2 Computerized tomography scan in a heparinized patient with an intracerebral hematoma. There are two blood-fluid levels in the clot with minimal surrounding brain edema (hypodensity ring around the clot). A ventriculostomy had been placed at the site of the ICH prior to coiling of a basilar apex aneurysm. (From Xi and Hoff [107], with permission)

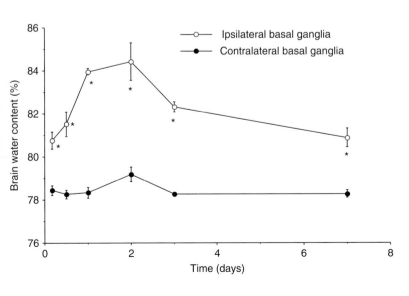

Fig. 18.3 Time courses of brain edema in the basal ganglia after intracerebral thrombin (5 U) infusion. Values are expressed as the mean ± SEM in five or six rats. *p < 0.01 vs. contralateral side. (Data from Xi et al. [108], with permission)

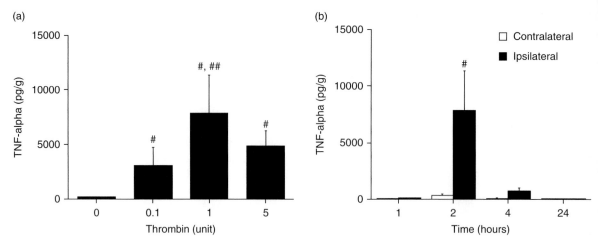

Fig. 18.4 (a) Ipsilateral basal ganglia TNF- content two hours after intracerebral infusion of different doses of thrombin. Values are mean ± SD, n = 6, #p < 0.01 vs. saline infusion, ##p < 0.05 vs. thrombin 0.1 U. (b) Time course of TNF- content in the contra- and ipsilateral basal ganglia after 1 U thrombin infusion. Values are mean ± SD, n = 6, #p < 0.01 vs. other time points. (From Hua *et al.* [75], with permission.)

suggest that there is a very close relationship between thrombin and complement. For example, consumption of complement, which is measured by total complement activity (CH50), is extensive. About 50% of C3 is cleaved during clot formation [64]. Thrombin can cleave and activate C3 [65]. Thrombin-cleaved C3a-like fragments are chemotactic for leukocytes and induce enzyme release from neutrophils [66]. Thrombin can also cleave C5 to produce C5a-like fragments which are leukotactic [66].

Much less is known about the interaction between the activation of PARs and the complement system. It is known that thrombin stimulates decay-accelerating factor (DAF) production through PAR-1 [67]. Decay-accelerating factor is also induced by tumor necrosis factor-alpha (TNF-α) [68]. However, the overall role of PARs in the effects of thrombin on the complement system is uncertain.

Inflammation aggravates hemorrhagic brain injury. An inflammatory response in the surrounding brain occurs shortly after ICH and peaks several days later in humans and in animals [69–72]. Thrombin contributes to the inflammatory response after ICH [73]. Tumor necrosis factor-alpha and interleukin-1 (IL-1) are two major pro-inflammatory cytokines, which are elevated after many central nervous system diseases such as cerebral ischemia and brain trauma [74]. Overexpression of interleukin-1 receptor

antagonist (IL-1ra) by using an adenovirus vector attenuated brain edema formation and thrombin-induced intracerebral inflammation following ICH. The reduction in ICH-induced edema with IL-1ra may result from reduction of thrombin-induced brain inflammation.

Our recent study also indicates that TNF-α levels in the brain are increased after thrombin infusion and ICH [75] (Fig. 18.4). Tumor necrosis factor-alpha recruits neutrophils by stimulating endothelial cells to produce intercellular adhesion molecule 1 (ICAM-1) and E-selectin [76]. Neutrophils can migrate into the brain parenchyma [77], release proteases and oxidases, and cause secondary brain injury. Barone *et al.* [78] reported that exogenous TNF-α exacerbates brain injury and that blocking TNF-α activity, with anti-TNF-α monoclonal antibody or soluble TNF receptor I, reduces infarct volume after middle cerebral artery occlusion in the rat. Tumor necrosis factor-alpha itself also increases MMP production and BBB permeability [79].

Microglia activation contributes to brain injury after ICH [80–82]. Thrombin can induce microglial proliferation and activation in vitro and in vivo [83,84]. While PAR-1 can induce microglial proliferation, it appears that it is PAR-4 that mediates microglial activation and the potentially detrimental effects (e.g., increased TNF-α production) associated with activation [36,37].

Thrombin, cell death, and neurological deficits after intracerebral hemorrhage

Necrotic and apoptotic cell death occurs in the brain after ICH [20,85,86]) and thrombin may play an important role [1]. Thrombin can activate potentially harmful pathways. For example, thrombin induces apoptosis in cultured neurons and astrocytes [87], potentiates NMDA receptor function [88], and kills neurons in vivo [89,90].

Necrotic brain tissue appears adjacent to the hematoma within six hours of the ICH [91]. Necrotic injury may result from either mechanical forces during hematoma formation or chemical toxicity from the clot components such as thrombin. Thrombin results in neuronal death in vitro and in vivo [89,90,92]. Cell culture experiments were performed to determine whether thrombin has a direct toxic effect on brain cells. To ascertain the effect of thrombin on cell viability in mixed rat neuron/astrocyte cultures, different doses of thrombin (1, 2, 5, 10, 20, 50, or 100 U/ml) were added to the cell cultures and media lactate dehydrogenase (LDH; an indicator of cell viability) concentrations were determined 24 hours later. Low doses of thrombin (1 and 2 U/ml) did not induce cell death. However, doses greater than 5 U/ml resulted in dose-dependent LDH release [92].

Apoptosis also occurs in brain adjacent to an ICH in animal studies [72,93–96]. Hickenbottom *et al.* detected nuclear factor-κB protein and TUNEL in cells around the hematoma eight hours to four days after the ICH, suggesting that cells were dying by apoptosis or necrosis, or both [94]. Matsushita *et al.* also found TUNEL-positive cells in and around the clot as well as DNA "laddering." A caspase inhibitor, zVADfmk, reduced the density of TUNEL-positive cells markedly [95]. Recently, ICH-induced apoptosis was also detected in humans [85].

Thrombin formation plays an important role in ICH-induced neurological deficits because thrombin inhibition with hirudin reduces the deficits [7]. In addition, intra-caudate infusion of thrombin caused severe neurological deficits [7]. For example, thrombin-induced forelimb placing deficits recover slowly after two weeks. Injection of saline also caused a slight forelimb placing deficit on day 1, but there was full recovery by three days. Thrombin injection also resulted in significant forelimb use asymmetry. This was present on day 1 and lasted at least four weeks. There were significant differences between thrombin and saline groups in this parameter at all time points. With the corner test, thrombin-treated rats showed an increased percentage of right (ipsiversive) turns compared to saline-treated rats at all time points.

Thrombin exacerbates iron-induced brain damage

Investigations suggest that delayed release of hemoglobin degradation products, particularly iron, is involved in ICH-induced brain injury [20,97,98]. We also found evidence of iron-induced brain injury soon after ICH [99,100]. Intracerebral caudate injections of high doses of thrombin or ferrous iron cause marked edema formation in rats [6,58,101].

In a recent study, we found that the toxic effects of thrombin are enhanced by a low dose of iron. Rats received an intracerebral infusion of holo-transferrin (holo-Tf, iron load), apo (non-iron loaded)-Tf, thrombin, or a combination of Tf with thrombin into the right basal ganglia. The rats were sacrificed 24 hours later for measurement of brain edema and assessment of DNA damage (single and double strand breaks of DNA and 8-hydroxyl-2'-deoxyguanosine immunohistochemistry). Iron distribution was examined histochemically. Holo-Tf, apo-Tf and the dose of thrombin used (1 U) all failed to induce brain edema when administered alone. However, the combination of holo-Tf with thrombin (but not apo-Tf with thrombin) caused brain edema, DNA damage, and intracellular iron accumulation in the ipsilateral basal ganglia. These results suggest that in addition to hemoglobin-bound iron, transferrin-bound iron may contribute to ICH-induced brain injury and that thrombin may contribute to the latter by facilitating cellular iron uptake [102].

Antithrombin therapy in ICH

To examine whether delayed and systemic administration of a thrombin inhibitor could reduce ICH-induced injury, experiments were performed with argatroban. Intracerebral infusion of blood caused a marked increase in perihematomal water content. Intracerebral injection of argatroban three hours after ICH caused a significant reduction in edema measured at 48 hours [8]. The systemic administration of high-dose argatroban (i.p. 0.9 mg/[h rat]) starting six hours after ICH also significantly reduced edema [8]. Nagatsuna *et al.* [9] have also found that argatroban

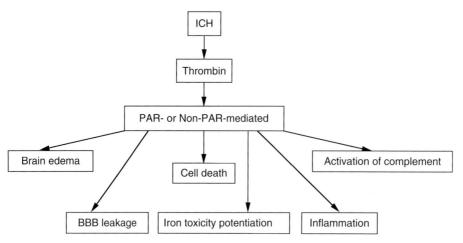

Fig. 18.5 Mechanisms of thrombin-induced brain injury after intracerebral hemorrhage. While thrombin may limit hematoma size, it may cause a variety of potentially harmful effects.

could reduce cerebral edema formation and brain inflammation in a rat collagenase ICH model. In very preliminary data, Hamada *et al.* [103] found that argatroban improved ICH outcome in patients when administered 24 hours after ictus.

The beneficial effects are not limited to argatroban. Intracerebral injection of hirudin, another thrombin inhibitor, reduced perihematomal brain edema and improved ICH-induced neurological deficits [2,7].

Thrombin-induced neuroprotection

Low concentrations of thrombin are neuroprotective in vitro and in vivo. In vitro studies have shown that thrombin protects rat primary astrocytes from hypoglycemia or oxidative stress induced cell death. Thrombin also protects rat primary hippocampal neurons from cell death produced by hypoglycemia, hypoxia, or growth supplement deprivation [11,12]. In addition, thrombin attenuates neuronal cell death and modulates astrocyte reactivity induced by β-amyloid in vitro. The effect of thrombin on both neurons and astrocytes is mimicked by thrombin receptor-activating peptide and inhibited by two potent thrombin inhibitors, hirudin and PN-1 [104]. Furthermore, thrombin pretreatment prevents cell damage induced by a large dose of thrombin in vitro [92].

In-vivo studies have shown that prior intracerebral infusion of a low dose of thrombin (thrombin preconditioning; TPC) reduces brain injury that follows a subsequent intracerebral infusion of a high dose of thrombin, an ICH, or cerebral ischemia [10,13,14]. Thrombin pretreatment significantly attenuated the brain edema which normally follows the infusion of a large dose of thrombin. This effect was abolished by a thrombin inhibitor, hirudin [14]. Thrombin preconditioning may also be an important component of ischemic preconditioning as the thrombin inhibitor, hirudin, can block ischemic brain tolerance [11].

Although the precise mechanisms of thrombin-induced brain tolerance to hemorrhagic and ischemic stroke are not known, activation of thrombin receptors, upregulation of thrombin inhibitors, iron handling proteins, and heat shock proteins in the brain may be associated with the induced tolerance [13,14,92,105,106].

Summary

Thrombin activates multiple pathways during ICH which can have both deleterious (Fig. 18.5) and protective effects. Modulating thrombin activity in the brain may establish novel therapeutic strategies for ICH. However, because of the dichotomy in the effects of thrombin on brain injury, it is essential to delineate the pathways involved in both the deleterious and the beneficial effects of thrombin on brain injury.

Acknowledgements

This study was supported by grants NS-17760, NS-34709, NS-39866 and NS-47245 from the National Institutes of Health.

References

1. Xi G, Reiser G, Keep RF. The role of thrombin and thrombin receptors in ischemic, hemorrhagic and traumatic brain injury: deleterious or protective? *J Neurochem* 2003; **84**: 3–9.

2. Lee KR, Colon GP, Betz AL, *et al*. Edema from intracerebral hemorrhage: the role of thrombin. *J Neurosurg* 1996; **84**: 91–96.

3. Lee KR, Drury I, Vitarbo E, Hoff JT. Seizures induced by intracerebral injection of thrombin: a model of intracerebral hemorrhage. *J Neurosurg* 1997; **87**: 73–78.

4. Lee KR, Kawai N, Kim S, Sagher O, Hoff JT. Mechanisms of edema formation after intracerebral hemorrhage: effects of thrombin on cerebral blood flow, blood-brain barrier permeability, and cell survival in a rat model. *J Neurosurg* 1997; **86**: 272–278.

5. Nishino A, Suzuki M, Ohtani H, *et al*. Thrombin may contribute to the pathophysiology of central nervous system injury. *J Neurotrauma* 1993; **10**: 167–179.

6. Xi G, Wagner KR, Keep RF, *et al*. The role of blood clot formation on early edema development following experimental intracerebral hemorrhage. *Stroke* 1998; **29**: 2580–2586.

7. Hua Y, Schallert T, Keep RF, *et al*. Behavioral tests after intracerebral hemorrhage in the rat. *Stroke* 2002; **33**: 2478–2484.

8. Kitaoka T, Hua Y, Xi G, Hoff JT, Keep RF. Delayed argatroban treatment reduces edema in a rat model of intracerebral hemorrhage. *Stroke* 2002; **33**: 3012–3018.

9. Nagatsuna T, Nomura S, Suehiro E, *et al*. Systemic administration of argatroban reduces secondary brain damage in a rat model of intracerebral hemorrhage: histopathological assessment. *Cerebrovasc Dis* 2005; **19**: 192–200.

10. Masada T, Xi G, Hua Y, Keep RF. The effects of thrombin preconditioning on focal cerebral ischemia in rats. *Brain Res* 2000; **867**: 173–179.

11. Striggow F, Riek M, Breder J, *et al*. The protease thrombin is an endogenous mediator of hippocampal neuroprotection against ischemia at low concentrations but causes degeneration at high concentrations. *Proc Natl Acad Sci USA* 2000; **97**: 2264–2269.

12. Vaughan PJ, Pike CJ, Cotman CW, Cunningham DD. Thrombin receptor activation protects neurons and astrocytes from cell death produced by environmental insults. *J Neurosci* 1995; **15**: 5389–5401.

13. Xi G, Hua Y, Keep RF, Hoff JT. Induction of colligin may attenuate brain edema following intracerebral hemorrhage. *Acta Neurochir Suppl* 2000; **76**: 501–505.

14. Xi G, Keep RF, Hua Y, Xiang JM, Hoff JT. Attenuation of thrombin-induced brain edema by cerebral thrombin preconditioning. *Stroke* 1999; **30**: 1247–1255.

15. Lewczuk P, Reiber H, Ehrenreich H. Prothrombin in normal human cerebrospinal fluid originates from the blood. *Neurochem Res* 1998; **23**: 1027–1030.

16. Smirnova IV, Salazar A, Arnold PM, *et al*. Thrombin and its precursor in human cerebrospinal fluid. *Thromb Haemost* 1997; **78**: 1473–1479.

17. Dihanich M, Kaser M, Reinhard E, Cunningham D, Monard D. Prothrombin mRNA is expressed by cells of the nervous system. *Neuron* 1991; **6**: 575–581.

18. Citron BA, Smirnova IV, Arnold PM, Festoff BW. Upregulation of neurotoxic serine proteases, prothrombin, and protease-activated receptor 1 early after spinal cord injury. *J Neurotrauma* 2000; **17**: 1191–1203.

19. Hua Y, Wu J, Keep RF, Hoff JT, Xi G. Thrombin exacerbates brain edema in focal cerebral ischemia. *Acta Neurochir Suppl* 2003; **86**: 163–166.

20. Xi G, Keep RF, Hoff JT. Mechanisms of brain injury after intracerebral hemorrhage. *Lancet Neurol* 2005; **5**(1): 56–63.

21. Shikamoto Y, Morita T. Expression of factor X in both the rat brain and cells of the central nervous system. *FEBS Lett* 1999; **463**: 387–389.

22. Neveu I, Jehan F, Jandrot-Perrus M, Wion D, Brachet P. Enhancement of the synthesis and secretion of nerve growth factor in primary cultures of glial cells by proteases: a possible involvement of thrombin. *J Neurochem* 1993; **60**: 858–867.

23. Gurwitz D, Cunningham DD. Thrombin modulates and reverses neuroblastoma neurite outgrowth. *Proc Natl Acad Sci U S A* 1988; **85**: 3440–3444.

24. Cavanaugh KP, Gurwitz D, Cunningham DD, Bradshaw RA. Reciprocal modulation of astrocyte stellation by thrombin and protease nexin-1. *J Neurochem* 1990; **54**: 1735–1743.

25. Loret C, Sensenbrenner M, Labourdette G. Differential phenotypic expression induced in cultured rat astroblasts by acidic fibroblast growth factor, epidermal growth factor, and thrombin. *J Biol Chem* 1989; **264**: 8319–8327.

26. Perraud F, Besnard F, Sensenbrenner M, Labourdette G. Thrombin is a potent mitogen for rat astroblasts but not for oligodendroblasts and neuroblasts in primary culture. *Int J Dev Neurosci* 1987; **5**: 181–188.

27. Carney DH, Cunningham DD. Role of specific cell surface receptors in thrombin-stimulated cell division. *Cell* 1978; **15**: 1341–1349.

28. Rasmussen UB, Vouret-Craviari V, Jallat S, *et al*. cDNA cloning and expression of a hamster

alpha-thrombin receptor coupled to Ca2+ mobilization. *FEBS Lett* 1991; **288**: 123–128.

29. Vu TK, Hung DT, Wheaton VI, Coughlin SR. Molecular cloning of a functional thrombin receptor reveals a novel proteolytic mechanism of receptor activation. *Cell* 1991; **64**: 1057–1068.

30. Coughlin SR. How the protease thrombin talks to cells. *Proc Natl Acad Sci U S A* 1999; **96**: 11023–11027.

31. Coughlin SR. Thrombin signalling and protease-activated receptors. *Nature* 2000; **407**: 258–264.

32. Dery O, Corvera CU, Steinhoff M, Bunnett NW. Proteinase-activated receptors: novel mechanisms of signaling by serine proteases. *Am J Physiol* 1998; **274**: C1429–1452.

33. Niclou S, Suidan HS, Brown-Luedi M, Monard D. Expression of the thrombin receptor mRNA in rat brain. *Cell Mol Biol* 1994; **40**: 421–428.

34. Weinstein JR, Gold SJ, Cunningham DD, Gall CM. Cellular localization of thrombin receptor mRNA in rat brain: expression by mesencephalic dopaminergic neurons and codistribution with prothrombin mRNA. *J Neurosci* 1995; **15**: 2906–2919.

35. Wang H, Reiser G. Thrombin signaling in the brain: the role of protease-activated receptors. *Biol Chem* 2003; **384**: 193–202.

36. Suo Z, Wu M, Ameenuddin S, *et al.* Participation of protease-activated receptor-1 in thrombin-induced microglial activation. *J Neurochem* 2002; **80**: 655–666.

37. Suo Z, Wu M, Citron BA, Gao C, Festoff BW. Persistent protease-activated receptor 4 signaling mediates thrombin-induced microglial activation. *J Biol Chem* 2003; **278**: 31177–31183.

38. Wang Y, Richter-Landsberg C, Reiser G. Expression of protease-activated receptors (PARs) in OLN-93 oligodendroglial cells and mechanism of PAR-1-induced calcium signaling. *Neuroscience* 2004; **126**: 69–82.

39. Junge CE, Sugawara T, Mannaioni G, *et al.* The contribution of protease-activated receptor 1 to neuronal damage caused by transient focal cerebral ischemia. *Proc Natl Acad Sci U S A* 2003; **100**: 13019–13024.

40. Debeir T, Benavides J, Vige X. Dual effects of thrombin and a 14-amino acid peptide agonist of the thrombin receptor on septal cholinergic neurons. *Brain Res* 1996; **708**: 159–166.

41. Suidan HS, Stone SR, Hemmings BA, Monard D. Thrombin causes neurite retraction in neuronal cells through activation of cell surface receptors. *Neuron* 1992; **8**: 363–375.

42. Noorbakhsh F, Vergnolle N, Hollenberg MD, Power C. Proteinase-activated receptors in the nervous system. *Nat Rev Neurosci* 2003; **4**: 981–990.

43. Vogel SM, Gao X, Mehta D, *et al.* Abrogation of thrombin-induced increase in pulmonary microvascular permeability in PAR-1 knockout mice. *Physiol Genomics* 2000; **4**: 137–145.

44. Ossovskaya VS, Bunnett NW. Protease-activated receptors: contribution to physiology and disease. *Physiol Rev* 2004; **84**: 579–621.

45. Guenther J, Nick H, Monard D. A glia-derived neurite-promoting factor with protease inhibitory activity. *EMBO J* 1985; **4**: 1963–1966.

46. Stone SR, Nick H, Hofsteenge J, Monard D. Glial-derived neurite-promoting factor is a slow-binding inhibitor of trypsin, thrombin, and urokinase. *Arch Biochem Biophys* 1987; **252**: 237–244.

47. Mutch NJ, Robbie LA, Booth NA. Human thrombi contain an abundance of active thrombin. *Thromb Haemost* 2001; **86**: 1028–1034.

48. Pindon A, Berry M, Hantai D. Thrombomodulin as a new marker of lesion-induced astrogliosis: involvement of thrombin through the G-protein-coupled protease-activated receptor-1. *J Neurosci* 2000; **20**: 2543–2550.

49. Sarker KP, Abeyama K, Nishi J, *et al.* Inhibition of thrombin-induced neuronal cell death by recombinant thrombomodulin and E5510, a synthetic thrombin receptor signaling inhibitor. *Thromb Haemost* 1999; **82**: 1071–1077.

50. Brott T, Broderick J, Kothari R, *et al.* Early hemorrhage growth in patients with intracerebral hemorrhage. *Stroke* 1997; **28**: 1–5.

51. Mayer SA, Brun NC, Begtrup K, *et al.* Recombinant Activated Factor VII Intracerebral Hemorrhage Trial Investigators. Recombinant activated factor VII for acute intracerebral hemorrhage. *N Engl J Med* 2005; **352**: 777–785.

52. Hsieh K. Thrombin interaction with fibrin polymerization sites. *Thromb Res* 1997; **86**: 301–316.

53. Wagner KR, Xi G, Hua Y, *et al.* Lobar intracerebral hemorrhage model in pigs: rapid edema development in perihematomal white matter. *Stroke* 1996; **27**: 490–497.

54. Yang GY, Betz AL, Chenevert TL, Brunberg JA, Hoff JT. Experimental intracerebral hemorrhage: relationship between brain edema, blood flow, and blood-brain barrier permeability in rats. *J Neurosurg* 1994; **81**: 93–102.

55. Gebel JM, Brott TG, Sila CA, *et al.* Decreased perihematomal edema in thrombolysis-related intracerebral hemorrhage compared with spontaneous intracerebral hemorrhage. *Stroke* 2000; **31**: 596–600.

56. Lee KR, Betz AL, Kim S, Keep RF, Hoff JT. The role of the coagulation cascade in brain edema formation after

intracerebral hemorrhage. *Acta Neurochir (wien)* 1996; **138**: 396–400; discussion 400–391.

57. Gebel JM, Sila CA, Sloan MA, *et al.* Thrombolysis-related intracranial hemorrhage: a radiographic analysis of 244 cases from the GUSTO-1 trial with clinical correlation. Global Utilization of Streptokinase and Tissue Plasminogen Activator for Occluded Coronary Arteries. *Stroke* 1998; **29**: 563–569.

58. Lee KR, Betz AL, Keep RF, *et al.* Intracerebral infusion of thrombin as a cause of brain edema. *J Neurosurg* 1995; **83**: 1045–1050.

59. Nguyen M, Arkell J, Jackson CJ. Thrombin rapidly and efficiently activates gelatinase A in human microvascular endothelial cells via a mechanism independent of active MT1 matrix metalloproteinase. *Lab Invest* 1999; **79**: 467–475.

60. Lapchak PA, Chapman DF, Zivin JA. Metalloproteinase inhibition reduces thrombolytic (tissue plasminogen activator)-induced hemorrhage after thromboembolic stroke. *Stroke* 2000; **31**: 3034–3040.

61. Gong Y, Xi G, Keep R, Hoff J, Hua Y. Complement inhibition attenuates brain edema and neurological deficits induced by thrombin. *Acta Neurochir Suppl* 2005; **95**: 389–392.

62. Johnson A, Blumenstock FA, Malik AB. Effect of complement depletion on lung fluid balance after thrombin. *J Appl Physiol* 1983; **55**: 1480–1485.

63. Johnson A, Lo SK, Blumenstock FB, Malik AB. CVF-induced decomplementation: effect on lung transvascular protein flux after thrombin. *J Appl Physiol* 1987; **62**: 863–869.

64. Fareed J, Messmore HL, Fenton JW, Brinkhous KM. *Perspectives in Hemostasis.* New York, Pergamon Press, 1981.

65. Bokisch VA, Muller-Eberhard HJ, Cochrane CG. Isolation of a fragment (C3a) of the third component of human complement containing anaphylatoxin and chemotactic activity and description of an anaphylatoxin inactivator of human serum. *J Exp Med* 1969; **129**: 1109–1130.

66. Hugli TE. Complement factors and inflammation: effects of thrombin on components of C3 and C5. In: Lundblad RL, Fenton JW, Mann KG, eds. *Chemistry and Biology of Thrombin.* Ann Arbor, Ann Arbor Science Publishers. 1977; 345–360.

67. Lidington EA, Haskard DO, Mason JC. Induction of decay-accelerating factor by thrombin through a protease-activated receptor 1 and protein kinase C-dependent pathway protects vascular endothelial cells from complement-mediated injury. *Blood* 2000; **96**: 2784–2792.

68. Ahmad SR, Lidington EA, Ohta R, *et al.* Decay-accelerating factor induction by tumour necrosis factor-alpha, through a phosphatidylinositol-3 kinase and protein kinase C-dependent pathway, protects murine vascular endothelial cells against complement deposition. *Immunology* 2003; **110**: 258–268.

69. Enzmann DR, Britt RH, Lyons BE, Buxton JL, Wilson DA. Natural history of experimental intracerebral hemorrhage: sonography, computed tomography and neuropathology. *AJNR Am J Neuroradiol* 1981; **2**: 517–526.

70. Gong C, Hoff JT, Keep RF. Acute inflammatory reaction following experimental intracerebral hemorrhage. *Brain Res* 2000; **871**: 57–65.

71. Jenkins A, Maxwell W, Graham D. Experimental intracerebral hematoma in the rat: sequential light microscopic changes. *Neuropathol Appl Neurobiol* 1989; **15**: 477–486.

72. Xue M, Del Bigio MR. Intracerebral injection of autologous whole blood in rats: time course of inflammation and cell death. *Neurosci Lett* 2000; **283**: 230–232.

73. Masada T, Hua Y, Xi G, *et al.* Overexpression of interleukin-1 receptor antagonist reduces brain edema induced by intracerebral hemorrhage and thrombin. *Acta Neurochir Suppl* 2003; **86**: 463–467.

74. Barone FC, Feuerstein GZ. Inflammatory mediators and stroke: new opportunities for novel therapeutics. *J Cereb Blood Flow Metab* 1999; **19**: 819–834.

75. Hua Y, Wu J, Keep R, *et al.* Tumor necrosis factor-alpha increases in the brain after intracerebral hemorrhage and thrombin stimulation. *Neurosurgery* 2005; **58**(3): 542–550.

76. Thorp KM, Southern C, Bird IN, Matthews N. Tumour necrosis factor induction of ELAM-1 and ICAM-1 on human umbilical vein endothelial cells–analysis of tumour necrosis factor-receptor interactions *Cytokine* 1992; **4**: 313–319. Erratum in: *Cytokine* 1992; **4**(5): following 409.

77. Del Bigio MR, Yan HJ, Buist R, Peeling J. Experimental intracerebral hemorrhage in rats. Magnetic resonance imaging and histopathological correlates. *Stroke* 1996; **27**: 2312–2319; discussion 2319–2320.

78. Barone FC, Arvin B, White RF, *et al.* Tumor necrosis factor-alpha. A mediator of focal ischemic brain injury. *Stroke* 1997; **28**: 1233–1244.

79. Rosenberg GA, Estrada EY, Dencoff JE, Stetler-Stevenson WG. Tumor necrosis factor-alpha-induced gelatinase B causes delayed opening of the blood-brain barrier: an expanded therapeutic window. *Brain Res* 1995; **703**: 151–155.

80. Gong Y, Hua Y, Keep RF, Hoff JT, Xi G. Intracerebral hemorrhage: effects of aging on brain edema and neurological deficits. *Stroke* 2004; **35**: 2571–2575.

81. Wang J, Rogove AD, Tsirka AE, Tsirka SE. Protective role of tuftsin fragment 1–3 in an animal model of intracerebral hemorrhage. *Ann Neurol* 2003; **54**: 655–664.

82. Wang J, Tsirka SE. Tuftsin fragment 1–3 is beneficial when delivered after the induction of intracerebral hemorrhage. *Stroke* 2005; **36**: 613–618.

83. Choi SH, Lee da Y, Kim SU, Jin BK. Thrombin-induced oxidative stress contributes to the death of hippocampal neurons in vivo: role of microglial NADPH oxidase. *J Neurosci* 2005; **25**: 4082–4090.

84. Moller T, Hanisch UK, Ransom BR. Thrombin-induced activation of cultured rodent microglia. *J Neurochem* 2000; **75**: 1539–1547.

85. Qureshi AI, Suri MF, Ostrow PT, *et al.* Apoptosis as a form of cell death in intracerebral hemorrhage. *Neurosurgery* 2003; **52**: 1041–1047.

86. Qureshi AI, Tuhrim S, Broderick JP, *et al.* Spontaneous intracerebral hemorrhage. *N Engl J Med* 2001; **344**: 1450–1460.

87. Donovan FM, Pike CJ, Cotman CW, Cunningham DD. Thrombin induces apoptosis in cultured neurons and astrocytes via a pathway requiring tyrosine kinase and RhoA activities. *J Neurosci* 1997; **17**: 5316–5326.

88. Gingrich MB, Junge CE, Lyuboslavsky P, Traynelis SF. Potentiation of NMDA receptor function by the serine protease thrombin. *J Neurosci* 2000; **20**: 4582–4595.

89. Choi SH, Joe EH, Kim SU, Jin BK. Thrombin-induced microglial activation produces degeneration of nigral dopaminergic neurons in vivo. *J Neurosci* 2003; **23**: 5877–5886.

90. Choi SH, Lee da Y, Ryu JK, *et al.* Thrombin induces nigral dopaminergic neurodegeneration in vivo by altering expression of death-related proteins. *Neurobiol Dis* 2003; **14**: 181–193.

91. Suzuki J, Ebina T. Sequential changes in tissue surrounding ICH. In: Pia HW, Longmaid C, Zierski J, eds. *Spontaneous Intracerebral Hematomas*. Berlin, Springer. 1980; 121–128.

92. Jiang Y, Wu J, Hua Y, *et al.* Thrombin-receptor activation and thrombin-induced brain tolerance. *J Cereb Blood Flow Metab* 2002; **22**: 404–410.

93. Gong C, Boulis N, Qian J. Intracerebral hemorrhage-induced neuronal death. *Neurosurgery* 2001; **48**: 875–883.

94. Hickenbottom SL, Grotta JC, Strong R, Denner LA, Aronowski J. Nuclear factor-kappaB and cell death after experimental intracerebral hemorrhage in rats. *Stroke* 1999; **30**: 2472–2477; discussion 2477–2478.

95. Matsushita K, Meng W, Wang X, *et al.* Evidence for apoptosis after intercerebral hemorrhage in rat striatum. *J Cereb Blood Flow Metab* 2000; **20**: 396–404.

96. Qureshi AI, Ling GS, Khan J, *et al.* Quantitative analysis of injured, necrotic, and apoptotic cells in a new experimental model of intracerebral hemorrhage. *Crit Care Med* 2001; **29**: 152–157.

97. Hua Y, Nakamura T, Keep R, *et al.* Long-term effects of experimental intracerebral hemorrhage: the role of iron. *J Neurosurg* 2005; **104**(2): 305–312.

98. Xi G, Keep RF, Hoff JT. Erythrocytes and delayed brain edema formation following intracerebral hemorrhage in rats. *J Neurosurg* 1998; **89**: 991–996.

99. Nakamura T, Keep R, Hua Y, *et al.* Deferoxamine-induced attenuation of brain edema and neurological deficits in a rat model of intracerebral hemorrhage. *J Neurosurg* 2004; **100**: 672–678.

100. Wu J, Hua Y, Keep RF, *et al.* Iron and iron-handling proteins in the brain after intracerebral hemorrhage. *Stroke* 2003; **34**: 2964–2969.

101. Huang F, Xi G, Keep RF, *et al.* Brain edema after experimental intracerebral hemorrhage: role of hemoglobin degradation products. *J Neurosurg* 2002; **96**: 287–293.

102. Nakamura T, Xi G, Park JW, *et al.* Holo-transferrin and thrombin can interact to cause brain damage. *Stroke* **36**: 348–352.

103. Hamada R, Matsuoka H, Wagner KR, *et al.* Antithrombin therapy for intracerebral hemorrhage. *Stroke* 2000; **31**: 794–795.

104. Pike CJ, Vaughan PJ, Cunningham DD, Cotman CW. Thrombin attenuates neuronal cell death and modulates astrocyte reactivity induced by beta-amyloid in vitro. *J Neurochem* 1996; **66**: 1374–1382.

105. Hua Y, Keep RF, Hoff JT, Xi G. Thrombin preconditioning attenuates brain edema induced by erythrocytes and iron. *J Cereb Blood Flow Metab* 2003; **23**: 1448–1454.

106. Hua Y, Xi G, Keep RF, *et al.* Plasminogen activator inhibitor-1 induction after experimental intracerebral hemorrhage. *J Cereb Blood Flow Metab* 2002; **22**: 55–61.

107. Xi G, Hoff JT. The pathophysiology of hemorrhagic lesions. In: Latchaw RE, Kucharczyk J, Moseley ME, eds. *Imaging of the Nervous System: Diagnosis and Therapeutic Applications*. Philadelphia, Elsevier Mosby. 2005; 519–534.

108. Xi G, Keep RF, Hoff JT. Pathophysiology of brain edema formation. *Neurosurg Clin N Am* 2002; **13**: 371–383.

Chapter 9

Cytoprotection strategies for experimental intracerebral hemorrhage

Crystal MacLellan, James Peeling, and Frederick Colbourne

Introduction

A surge in studies examining the pathophysiology of intracerebral hemorrhagic stroke (ICH) has garnered interest and hope that an effective cytoprotective (cell saving) treatment is on the horizon. This chapter critically reviews some of the cytoprotection strategies and methodologies that have been used in an effort to improve outcome in experimental models of ICH. We prefer the term "cytoprotection" to "neuroprotection" as it highlights the need for treatments that target and rescue more than just neurons, for instance glia and the vasculature. Besides treatments that directly target mechanisms of cell death, such as caspase inhibitors, we review interventions that counteract inflammation and edema, and other treatments that may have unrealized cytoprotective benefits. This chapter does not cover in detail those treatments that affect bleeding, such as blood pressure management and hemostatic therapy (e.g., recombinant activated factor VII [rFVIIa]), although it is anticipated that these should also be cytoprotective by limiting the hematoma size.

The development of effective therapies depends upon an understanding of the pathophysiology of ICH. While much progress has occurred, ICH remains a complex problem that is incompletely understood. Nonetheless, a number of therapeutic targets have been identified. Tissue at the epicenter of the ICH is unlikely to be salvaged because the immediate dissection of blood through this area causes direct and rapid tissue destruction. However, the degenerative cascades and secondary events in regions adjacent or distal to the hematoma are feasible targets, as recent studies show that injury occurs in these regions over hours to weeks [1–3]. Thus, this tissue is potentially salvageable by countering degenerative events, which include neurotoxicity induced by the coagulation cascade (e.g., thrombin production) and degenerating red blood cells (RBC), oxidative damage, disruption of the blood–brain barrier (BBB), edema formation, and inflammation. Notably, ICH and ischemia share many mechanisms of injury and thus it is not surprising that many treatments found to be effective in ischemia are being tested for treating ICH. However, there are fundamental differences between ischemia and hemorrhage. For instance, intracerebral blood has direct and indirect toxic effects, such as through the production of thrombin, which stimulates edema, inflammation, and the generation of free radicals. Another difference is that the evidence for an ischemic penumbra surrounding the hematoma core is controversial [4,5], whereas it is well established to follow ischemia. Perhaps this is because reductions in cerebral blood flow (CBF) in perihematomal tissue may indicate reduced metabolic demand, and not necessarily ischemia. Thus, treatments that are efficacious in ischemia may fail to improve outcome after ICH. Accordingly, alternative approaches to ICH must be investigated, rather than simply replicating what has been done in ischemia. In this chapter we review prospective cytoprotectants that aim to preserve parenchymal and vascular integrity by inhibiting a variety of deleterious processes.

The pathophysiology of an ICH and the efficacy of putative treatments are assessed using a number of experimental models (for review, see Chapter 17). The majority of cytoprotection studies use rodent models of ICH, but other species, such as pig [6], are also used. A hematoma may be created by injecting autologous whole blood directly into the striatum [7] or cortex [8], mimicking the single large bleed that occurs in most ICH patients [9]. Alternatively,

Intracerebral Hemorrhage, ed. J. R. Carhuapoma, S. A. Mayer, and D. F. Hanley. Published by Cambridge University Press.
© J. R. Carhuapoma, S. A. Mayer, and D. F. Hanley 2010.

infusion of bacterial collagenase into the striatum disrupts the basal lamina of cerebral capillaries and causes bleeding into brain tissue [10]. The progression of cell death [1,2] and neurological deficits [11,12] are well characterized in these models. Other models of ICH, such as implanting an inflatable balloon [13], or injecting components of blood into the parenchyma [14], are used principally to characterize pathological processes of ICH, and less often for evaluating cytoprotectants.

A number of recommendations have been made to improve the quality of experimental ischemia cytoprotection studies [15,16], and many of these are relevant to evaluating cytoprotection in ICH. For instance, the optimal dose and duration of treatment must be identified. Furthermore, longer delays to initiation of drug administration for up to several hours after stroke should be examined. Whereas most cytoprotection studies use young-adult, male, healthy animals, efficacy should also be assessed in aged animals of both sexes, and with comorbid conditions such as hypertension and diabetes. Studies in neonates mimicking periventricular/intraventricular hemorrhage are also needed [17]. Most studies rely only on histological measures to assess outcome, yet few examine both white matter and gray matter injury. In addition to histological outcome, functional assessment is a priority as it is the clinical endpoint of greatest concern. Thus, a battery of functional tests appropriate for each model should be used. As cytoprotectants may provide only transient benefit, late assessment of histological and functional outcome should be performed. Finally, rigorous preclinical testing requires the evaluation of cytoprotectants using multiple clinically relevant models and several species, for instance in both rodent and porcine, and eventually primate models. The identification of truly effective cytoprotectants for ICH warrants a similar approach.

Approaches that target cell death
Anti-apoptotic agents
Although most tissue in the hematoma undergoes necrotic cell death and will not likely be salvaged by any cytoprotectant, apoptotic pathways may mediate cell death in the tissue surrounding the hematoma. Accordingly, several anti-apoptotic agents have been administered after experimental ICH with encouraging results. For example, the caspase inhibitor zVADfmk transiently reduced the density of TUNEL positive cells at 24 hours [18]. Additionally, tauroursodeoxycholic acid (TUDCA), an endogenous bile acid that blocks apoptotic pathways, reduced lesion volume and cell death in the perihematomal region by approximately 50% at two days after ICH [19]. Notably, TUDCA also improved neurological function. While these studies suggest a role for apoptosis in the pathophysiology of ICH, further studies must confirm the existence of neuronal apoptosis with additional measures (e.g., electron microscopy), and determine the pathological processes responsible for initiating the apoptotic cascade. Given that necrotic injury undoubtedly occurs as well, it seems prudent to combine therapeutic approaches to maximally reduce cell death. Finally, inhibiting apoptotic or necrotic cellular cascades must be shown to provide long-term histological and functional benefit.

Free radical scavengers
Cell death, edema, and neurological deficits after ICH occur, at least in part, by DNA damage caused by oxidative stress [20,21]. Free radicals are generated in the region surrounding the hematoma [1,20] through mechanisms involving iron compounds released from lysed blood cells [21–24]. Because iron compounds are present in high concentrations after ICH, targeting them to prevent oxidative damage may be a valuable therapeutic approach. For instance, iron chelators such as deferoxamine reduce oxidative stress after ICH in rats, in addition to reducing edema and neurological deficits [25]. Furthermore, inhibiting heme oxygenase with tin-mesoporphyrin reduced neuronal loss after ICH in rabbits [26] and decreased edema in pigs [27] and rats [23]. Peeling and colleagues have tested whether reducing free radical production provides benefit for ICH in rats. The hydroxyl radical scavenger, 1,3-dimethyl-2-thiourea (DMTU), and the free radical spin trap agent, α-phenyl-N-tert-butyl nitrone (PBN) failed to affect edema formation, volume of tissue lost, or neuronal injury in tissue surrounding the hematoma, but did provide some long-term functional benefit (neurological deficit score test; [28]). Administration of a water soluble spin-trapping nitrone compound, NXY-059 (disodium 4-[(tert-butylimino)methyl]benzene-1.3-disulfonate N-oxide) reduced perihematomal cell death and infiltration of neutrophils two days after

ICH, and significantly reduced neurological deficits [29]. Thus, free radical scavengers hold promise for treating ICH.

Excitotoxicity

Contrary to ischemia and traumatic brain injury studies, the role of excitatory amino acids (EAAs) has not been well defined in ICH. Elevated levels of EAAs, such as glutamate, have been detected in tissue surrounding the hematoma shortly after ICH in humans [30] and rabbits [31]. However, to date, only two studies have examined whether blocking glutamate accumulation will provide benefit for ICH. Mendelow [32] found that the NMDA receptor antagonist D-(E)-4-(3-phosphonoprop-2-enyl) piperazine-2-carboxylic acid reduced edema in rats, but the effects on cell death were not assessed. More recently, Lee and colleagues [33] showed that the NMDA receptor antagonist memantine reduced cell death (presumed to be apoptotic) and infiltration of inflammatory cells after ICH in rats, and reduced neurological deficits. Surprisingly, memantine also decreased hematoma size. These findings suggest that excitotoxicity may be an important mediator of cell death, and targeting EAAs may be a useful therapeutic approach for ICH. Further study is clearly needed.

Surgical removal of the hematoma

Surgical removal of the hematoma may limit the extent of cell death and secondary degenerative processes after ICH by reducing space-occupying effects of the hematoma and subsequent elevations in intracranial pressure (ICP), by improving CBF, and by removing potentially toxic blood breakdown products. Although some benefit was obtained in rats [34], findings in pigs are contradictory [35,36]. Importantly, the recently failed Surgical Trial in ICH suggests that surgery does not benefit ICH patients [37]. However, surgical removal of the hematoma may be more effective for some types of hemorrhagic stroke, such as a lobar or cerebellar ICH.

Approaches that target secondary consequences of an ICH

Although cytoprotectants can directly target cell death after ICH, they can also limit injury by attenuating secondary deleterious processes, such as edema and inflammation. Alternatively, improved recovery may occur despite failing to lessen cell death, reducing inflammation, or affecting edema. Indeed, it is difficult to disentangle such effects on promoting recovery from cytoprotection as many treatments may broadly affect outcome after an ICH.

Blood–brain barrier disruption

The degree of BBB breakdown is directly correlated with late functional recovery in patients with ICH [38]. Furthermore, the temporal pattern of BBB disruption is similar to the pattern of edema formation in animal models of ICH. Xi and colleagues found that in rats intracerebral infusion of lysed RBCs caused marked BBB disruption and edema 24 hours later, whereas after infusion of packed RBCs, these events were delayed until 72 hours [39]. Therefore, therapies that limit BBB disruption should also reduce edema and improve recovery. Indeed, granulocyte colony-stimulating factor reduced BBB permeability, as well as edema, inflammation, and perihematomal cell death after ICH in adult rats [40]. Lesion volume and functional outcome were also improved. Albumin therapy reduced BBB permeability two days after ICH in rats and was associated with a modest, but transient, reduction in neurological deficits [41]. Few cytoprotection studies actually measure BBB disruption. Instead, because BBB permeability leads to vasogenic edema, many researchers test therapies expected to reduce edema (as discussed below).

Edema

Clinical studies have confirmed that many ICH-induced deaths occur within the first few days following onset, and are likely to be associated with progressively worsening edema [42]. Thus, understanding the causes of edema is necessary for the development of therapies that limit it, and consequently limit secondary brain injury and death. Indeed, much attention has focused on identifying the temporal progression of edema after ICH and the mechanisms of edema formation (for review, see Chapter 20). Specifically, the role of components of the coagulation cascade, such as thrombin [14,42–48], and toxic substances released from lysed RBCs including hemoglobin [14,23,49] and heme oxygenase [24,26,27,50], has been extensively studied. This work has identified contributors to edema that could be useful therapeutic targets. A number of compounds have been shown to reduce edema after experimental ICH, including granulocyte colony-stimulating factor [40], the cyclooxygenase (COX)-2 inhibitor celecoxib [51], atorvastatin [52,53], thrombin inhibitors such as argatroban [54–56], iron chelators such as deferoxamine [25], hypothermia [57,58], estrogen [59], the calcium channel blocker S-emopamil [60], and the heme-oxygenase inhibitor tin-mesoporphyrin [24,26,27].

Unlike clinical ICH, the mortality rate in experimental ICH studies tends to be very low, and is not commonly used as an endpoint to gauge efficacy. Therefore, it is important to determine whether reductions in edema found in rodent models translate into improved long-term histological and functional protection in animals as well as predict morbidity and mortality in humans. Fortunately, many rodent studies show that reductions in edema are associated with long-term sensorimotor recovery [40,51–53].

Inflammation

The robust inflammatory response that follows experimental ICH likely contributes to injury (for review see [61]). Many experimental studies have attempted to understand the time course and significance of the inflammatory response and its contribution to injury after ICH [1,62–64]. Furthermore, studies have also defined the role of inflammatory mediators, including cytokines such as tumor necrosis factor-alpha (TNF-α [65]) and interleukin-1β [46,66], enzymes associated with inflammation such as matrix metalloproteinases (MMPs, [67–72]), and transcription factors such as nuclear factor (NF)-κB [73,74]. Limiting the cascade of deleterious inflammatory processes after ICH is thought to reduce ICH injury and promote improved outcome.

Accordingly, a broad range of anti-inflammatory agents has been tested after experimental ICH. A number of drugs reduce neutrophil and/or macrophage infiltration, including FK-506 [75], fucoidan [76], granulocyte colony-stimulating factor [40], atorvastatin [52], and the peroxisome proliferator-activated receptor-γ (PPARγ) agonist, 15-deoxy-$\Delta^{12,14}$-prostaglandin J$_2$ (15d-PGJ$_2$) [77]. Furthermore, inhibiting microglia activation with tuftsin fragment 1–3 significantly reduced hematoma size and improved neurological outcome in mice [78]. Other

agents target specific cytokines. For example, after ICH in rats, inhibition of TNF-α lessened perihematomal cell death and persistently reduced neurological deficits [65]; interleukin-1 receptor antagonists decreased neutrophil infiltration and edema [46,66]; and reduction of NF-κB activity and neutrophil infiltration by 15d-PGJ$_2$ predicted reduced neuronal cell death and behavioral deficits [77]. Targeting inflammatory enzymes also appears to provide significant benefit. Chu and colleagues demonstrated that the COX-2 inhibitor, celecoxib, decreased inflammation, edema, and neurological deficits after ICH [51]. Furthermore, reducing MMP-12 expression with minocycline provided significant functional benefit [70] (but see [79]), and the broad spectrum MMP inhibitor GM6001 reduced oxidative stress, edema, cell death, and neurological impairments after ICH in rats [71]. In most cases, decreased infiltration of leukocytes or cytokine expression was associated with persistent improvements in sensorimotor outcome, which may be of great clinical value. However, only a few studies show that inhibiting inflammation actually leads to decreased brain injury (e.g., [40,51,71,72]). Therefore, it is possible that inflammation promotes functional recovery independently of any effects on cell death.

Although a pathological role for inflammation is assumed, one should not lose sight of the necessity of cytokines and inflammation. For example, microglia may contribute to ICH injury, but they also participate in limiting and clearing the hematoma [78]. Acute elevations in TNF-α appear to be pathological and should be mitigated, but basal levels of TNF-α are essential for normal neuronal and glial development and survival [80]. Furthermore, TNF-α is neuroprotective during ischemic stress [81]. Thus, prior to clinical investigation of potent and/or broad-spectrum anti-inflammatory agents for ICH, further research is needed to increase our understanding of the positive and negative roles of the inflammatory response. Finally, there are notable weaknesses in current experimental studies. For instance, many investigators assess inflammation at one time point, and treatments may simply alter the time course of inflammation, for instance shifting the time or magnitude of the peak response [82]. Thus, the progression of inflammation should be assessed at multiple times to verify whether a putative cytoprotectant does indeed inhibit these processes.

Overview and considerations for cytoprotection studies

In the past decade, the efficacy of many cytoprotective agents has been tested in treating ICH. Some of these therapies directly target cell death mediated by oxidative stress or caspases. Others aim to reduce secondary degenerative processes like edema and inflammation, which are also thought to contribute to brain injury and functional impairment. Many of the experimental studies discussed above report positive results, which have increased hope in developing effective cytoprotective strategies for ICH. Before putative cytoprotectants are tested in ICH patients, however, efficacy must be rigorously evaluated in experimental studies. There are a number of limitations to how cytoprotective agents are typically assessed, and we offer suggestions as to how these shortcomings can be overcome in future studies. Such advances are needed if we are to identify truly effective treatments for ICH, and gain adequate support for them prior to clinical testing.

First, rodent models of ICH are most commonly used in experimental cytoprotection studies. However, creating animal models that better reflect aspects of human ICH such as hemorrhagic transformation [83] or the rebleeding that occurs in ~ 30% of ICH patients [84] should be a priority for ICH investigators [85]. Furthermore, there are substantial differences in the amount of gray and white matter in rodent and human brains [86]. Thus, efficacy of potential cytoprotectants should be assessed in larger, gyrencephalic animals, such as pigs and primates, before being used in humans. Despite the limitations of animal models of ICH, there is hope that such models will have better clinical predictive value if the experimental conditions more precisely reproduce the clinical setting, for instance through including realistic delays before commencing treatment. An additional concern is that many cytoprotection studies fail to measure or regulate physiological variables that could affect outcome after ICH, including blood gases, hematocrit, blood pressure [87,88], glucose levels [89,90], and postoperative temperature [88,91].

Functional outcome is the endpoint of greatest clinical concern, yet, surprisingly, many investigators either do not assess recovery or use tests of gross neurological function over the first few days after ICH. Other behaviors such as reaching and walking are often severely and persistently disrupted after ICH, and should also be assessed [12]. Recent studies have identified tests sensitive to a striatal ICH, and have demonstrated that a battery of tests sensitive to a range of deficits is preferred over a single test [11,12]. Functional testing should be conducted throughout an experiment to track recovery, and to determine whether a cytoprotectant provides significant long-term functional benefit. Furthermore, a reduction in brain injury does not necessarily translate into functional improvement (for review, see [92]). Accordingly, histological protection in the absence of functional improvement is not a sufficient indicator of treatment efficacy.

Importantly, functional or histological outcome should be assessed using long survival times, as a cytoprotectant may improve outcome only transiently. Markers of injury such as the size of the hematoma or amount of edema are often used to gauge treatment efficacy. However, reductions in edema, for instance, may not result in improved long-term functional outcome or permanently reduced injury. Thus, further research is needed to determine how biochemical markers of injury relate to cell death, and whether targeting these processes improves long-term histological and functional outcome. Investigators should also strive to supplement non-specific histological procedures or to use more specific measures. For example, a marker specific to degenerating neurons, such as Fluoro Jade B [93], can be used to distinguish neurons from other types of degenerating cells after ICH. Furthermore, electron microscopic evaluation of morphological features could be coupled with TUNEL staining to confirm apoptosis.

Very few ICH studies assess cytoprotective therapies on very young (e.g., neonates [17]) or aged animals, despite the fact that significant differences in edema and neurological deficits occur in aged (vs. young) rats [94]. Furthermore, differences between males and females are rarely assessed, but recent data show that edema formation following ICH is lower in female rats [59]. These and other data suggest that hormones such as estrogen can modulate ICH damage [59,95], through effects on estrogen receptors in the brain, through bleeding, and perhaps through more subtle physiological differences such as hemoglobin and hematocrit levels.

The therapeutic window of a potential cytoprotectant is often not assessed. Instead, drugs are commonly administered prior to, during, or immediately after ICH in order to maximize efficacy. As in ischemia studies, the earliest intervention will likely provide the greatest benefit. However, clinically realistic intervention delays should be used, which may greatly affect outcome. For example, minocycline improves neurological outcome when administered starting one hour after ICH [70], but not at three hours [79]. Prior to clinical investigation, the efficacy of putative cytoprotectants should be assessed when administered many hours after ICH. Current recommendations are that treatments for ICH should be initiated as soon as possible after onset. However, it is possible that the therapeutic window is longer than predicted, and it would be of great clinical benefit to have this clearly established.

Future directions

In studies of both ischemic and hemorrhagic stroke, investigators often target the acute phase of the insult and administer cytoprotectants within a few hours of stroke onset. However, the cell death that continues over days to weeks [1,2] may be an additional therapeutic target that has a wider treatment time window. For instance, rehabilitation therapies improve outcome in ischemia and ICH patients, even if applied weeks or months after stroke [96] and this may involve subtle modulation of ongoing cell death. Rodent studies also show that rehabilitation therapies reduce brain injury after ICH [89,97,98].

Single drug treatments have generally failed to benefit ischemia and have so far failed to provide substantial protection for ICH. Due to the complex nature of ICH, it is reasonable to expect that therapies targeting several components of injury would be more efficacious than a single therapy. Indeed, a combination of cytoprotectants with different mechanisms of action might be expected to act synergistically to provide maximal benefit for ICH. Furthermore, non-pharmacological interventions such as rehabilitation should also be tested in combination with cytoprotectants. Notably, a recent study of severe ICH demonstrated that the combination of hypothermia and rehabilitation improved outcome more so than either treatment alone [99]. Finally, any potential cytoprotectant must be compatible with other drugs that are given to ICH patients, which may include rFVIIa, as it appears to provide clinical benefit in some ICH patients [100].

Several other treatment approaches have recently gained much interest. For instance, investigation of genomic responses after experimental ICH [101,102] has generated information on signaling pathways that contribute to the pathology of ICH, and may represent novel therapeutic targets. Likewise, investigators could take advantage of the capacity for neuroplasticity and repair after ICH. Interestingly, administration of a cytoprotectant may augment plasticity and contribute to improved outcome [53]. It has been shown recently that endogenous stem cells are activated after ICH [103]. Accordingly, therapies such as exercise that increase cell proliferation [90] may be of great use for treating ICH. Furthermore, the prospect of using transplanted stem cells to treat ICH has also gathered much attention. Initial studies have yielded promising results [104–106] (but see [107]), but before these therapies can be applied clinically, many basic questions must be answered regarding the optimal timing and site of administration, type of cells used, and safety of such treatments.

Summary

Over the past decade, the number of experimental cytoprotection studies for ICH has increased dramatically. These efforts have produced encouraging results. For instance, a number of putative cytoprotectants attenuate such pathological consequences of an ICH as edema or inflammation, reduce hematoma size, and improve motor recovery in animal models. Despite these successes, cytoprotective agents have yet to benefit ICH patients. Other than rFVIIa, no treatment has been shown to improve outcome in clinical trials of ICH. Reasons for failed cytoprotectants in ischemic stroke have been reviewed, and include limitations with animal models, choice of end points, and failure to accurately apply information obtained from experimental studies to the clinical trials [15,108–110]. Here we have highlighted the need to re-evaluate both experimental and clinical practices in ICH, so the mistakes made in studies of ischemic stroke are not repeated. Using knowledge gained from previous failures, a better understanding of the pathophysiology of ICH, and continued preclinical success, it is reasonable to expect that truly effective cytoprotectants will be identified.

References

1. Del Bigio MR, Yan HJ, Buist R, Peeling J. Experimental intracerebral hemorrhage in rats. Magnetic resonance imaging and histopathological correlates. *Stroke* 1996: **27**: 2312–2319.

2. Felberg RA, Grotta JC, Shirzadi AL, *et al.* Cell death in experimental hemorrhage: the "black hole" model of hemorrhagic damage. *Ann Neurol* 2002; **51**: 517–524.

3. Qureshi AI, Ling GS, Khan J, *et al.* Quantitative analysis of injured, necrotic, and apoptotic cells in a new experimental model of intracerebral hemorrhage. *Crit Care Med* 2001; **29**: 152–157.

4. Kidwell CS, Saver JL, Mattiello J, *et al.* Diffusion-perfusion MR evaluation of perihematomal injury in hyperacute intracerebral hemorrhage. *Neurology* 2001; **57**: 1611–1617.

5. Schellinger PD, Fiebach JB, Hoffmann K, *et al.* Stroke MRI in intracerebral hemorrhage: is there a perihemorrhagic penumbra? *Stroke* 2003; **34**: 1674–1679.

6. Wagner KR, Xi G, Hua Y, *et al.* Lobar intracerebral hemorrhage model in pigs: rapid edema development in perihematomal white matter. *Stroke* 1996; **27**: 490–497.

7. Nath FP, Jenkins A, Mendelow AD, Graham DI, Teasdale GM. Early hemodynamic changes in experimental intracerebral hemorrhage. *J Neurosurg* 1986; **65**: 697–703.

8. Xue M, Del Bigio MR. Intracortical hemorrhage injury in rats: relationship between blood fractions and brain cell death. *Stroke* 2000; **31**: 1721–1727.

9. Herbstein DJ, Schaumberg HH. Hypertensive intracerebral hematoma. An investigation of the initial hemorrhage and rebleeding using chromium Cr 51-labeled erythrocytes. *Arch Neurol* 1974; **30**: 412–414.

10. Rosenberg GA, Mun-Bryce S, Wesley M, Kornfeld M. Collagenase-induced intracerebral hemorrhage in rats. *Stroke* 1990; **21**: 801–807.

11. Hua Y, Schallert T, Keep RF, *et al.* Behavioral tests after intracerebral hemorrhage in the rat. *Stroke* 2002; **33**: 2478–2484.

12. MacLellan C, Auriat A, McGie S, *et al.* Gauging recovery after hemorrhagic stroke in rats: implications for cytoprotection studies. *J Cereb Blood Flow Metab* 2006; **26**(8): 1031–1042.

13. Bullock R, Mendelow AD, Teasdale GM, Graham DI. Intracranial haemorrhage induced at arterial pressure in the rat. Part 1: Description of technique, ICP changes and neuropathological findings. *Neurol Res* 1984; **6**: 184–188.

14. Xi G, Keep RF, Hoff JT. Erythrocytes and delayed brain edema formation following intracerebral hemorrhage in rats. *J Neurosurg* 1998; **89**: 991–996.

15. Gladstone DJ, Black SE, Hakim AM. Toward wisdom from failure: lessons from neuroprotective stroke trials and new therapeutic directions. *Stroke* 2002; **33**: 2123–2136.

16. Stroke Therapy Academic Industry Roundtable (STAIR). Recommendations for standards regarding preclinical neuroprotective and restorative drug development. *Stroke* 1999; **30**: 2752–2758.

17. Xue M, Balasubramaniam J, Buist RJ, Peeling J, Del Bigio MR. Periventricular/intraventricular hemorrhage in neonatal mouse cerebrum. *J Neuropathol Exp Neurol* 2003; **62**: 1154–1165.

18. Matsushita K, Meng W, Wang X, *et al.* Evidence for apoptosis after intercerebral hemorrhage in rat striatum. *J Cereb Blood Flow Metab* 2000; **20**: 396–404.

19. Rodrigues CM, Sola S, Nan Z, *et al.* Tauroursodeoxycholic acid reduces apoptosis and protects against neurological injury after acute hemorrhagic stroke in rats. *Proc Natl Acad Sci U S A* 2003; **100**: 6087–6092.

20. Nakamura T, Keep RF, Hua Y, Hoff JT, Xi G. Oxidative DNA injury after experimental intracerebral hemorrhage. *Brain Res* 2005; **1039**: 30–36.

21. Wu J, Hua Y, Keep RF, *et al.* Oxidative brain injury from extravasated erythrocytes after intracerebral hemorrhage. *Brain Res* 2002; **953**: 45–52.

22. Halliwell B, Gutteridge JM. Biologically relevant metal ion-dependent hydroxyl radical generation. An update. *FEBS Lett* 1992; **307**: 108–112.

23. Huang FP, Xi G, Keep RF, *et al.* Brain edema after experimental intracerebral hemorrhage: role of hemoglobin degradation products. *J Neurosurg* 2002; **96**: 287–293.

24. Wagner KR, Packard BA, Hall CL, *et al.* Protein oxidation and heme oxygenase-1 induction in porcine white matter following intracerebral infusions of whole blood or plasma. *Dev Neurosci* 2002; **24**: 154–160.

25. Nakamura T, Keep RF, Hua Y, *et al.* Deferoxamine-induced attenuation of brain edema and neurological deficits in a rat model of intracerebral hemorrhage. *J Neurosurg* 2004; **100**: 672–678.

26. Koeppen AH, Dickson AC, Smith J. Heme oxygenase in experimental intracerebral hemorrhage: the benefit of tin-mesoporphyrin. *J Neuropathol Exp Neurol* 2004; **63**: 587–597.

27. Wagner KR, Hua Y, de Courten-Myers GM, *et al.* Tin-mesoporphyrin, a potent heme oxygenase inhibitor, for treatment of intracerebral hemorrhage: in vivo and in vitro studies. *Cell Mol Biol (Noisy-le-grand)* 2000; **46**: 597–608.

28. Peeling J, Yan HJ, Chen SG, Campbell M, Del Bigio MR. Protective effects of free radical inhibitors in intracerebral hemorrhage in rat. *Brain Res* 1998; **795**: 63–70.

29. Peeling J, Del Bigio MR, Corbett D, Green AR, Jackson DM. Efficacy of disodium 4-[(tert-butylimino)

methyl]benzene-1,3-disulfonate N-oxide (NXY-059), a free radical trapping agent, in a rat model of hemorrhagic stroke. *Neuropharmacology* 2001; **40**: 433–439.

30. Castillo J, Davalos A, Alvarez-Sabin J, *et al*. Molecular signatures of brain injury after intracerebral hemorrhage. *Neurology* 2002; **58**: 624–629.

31. Qureshi AI, Ali Z, Suri MF, *et al*. Extracellular glutamate and other amino acids in experimental intracerebral hemorrhage: an in vivo microdialysis study. *Crit Care Med* 2003; **31**: 1482–1489.

32. Mendelow AD. Mechanisms of ischemic brain damage with intracerebral hemorrhage. *Stroke* 1993; **24** (12 Suppl): I115–117.

33. Lee ST, Chu K, Jung KH, *et al*. Memantine reduces hematoma expansion in experimental intracerebral hemorrhage, resulting in functional improvement. *J Cereb Blood Flow Metab* 2006; **26**(4): 536–544.

34. Altumbabic M, Peeling J, Del Bigio MR. Intracerebral hemorrhage in the rat: effects of hematoma aspiration. *Stroke* 1998; **29**: 1917–1922.

35. Thiex R, Kuker W, Muller HD, *et al*. The long-term effect of recombinant tissue-plasminogen-activator (rt-PA) on edema formation in a large-animal model of intracerebral hemorrhage. *Neurol Res* 2003; **25**: 254–262.

36. Wagner KR, Xi G, Hua Y, *et al*. Ultra-early clot aspiration after lysis with tissue plasminogen activator in a porcine model of intracerebral hemorrhage: edema reduction and blood-brain barrier protection. *J Neurosurg* 1999; **90**: 491–498.

37. Mendelow AD, Gregson BA, Fernandes HM, *et al*. STICH investigatiors. Early surgery versus initial conservative treatment in patients with spontaneous supratentorial intracerebral haematomas in the International Surgical Trial in Intracerebral Haemorrhage (STICH): a randomised trial. *Lancet* 2005; **365**: 387–397.

38. Lampl Y, Shmuilovich O, Lockman J, Sadeh M, Lorberboym M. Prognostic significance of blood brain barrier permeability in acute hemorrhagic stroke. *Cerebrovasc Dis* 2005; **20**: 433–437.

39. Xi G, Hua Y, Bhasin RR, *et al*. Mechanisms of edema formation after intracerebral hemorrhage: effects of extravasated red blood cells on blood flow and blood-brain barrier integrity. *Stroke* 2001; **32**: 2932–2938.

40. Park HK, Chu K, Lee ST, *et al*. Granulocyte colony-stimulating factor induces sensorimotor recovery in intracerebral hemorrhage. *Brain Res* 2005; **1041**: 125–131.

41. Belayev L, Saul I, Busto R, *et al*. Albumin treatment reduces neurological deficit and protects blood-brain

42. Broderick JP, Brott TG, Duldner JE, Tomsick T, Huster G. Volume of intracerebral hemorrhage. A powerful and easy-to-use predictor of 30-day mortality. *Stroke* 1993; **24**: 987–993.

43. Lee KR, Betz AL, Keep RF, *et al*. Intracerebral infusion of thrombin as a cause of brain edema. *J Neurosurg* 1995; **83**: 1045–1050.

44. Lee KR, Colon GP, Betz AL, *et al*. Edema from intracerebral hemorrhage: the role of thrombin. *J Neurosurg* 1996; **84**: 91–96.

45. Lee KR, Kawai N, Kim S, Sagher O, Hoff JT. Mechanisms of edema formation after intracerebral hemorrhage: effects of thrombin on cerebral blood flow, blood-brain barrier permeability, and cell survival in a rat model. *J Neurosurg* 1997; **86**: 272–278.

46. Masada T, Hua Y, Xi G, *et al*. Attenuation of intracerebral hemorrhage and thrombin-induced brain edema by overexpression of interleukin-1 receptor antagonist. *J Neurosurg* 2001; **95**: 680–686.

47. Xi G, Wagner KR, Keep RF, *et al*. Role of blood clot formation on early edema development after experimental intracerebral hemorrhage. *Stroke* 1998; **29**: 2580–2586.

48. Xue M, Del Bigio MR. Acute tissue damage after injections of thrombin and plasmin into rat striatum. *Stroke* 2001; **32**: 2164–2169.

49. Bhasin RR, Xi G, Hua Y, Keep RF, Hoff JT. Experimental intracerebral hemorrhage: effect of lysed erythrocytes on brain edema and blood-brain barrier permeability. *Acta Neurochir Suppl* 2002; **81**: 249–251.

50. Wagner KR, Dwyer BE. Hematoma removal, heme, and heme oxygenase following hemorrhagic stroke. *Ann N Y Acad Sci* 2004; **1012**: 237–251.

51. Chu K, Jeong SW, Jung KH, *et al*. Celecoxib induces functional recovery after intracerebral hemorrhage with reduction of brain edema and perihematomal cell death. *J Cereb Blood Flow Metab* 2004; **24**: 926–933.

52. Jung KH, Chu K, Jeong SW, *et al*. HMG-CoA reductase inhibitor, atorvastatin, promotes sensorimotor recovery, suppressing acute inflammatory reaction after experimental intracerebral hemorrhage. *Stroke* 2004; **35**: 1744–1749.

53. Seyfried D, Han Y, Lu D, *et al*. Improvement in neurological outcome after administration of atorvastatin following experimental intracerebral hemorrhage in rats. *J Neurosurg* 2004; **101**: 104–107.

54. Kitaoka T, Hua Y, Xi G, Hoff J, Keep R. Delayed argatroban treatment reduces edema in a rat model of intracerebral hemorrhage. *Stroke* 2002; **33**: 3012–3018.

55. Kitaoka T, Hua Y, Xi G, *et al.* Effect of delayed argatroban treatment on intracerebral hemorrhage-induced edema in the rat. *Acta Neurochir Suppl* 2003; **86**: 457–461.

56. Nagatsuna T, Nomura S, Suehiro E, *et al.* Systemic administration of argatroban reduces secondary brain damage in a rat model of intracerebral hemorrhage: histopathological assessment. *Cerebrovasc Dis* 2005; **19**: 192–200.

57. Kawai N, Nakamura T, Nagao S. Effects of brain hypothermia on brain edema formation after intracerebral hemorrhage in rats. *Acta Neurochir Suppl* 2002; **81**: 233–235.

58. Kawanishi M. Effect of hypothermia on brain edema formation following intracerebral hemorrhage in rats. *Acta Neurochir Suppl* 2003; **86**: 453–456.

59. Nakamura T, Hua Y, Keep RF, *et al.* Estrogen therapy for experimental intracerebral hemorrhage in rats. *J Neurosurg* 2005; **103**: 97–103.

60. Rosenberg GA, Navratil MJ. (S)-emopamil reduces brain edema from collagenase-induced hemorrhage in rats. *Stroke* 1994; **25**: 2067–2071.

61. Aronowski J, Hall CE. New horizons for primary intracerebral hemorrhage treatment: experience from preclinical studies. *Neurol Res* 2005; **27**: 268–279.

62. Jenkins A, Maxwell WL, Graham DI. Experimental intracerebral haematoma in the rat: sequential light microscopical changes. *Neuropathol Appl Neurobiol* 1989; **15**: 477–486.

63. Kowianski P, Karwacki Z, Dziewiatkowski J, *et al.* Evolution of microglial and astroglial response during experimental intracerebral haemorrhage in the rat. *Folia Neuropathol* 2003; **41**: 123–130.

64. Xue M, Del Bigio MR. Intracerebral injection of autologous whole blood in rats: time course of inflammation and cell death. *Neurosci Lett* 2000; **283**: 230–232.

65. Mayne M, Ni W, Yan HJ, *et al.* Antisense oligodeoxynucleotide inhibition of tumor necrosis factor-alpha expression is neuroprotective after intracerebral hemorrhage. *Stroke* 2001; **32**: 240–248.

66. Masada T, Hua Y, Xi G, *et al.* Overexpression of interleukin-1 receptor antagonist reduces brain edema induced by intracerebral hemorrhage and thrombin. *Acta Neurochir Suppl* 2003; **86**: 463–467.

67. Abilleira S, Montaner J, Molina CA, *et al.* Matrix metalloproteinase-9 concentration after spontaneous intracerebral hemorrhage. *J Neurosurg* 2003; **99**: 65–70.

68. Lapchak PA, Chapman DF, Zivin JA. Metalloproteinase inhibition reduces thrombolytic (tissue plasminogen activator)-induced hemorrhage after thromboembolic stroke. *Stroke* 2000; **31**: 3034–3040.

69. Mun-Bryce S, Wilkerson A, Pacheco B, *et al.* Depressed cortical excitability and elevated matrix metalloproteinases in remote brain regions following intracerebral hemorrhage. *Brain Res* 2004; **1026**: 227–234.

70. Power C, Henry S, Del Bigio MR, *et al.* Intracerebral hemorrhage induces macrophage activation and matrix metalloproteinases. *Ann Neurol* 2003; **53**: 731–742.

71. Wang J, Tsirka SE. Neuroprotection by inhibition of matrix metalloproteinases in a mouse model of intracerebral haemorrhage. *Brain* 2005; **128**: 1622–1633.

72. Wells JE, Biernaskie J, Szymanska A, *et al.* Matrix metalloproteinase (MMP)-12 expression has a negative impact on sensorimotor function following intracerebral haemorrhage in mice. *Eur J Neurosci* 2005; **21**: 187–196.

73. Hickenbottom SL, Grotta JC, Strong R, Denner LA, Aronowski J. Nuclear factor-kappaB and cell death after experimental intracerebral hemorrhage in rats. *Stroke* 1999; **30**: 2472–2477; discussion 2477–2478.

74. Wagner KR, Sharp FR, Ardizzone TD, Lu A, Clark JF. Heme and iron metabolism: role in cerebral hemorrhage. *J Cereb Blood Flow Metab* 2003; **23**: 629–652.

75. Peeling J, Yan HJ, Corbett D, Xue M, Del Bigio MR. Effect of FK-506 on inflammation and behavioral outcome following intracerebral hemorrhage in rat. *Exp Neurol* 2001; **167**: 341–347.

76. Del Bigio MR, Yan HJ, Campbell TM, Peeling J. Effect of fucoidan treatment on collagenase-induced intracerebral hemorrhage in rats. *Neurol Res* 1999; **21**: 415–419.

77. Zhao X, Zhang Y, Strong R, Grotta JC, Aronowski J. 15d-Prostaglandin J(2) activates peroxisome proliferator-activated receptor-gamma, promotes expression of catalase, and reduces inflammation, behavioral dysfunction, and neuronal loss after intracerebral hemorrhage in rats. *J Cereb Blood Flow Metab* 2006; **26**(6): 811–820.

78. Wang J, Rogove AD, Tsirka AE, Tsirka SE. Protective role of tuftsin fragment 1–3 in an animal model of intracerebral hemorrhage. *Ann Neurol* 2003; **54**: 655–664.

79. Szymanska A, Biernaskie J, Laidley D, Granter-Button S, Corbett D. Minocycline and intracerebral hemorrhage: influence of injury severity and delay to treatment. *Exp Neurol* 2006; **197**(1): 189–196.

80. Bruce AJ, Boling W, Kindy MS, *et al.* Altered neuronal and microglial responses to excitotoxic and ischemic brain injury in mice lacking TNF receptors. *Nat Med* 1996; **2**: 788–794.

81. Nawashiro H, Martin D, Hallenbeck JM. Inhibition of tumor necrosis factor and amelioration of brain infarction in mice. *J Cereb Blood Flow Metab* 1997; **17**: 229–232.

82. Inamasu J, Suga S, Sato S, *et al*. Post-ischemic hypothermia delayed neutrophil accumulation and microglial activation following transient focal ischemia in rats. *J Neuroimmunol* 2000; **109**: 66–74.

83. Lyden PD, Zivin JA. Hemorrhagic transformation after cerebral ischemia: mechanisms and incidence. *Cerebrovasc Brain Metab Rev* 1993; **5**: 1–16.

84. Fujii Y, Tanaka R, Takeuchi S, *et al*. Hematoma enlargement in spontaneous intracerebral hemorrhage. *J Neurosurg* 1994; **80**: 51–57.

85. NINDS ICH workshop Participants. Priorities for clinical research in intracerebral hemorrhage: report from a National Institute of Neurological Disorders and Stroke workshop. *Stroke* 2005; **36**: e23–41.

86. Dewar D, Yam P, McCulloch J. Drug development for stroke: importance of protecting cerebral white matter. *Eur J Pharmacol* 1999; **375**: 41–50.

87. Benveniste H, Kim KR, Hedlund LW, Kim JW, Friedman AH. Cerebral hemorrhage and edema following brain biopsy in rats: significance of mean arterial blood pressure. *J Neurosurg* 2000; **92**: 100–107.

88. MacLellan CL, Girgis J, Colbourne F. Delayed onset of prolonged hypothermia improves outcome after intracerebral hemorrhage in rats. *J Cereb Blood Flow Metab* 2004; **24**: 432–440.

89. Lee HH, Shin MS, Kim YS, *et al*. Early treadmill exercise decreases intrastriatal hemorrhage-induced neuronal cell death and increases cell proliferation in the dentate gyrus of streptozotocin-induced hyperglycemic rats. *J Diabetes Complications* 2005; **19**: 339–346.

90. Song EC, Chu K, Jeong SW, *et al*. Hyperglycemia exacerbates brain edema and perihematomal cell death after intracerebral hemorrhage. *Stroke* 2003; **34**: 2215–2220.

91. MacLellan CL, Colbourne F. Mild to moderate hyperthermia does not worsen outcome after severe intracerebral hemorrhage in rats. *J Cereb Blood Flow Metab* 2005; **25**: 1020–1029.

92. Corbett D, Nurse S. The problem of assessing effective neuroprotection in experimental cerebral ischemia. *Prog Neurobiol* 1998; **54**: 531–548.

93. Schmued LC, Albertson C, Slikker W Jr. Fluoro-Jade: a novel fluorochrome for the sensitive and reliable histochemical localization of neuronal degeneration. *Brain Res* 1997; **751**: 37–46.

94. Gong Y, Hua Y, Keep RF, Hoff JT, Xi G. Intracerebral hemorrhage: effects of aging on brain edema and neurological deficits. *Stroke* 2004; **35**: 2571–2575.

95. Auriat A, Plahta WC, McGie SC, Yan R, Colbourne F. 17ß-Estradiol pretreatment reduces bleeding and brain injury after intracerebral hemorrhagic stroke in male rats. *J Cereb Blood Flow Metab* 2005; **25**: 247–256.

96. Kelly PJ, Furie KL, Shafqat S, *et al*. Functional recovery following rehabilitation after hemorrhagic and ischemic stroke. *Arch Phys Med Rehabil* 2003; **84**: 968–972.

97. DeBow SB, Davies ML, Clarke HL, Colbourne F. Constraint-induced movement therapy and rehabilitation exercises lessen motor deficits and volume of brain injury after striatal hemorrhagic stroke in rats. *Stroke* 2003; **34**: 1021–1026.

98. Lee HH, Kim H, Lee MH, *et al*. Treadmill exercise decreases intrastriatal hemorrhage-induced neuronal cell death via suppression on caspase-3 expression in rats. *Neurosci Lett* 2003; **352**: 33–36.

99. MacLellan C, Grams J, Adams K, Colbourne F. Combined use of a cytoprotectant and rehabilitation therapy after severe intracerebral hemorrhage in rats. *Brain Res* 2005; **1063**: 40–47.

100. Mayer SA, Brun NC, Begtrup K, *et al*. and the Recombinant Activated Factor VII Intracerebral Hemorrhage Trial Investigators. Recombinant activated factor VII for acute intracerebral hemorrhage. *N Engl J Med.* 2005; **352**: 777–785.

101. Lu A, Tang Y, Ran R, *et al*. Brain genomics of intracerebral hemorrhage. *J Cereb Blood Flow Metab* 2006; **26**(2): 230–252.

102. Tang Y, Lu A, Aronow BJ, Wagner KR, Sharp FR. Genomic responses of the brain to ischemic stroke, intracerebral haemorrhage, kainate seizures, hypoglycemia, and hypoxia. *Eur J Neurosci* 2002; **15**: 1937–1952.

103. Tang T, Li XQ, Wu H, *et al*. Activation of endogenous neural stem cells in experimental intracerebral hemorrhagic rat brains. *Chin Med J (Engl)* 2004; **117**: 1342–1347.

104. Jeong SW, Chu K, Jung KH, *et al*. Human neural stem cell transplantation promotes functional recovery in rats with experimental intracerebral hemorrhage. *Stroke* 2003; **34**(9): 2258–2263.

105. Nan Z, Grande A, Sanberg CD, Sanberg PR, Low WC. Infusion of human umbilical cord blood ameliorates neurologic deficits in rats with hemorrhagic brain injury. *Ann N Y Acad Sci* 2005; **1049**: 84–96.

106. Nonaka M, Yoshikawa M, Nishimura F, *et al*. Intraventricular transplantation of embryonic stem

cell-derived neural stem cells in intracerebral hemorrhage rats. *Neurol Res.* 2004; **26**: 265–72.

107. Altumbabic M, Del Bigio MR. Transplantation of fetal brain tissue into the site of intracerebral hemorrhage in rats. *Neurosci Lett* 1998; **257**: 61–64.

108. Fisher M, Albers GW, Donnan GA, *et al.* Enhancing the development and approval of acute stroke therapies. Stroke Therapy Academic Industry Roundtable. *Stroke* 2005; **36**(8): 1808–1813.

109. Green RA, Odergren T, Ashwood T. Animal models of stroke: do they have value for discovering neuroprotective agents? *Trends Pharmacol Sci* 2003; **24**: 402–408.

110. Wahlgren NG, Ahmed N. Neuroprotection in cerebral ischaemia: facts and fancies--the need for new approaches. *Cerebrovasc Dis* 2004; **17** Suppl 1: 153–166.

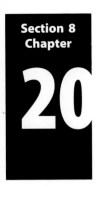

20 Natural history of perihematomal brain edema

Manuel Rodríguez-Yáñez, Antoni Dávalos, and José Castillo

Perihematomal brain edema (PHBE) plays an important role in secondary brain injury after intracerebral bleeding. The liquid accumulation surrounding intracerebral hemorrhage (ICH) is a common event, and it appears as hypodensity around the hematoma on CT scan and as hyperintensity on T2-weighted or FLAIR sequences [1]. Perihematomal brain edema development is associated with higher morbidity and mortality, since it can elevate intracranial pressure, leading to herniation, and causing brainstem compression and death [2].

The natural history and pathogenesis of PHBE are beginning to be understood. It has been postulated that the perihematomal region is hypoperfused, secondary to microvascular compression, resulting in ischemia and cytotoxic edema. Perihematomal brain edema has also been hypothesized to be of vascular origin, resulting from the oncotic effects of intrahematomal blood clotting [3]. The understanding of PHBE pathogenesis is important, since it will lead to a better therapeutic management of these patients. The knowledge about the predominance of ischemia or vasogenic edema may be important for the aggressive treatment of high blood pressure during the acute phase of ICH.

Epidemiology

Perihematomal brain edema is commonly observed during the acute and subacute phases in patients with ICH. Approximately one-third of patients with ICH lacked measurable edema on baseline CT scan, but nearly all had measurable edema at 20 hours of evolution. Perihematomal brain edema volume increases by approximately 75% during the first 24 hours after hyperacute spontaneous ICH, and patients with the least amounts of baseline relative edema volume are most likely to develop significant additional amounts of edema during the first 24 hours after spontaneous ICH [4].

Few studies have investigated what factors are associated with the development of PHBE. No clinical studies have been developed to establish PHBE-associated factors. In animal models, aging [5], gender, and hyperglycemia [6] have been related to an increase in PHBE.

Pathological features

The halo of hypodensity observed in the CT studies performed during the first week after ICH is mostly due to vasogenic edema [7], whereas cytotoxic edema in the peripheral tissue is limited, both in animal models [8] and in human clinical cases [9]. Vasogenic edema is due to an increase in blood–brain barrier permeability, causing water, electrolytes, and proteins to accumulate in extracellular space. The amount of edema is greatest in the white matter, but the same changes may take place in gray matter, but in a lesser extent. Cytotoxic edema is due to lack of adenosine triphosphate (ATP), leading to sodium and potassium pump failure, causing intracellular water accumulation.

Experimental studies in ICH demonstrated marked edema in white matter regions adjacent to hematoma [10]. Edema development was also observed in ipsilateral distal white matter regions, presumably due to fluid movement in the extracellular space along white matter fiber tracts. In animal models, 12 hours after hematoma development induced by injection of bacterial collagenase and heparin into the caudate nucleus, a diffuse halo around the hematoma and in white matter is observed by immunohistochemical techniques, indicating the presence of plasma-derived edema fluid, which persist at least hours [11].

Macroscopically, white and gray matter aspect differs not much from normal appearance, though effacement in their limit can be observed. If edema is more important, brain sulcal effacement, ventricular system compression, and even cerebral herniation can be produced.

In optic microscopy, edema is characterized by vacuolization or spongy change of the neuropil and pericellular vacuolization as well as pallor of the tissue and swollen astrocytes. When cytotoxic edema is produced, neurons and myelin sheaths may also be swollen. In electronic microscopy, an increase in extracellular space in white matter is observed, with separation between axons [12]. In the gray matter, the entry of water causes the relaxation of the prolongations of the astrocytes, which leads to empty perineuronal and perivascular spaces, without dilating extracellular space.

Chronology of PHBE

In animal models, PHBE increases gradually. At two hours from onset it is mild, and it increases over several hours, peaking at the third or fourth day. Subsequently, edema declines slowly, but still exists seven days after hemorrhage development [13,14]. In human studies, early CT scans demonstrate that PHBE develops within three hours of symptom onset [15]. The volume increases rapidly three days after hemorrhage and then slowly until day 14 after hemorrhage [16]. Perihematomal brain edema reaches its maximum between 10 and 20 days of evolution, and decreases thereafter.

Previous studies indicate that edema formation following ICH may involve several phases (Table 20.1). These include an early phase occurring in the first hours of evolution of the bleeding. This edema is interstitial in nature, and results from the accumulation of osmotically active substances and movement of water across an intact blood–brain barrier into the extracellular space [10]. This process involves hydrostatic pressure and clot retraction with secondary expulsion of serum from the clot that contributes to the creation of a low cerebral blood flow zone around the bleeding, causing transient ischemia around the clot. A second phase occurs in the next 24–48 hours, and involves the activation of the coagulation cascade, thrombin production, and induction of proteolytic enzymes that leads to an inflammatory response, resulting in direct cellular toxicity, blood–brain barrier disruption, depressed metabolic activity, and a secondary reduction in cerebral blood flow

Table 20.1. Different phases of PHBE formation

Phase	Time	Implicated mechanisms
Phase 1	First 8 hours	Hydrostatic pressure and clot retraction with secondary expulsion of serum from the clot
Phase 2	24 to 48 hours	Activation of the coagulation cascade, thrombin production, and induction of proteolytic enzymes
Phase 3	More than 72 hours	Red blood cell lysis and hemoglobin-induced neuronal toxicity

[17–20]. A third phase, after three days of evolution, is mainly mediated by red blood cell lysis and hemoglobin-induced neuronal toxicity [21].

Pathophysiology of PHBE

In Figure 20.1 we can see the different mechanisms implicated in the pathophysiology of PHBE. After an ICH, a decrease of cerebral blood flow to ischemic levels occurs immediately in brain tissue surrounding the hematoma [8,22]. This initial decrease in cerebral blood flow is related to a microvascular compromise due to local brain tissue compression. Although perihematomal oligemia occurs in acute ICH, it is not associated with MRI markers of ischemia [23], and this perihemorrhagic hypoperfusion probably is a consequence of reduced metabolic demand [24]. The cytotoxic edema produced by this mechanism, however, is minimal [1]. Later reperfusion of the brain damaged tissue may contribute to further edema growth [25].

In considering the pathogenesis of hyperacute PHBE, it has been postulated to be vascular in origin, resulting from the oncotic effects of intrahematomal blood clotting [3]. There are many experimental studies that support the hypothesis that it is largely compounded of the remaining, peripherally exuded serum proteins after clotting of the hematoma and consumption of plasma clotting factors [10,19,26,27].

The activation of the coagulation cascade plays an important role in early PHBE formation [28]. Interventions that reduce thrombin generation can reduce PHBE. In this context, intrahematomal injection of heparin prevents the hyperacute PHBE formation [29], and intrahematomal tissue plasminogen activator instillation can reduce it in a porcine model of

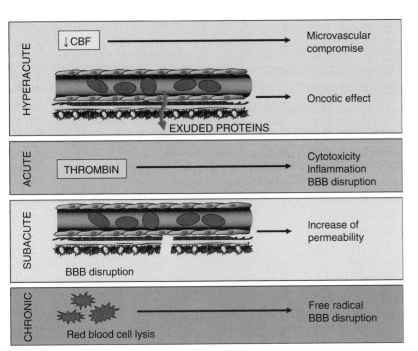

Fig. 20.1 Pathophysiology of PHBE. BBB, blood–brain barrier; CBF, cerebral blood flow.

ICH [30]. Clinical studies in humans support this hypothesis, for example Gebel *et al.* [3], found a lower relative edema volume in ICH related to thrombolytic or anticoagulant therapy compared with spontaneous ICH, a fact that was attributed to the lack of clot retraction in anticoagulated patients and lower thrombin production as a result of the blockade of the coagulation cascade. Thrombin is a serine protease derived from prothrombin and is essential in the coagulation cascade. It is produced immediately after bleeding at the same time as the blood clots. In addition, prothrombin from plasma may pass through the broken blood–brain barrier into the brain parenchyma, where it is converted into thrombin. Moreover, the clot formed during the coagulation process may retain some thrombin that can be released slowly into the surrounding bleeding area. The participation of thrombin in PHBE development has been demonstrated by experimental and clinical data. In fact, the administration of thrombin inhibitors decreases perihematomal edema both in experimental [19] and clinical studies [31]. Besides its participation in perihematomal edema formation, thrombin produces deleterious effects on the brain through cytotoxicity, inflammation, and blood–brain barrier breakdown [26,32,33], and also due to a direct proteolytic activity, causing necrosis and cell death in animal models after intracerebral injection, although the

doses required to cause damage are relatively great in consideration of the plasma content of this protein [34].

Blood–brain barrier disruption after ICH has been reported as contributing to brain edema formation. Blood–brain barrier permeability in the perihematomal region increases markedly approximately 8–12 hours after the beginning of ICH, and continues to increase for 48 hours [18]. As already mentioned, early blood–brain barrier disruption after ICH is related to thrombin generation [26].

Later in the evolution of pathogenic events, red blood cell lysis and hemoglobin toxicity further aggravate blood–brain barrier disruption and are responsible for delayed edema development [35]. The release of iron (a breakdown product of hemoglobin) after erythrocyte lysis may exert a potent lipid peroxidation by mediating free radical generation [36]. In fact, hemoglobin stimulates lipid peroxidation which in turn is inhibited by iron chelators [37]. Moreover, it has been reported that holo-transferrin, an iron-containing component of the hematoma, causes brain injury when combined with thrombin [38]. This seems to be related to an increased intracellular uptake of iron from holo-transferrin facilitated by thrombin. It has also been shown that oxyhemoglobin can induce apoptosis in cultured endothelial cells, possibly through free radical damage to the endothelial vessel wall tissue [39]. A second mechanism that might contribute to edema formation development after erythrocyte lysis is direct damage to neurons and astrocytes involved in maintaining extracellular homeostasis. Intracortical infusion of lysed blood but not unlysed blood, induced strong expression of heat shock protein 70, a neuronal injury marker, in experimental models [40]. There is a significant entry of prothrombin into the brain after erythrocyte lysis. If activated factor X is present, either because of the entry of factor X from the blood or through expression of factor X by brain parenchymal cells, an influx of prothrombin will result in the generation of thrombin within the brain, and consequently edema formation.

Complement, which is excluded from brain parenchyma in normal conditions by the intact blood–brain barrier, can enter into the brain after ICH as a result of the extravasation of blood or, later, as a result of blood–brain barrier disruption. Complement-related brain injury seems to be mediated by the membrane attack complex (MAC) formation which can cause the formation of pores in the cell membrane leading to cell lysis. The MAC also seems to be related to cytokine, oxygen radicals, and matrix proteins release. The complement cascade has been found to participate in PHBE formation in ICH experimental models which show the attenuation of PHBE after the administration of inhibitors of the complement cascade [41, 42].

Matrix metalloproteinases (MMPs), a group of proteolytic zinc-dependent enzymes that are able to degrade the endothelial basal lamina [43], may also play a key role in ICH brain injury, increasing capillary permeability and producing brain edema. In experimental models of cerebral ischemia, the inhibition of MMP has been reported as decreasing the PHBE. Different molecules have been implicated in the MMP-mediated injury, such as reactive oxygen species (ROS), nitric oxide (NO), and proteases. In experimental models of ICH, the expression of MMPs coincides with an increase in free radicals in cells and in the endothelium, and the treatment with an MMP inhibitor reduces both the production of the oxidative stress and brain edema formation [44].

Molecular signatures of PHBE

Pro-inflammatory molecules which are released as a result of the activation of clotting proteins [26,27,45]

and biomarkers of endothelial damage markers and blood–brain barrier disruption [20] have already been reported as associated with PHBE development in clinical studies.

A significant correlation has been found between high plasma levels of interleukin-6 (IL-6), tumor necrosis factor-alpha (TNF-α), and intercellular adhesion molecule-1 (ICAM-1) and the volume of PHBE developed 3–4 days after ICH [46]. These findings are in agreement with the notion of edema as an indicator of the inflammatory response induced by hematoma.

It has been also demonstrated that poor clinical outcome and increased volume of the residual cavity after ICH are associated with high concentrations of glutamate in blood within the first 24 hours from symptom onset [46], suggesting that excitotoxicity, as well as inflammation, may have an important role in causing secondary brain injury after cerebral hemorrhage.

Matrix metalloproteinases have also been reported to increase as a result of ICH [47–49]. More specifically, MMP-9 levels were demonstrated to positively correlate with the volume of PHBE as well as with the enlargement of PHBE within the first 48 hours of evolution [47, 49]. Significantly higher MMP-9 levels were found in patients with neurological worsening [47], whereas MMP-3 levels were associated with mortality at three months in patients with ICH [49]. It remains to be demonstrated whether other more specific markers of blood–brain barrier disruption, such as cellular fibronectin, which has recently been reported to be an independent predictor of early hematoma growth [50], could also be a marker of edema around the hematoma.

Neuroimaging features of PHBE

In the first hours of intraparenchymal hemorrhage, a hypodense ring in the periphery of the hematoma is observed in CT scan [51] (Fig. 20.2). The initial attenuation surrounding the high-density hemorrhage is caused by the serum extruded into the brain after clot retraction. Subsequently, the circumferential hypodensity increases and reaches maximum at approximately 3–4 days. This increment in PHBE is due to vasogenic edema, and can last several days.

Magnetic resonance imaging is playing an ever more important role in the evaluation of hyperacute cerebrovascular disease. In MRI, PHBE appears as a hypointense rim surrounding hematoma on T1-weighted imaging and hyperintense on T2-weighted imaging or FLAIR sequences (Fig. 20.3) [52]. Diffusion- and perfusion-weighted MRI (DWI and PWI) are useful techniques in the evaluation and management of acute ischemic stroke, as well as in the evaluation of perihematomal injury in hyperacute ICH. Diffusion-weighted MRI characterizes alterations in the diffusibility of water, which is thought to provide a measure of tissue bioenergetic compromise, and PWI provides a measure of relative cerebral perfusion. A perihematomal rim of increased apparent diffusion coefficient (ADC) in MRI studies in hyperacute phase of ICH is found in 25% of cases [53]. The elevated ADC indicates that perihematomal edema is highly diffusible, suggesting that it is a plasma-derived vasogenic edema [23].

Single-photon emission computerized tomography (SPECT) is useful in the study of PHBE evolution [25]. A primary reduction of cerebral blood flow occurs in immediately adjacent tissue surrounding hematoma, resolving within minutes to hours, leading to minimal edema. Perilesional blood flow normalizes from initially depressed levels during the first 72 hours, as edema forms, finding a correlation between extension of edema and the volume of reperfused tissue, indicating that the reperfusion injury is implicated in the pathogenesis of PHBE formation.

Clinical significance and prognosis of PHBE

Neurological deterioration is a common event after stroke. It occurs in 20–40% of patients, and is associated with poor prognosis, worsening functional outcome, and increasing mortality [54]. In patients with spontaneous ICH, neurological deterioration occurs in 22.9% of cases, and is more likely to happen within the first 48 hours from symptoms onset [55]. Several mechanisms are implicated in the development of neurological deterioration in patients with ICH. Early neurological deterioration is generally thought to be due to enlargement of the hemorrhage or development of hydrocephalus, whereas late deterioration is linked to delayed perilesional edema [56].

Several studies have evaluated the presence of PHBE and prognosis in patients with spontaneous ICH. Jauch et al. found that absolute edema volume is not independently associated with mortality [57]. Gebel et al. found that initial relative edema was strongly predictive of improved neurological outcome in patients with hyperacute supratentorial spontaneous ICH without intraventricular extension [58]. However, this paradox has not been replicated by

Fig. 20.2 Perihematomal edema as hypodensity around the hematoma on CT scan.

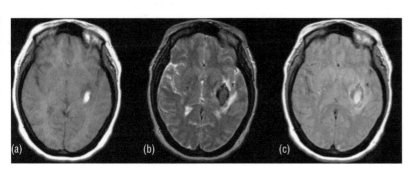

Fig. 20.3 Perihematomal edema appears as a hypointense rim in T1 sequences (a) and a hyperintense rim in T2 (b) and FLAIR (c) sequences.

(a)   (b)   (c)

others. In fact, Silva *et al.* found that the delayed increase in perihematomal edema was associated with poor neurological outcome, but not the initial perihematoma hypodensity [59]. Delayed edema growth that occurs days to weeks after spontaneous ICH may be associated with increased mass effect and clinical neurological deterioration [60].

Therapeutic management of PHBE

Several drugs have been used for the treatment of PHBE in ICH, with poor results. Glycerol has demonstrated no profit in management of PHBE [61], as well as corticosteroids, use of which is related in some occasions with higher number of infections [62]. Nowadays, mannitol is used when PHBE is associated with intracranial pressure increase, but its routine use is not accepted [63]. In a recent clinical trial, recombinant activated factor VII administered within the first four hours has been demonstrated to reduce mortality and improve functional outcome in patients with ICH, and also limits hematoma growth and reduces total lesion volume (hemorrhage plus edema), with small increase in the frequency of thromboembolic adverse events [64]. This drug opens new therapeutic options in the treatment of ICH.

Regarding surgical treatment, results are controversial. Stereotactic aspiration with local administration of urokinase has been demonstrated to be as effective as conventional craniotomy in reduction of brain edema volume caused by ICH [65]. However, other research found that despite significant reduction in the size of the hematoma, clot liquefaction with recombinant tissue plasminogen activator and aspiration invokes a substantial inflammatory response and does not result in a reduction of the PHBE [66]. Early surgical treatment of ICH, however, does not provide overall benefit compared with medical treatment [67].

Several drugs have demonstrated their benefit in PHBE treatment in animal models, and in the future may block PHBE development in clinical practice. Systemic administration within the first six hours of argatroban, an inhibitor of both free and fibrin-bound thrombin, in a rat model causes a significant reduction of edema and does not increase hematoma volume [68]. Deferoxamine and other iron chelators attenuate brain edema in ICH, and may be potential therapeutic agents for treating ICH, reducing the oxidative stress caused by the release of iron from the hematoma [69]. Celecoxib, a selective cyclooxygenase-2 inhibitor reduces inflammation and brain edema formation in patients with ICH, and induces better functional recovery in rats [70]. Besides diverse drugs, hypothermia also reduces the brain edema formation after ICH in rats [71].

References

1. Dul K, Drayer BP. CT and MR imaging of intracerebral hemorrhage. In: Kase CS, Caplan LR, eds. *Intracerebral Hemorrhage*. Boston, Butterworth-Heinemann. 1994; 73–98.

2. Diringer MN. Intracerebral hemorrhage: pathophysiology and management. *Crit Care Med* 1993; **21**: 1591–1603.

3. Gebel J, Brott T, Sila C, *et al.* Decreased perihematomal edema in thrombolysis-related intracerebral hemorrhage as compared to spontaneous intracerebral hemorrhage. *Stroke* 2000; **31**: 596–600.

4. Gebel JM, Jauch EC, Brott TG, *et al.* Natural history of perihematomal edema in patients with hyperacute spontaneous intracerebral hemorrhage. *Stroke* 2002; **33**: 2631–2635.

5. Gong Y, Hua Y, Keep RF, Hoff JT, Xi G. Intracerebral hemorrhage: effects of aging on brain edema and neurological deficits. *Stroke* 2004; **35**: 2571–2575.

6. Song EC, Chu K, Jeong SW, *et al.* Hyperglycemia exacerbates brain edema and perihematomal cell death after intracerebral hemorrhage. *Stroke* 2003; **34**: 2215–2220.

7. Herold S, von Kummer R, Jaeger CH. Follow-up of spontaneous intracerebral haemorrhage by computed tomography. *J Neurol* 1982; **228**: 267–276.

8. Sinar EJ, Mendelow AD, Graham DI, Teasdale GM. Experimental intracerebral hemorrhage; effects of a temporary mass lesion. *J Neurosurg* 1987; **66**: 568–576.

9. Carhuapoma JR, Wang PY, Beauchamp NJ, *et al.* Diffusion-weighted MRI, and proton MR spectroscopic imaging in the study of secondary neuronal injury after intracerebral hemorrhage. *Stroke* 2000; **31**: 726–732.

10. Wagner KR, Xi G, Hua Y, *et al.* Lobar intracerebral hemorrhage model in pigs: rapid edema development in perihematomal white matter. *Stroke* 1996; **27**: 490–497.

11. Del Bigio MR, Yan HJ, Buist R, Peeling J. Experimental intracerebral hemorrhage in rats. Magnetic resonance imaging and histopathological correlates. *Stroke* 1996; **27**: 2312–2319.

12. Fishman RA. Brain edema. *N Engl J Med* 1975; **293**: 706–711.

13. Enzmann DR, Britt RH, Lyons BE, Buxton JL, Wilson DA. Natural history of experimental intracerebral hemorrhage: sonography, computed sonography and neuropathology. *AJNR Am J Neuroradiol* 1981; **2**: 517–526.

14. Tomita H, Ito U, Ohno K, Hirakawa K. Chronological changes in brain edema induced by experimental intracerebral hematoma in cats. *Acta Neurochir Suppl (Wien)* 1994; **60**: 558–560.

15. Suzuki R, Ohno K, Hiratsuka H, Inaba Y. Chronological changes in brain edema in hypertensive intracerebral hemorrhage observed by CT and xenon-enhanced CT. In: Inaba Y, Klatzo I, Spatz M, eds. *Brain Edema*. Berlin, Springer. 1985; 613–620.

16. Inaji M, Tomita H, Tone O, *et al.* Chronological changes of perihematomal edema of human intracerebral hematoma. *Acta Neurochir Suppl* 2003; **86**: 445–448.

17. Nath FP, Kelly PT, Jenkins A, *et al.* Effects of experimental intracerebral hemorrhage on blood flow, capillary permeability, and histochemistry. *J Neurosurg* 1987; **66**: 555–562.

18. Yang GY, Betz AL, Chenevert TL, Brunberg JA, Hoff JT. Experimental intracerebral hemorrhage: relationship between brain edema, blood flow, and blood-brain barrier permeability in rats. *J Neurosurg* 1994; **81**: 93–102.

19. Lee KR, Colon GP, Betz AL, *et al.* Edema from intracerebral hemorrhage: the role of thrombin. *J Neurosurg* 1996; **84**: 91–96.

20. Rosenberg GA, Navratil M. Metalloproteinase inhibition blocks edema in intracerebral hemorrhage in rats. *Neurology* 1997; **48**: 921–926.

21. Xi G, Keep RF, Hoff JT. Erythrocytes and delayed brain edema formation following intracerebral hemorrhage in rats. *J Neurosurg* 1998; **89**: 991–996.

22. Kingman TA, Mendelow AD, Graham D, Teasdale G. Experimental intracerebral mass: time-related effects on local cerebral blood flow. *J Neurosurg* 1987; **67**: 732–738.

23. Butcher KS, Baird T, MacGregor L, *et al.* Perihematomal edema in primary intracerebral hemorrhage is plasma derived. *Stroke* 2004; **35**: 1879–1885.

24. Schellinger PD, Fiebach JB, Hoffmann K, *et al.* Stroke MRI in intracerebral hemorrhage: is there a perihemorrhagic penumbra? *Stroke* 2003; **34**: 1674–1680.

25. Mayer SA, Lignelli A, Fink ME, *et al.* Perilesional blood flow and edema formation in acute intracerebral hemorrhage: a SPECT study. *Stroke* 1998; **29**: 1791–1798.

26. Lee KR, Kawai N, Kim S, Sagher O, Hoff JT. Mechanisms of edema formation after intracerebral hemorrhage: effects of thrombin on cerebral blood flow, blood-brain barrier permeability, and cell survival in a rat model. *J Neurosurg* 1997; **86**: 272–278.

27. Xi G, Wagner KR, Keep RF, *et al.* Role of blood clot formation on early edema development after experimental intracerebral hemorrhage. *Stroke* 1998; **29**: 2580–2586.

28. Lee KR, Betz AL, Kim S, Keep RF, Hoff JT. The role of the coagulation cascade in brain edema formation after intracerebral hemorrhage. *Acta Neurochir (Wien)* 1996; **138**: 396–401.

29. Hua Y, Xi G, Keep RF, Hoff JT. Complement activation in the brain after experimental intracerebral hemorrhage. *J Neurosurg* 2000; **92**: 1016–1022.

30. Wagner KR, Xi G, Hua Y, *et al.* Ultra-early clot aspiration after lysis with tissue plasminogen activator in a porcine model of intracerebral hemorrhage: edema reduction and blood brain barrier protection. *J Neurosurg* 1999; **90**: 491–498.

31. Hamada R, Matsuoka H. Antithrombin therapy for intracerebral hemorrhage. *Stroke* 2000; **31**: 794–795.

32. Bar-Shavit R, Benezra M, Sabbah V, Bode W, Vlodavsky I. Thrombin as a multifunctinal protein: induction of cell adhesion and proliferation. *Am J Respir Cell Mol Biol* 1992; **6**: 123–130.

33. Malik AB, Fenton JW II. Thrombin-mediated increase in vascular endothelium permeability. *Semin Thromb Hemost* 1992; **18**: 193–199.

34. Xue M, Del Bigio MR. Acute tissue damage after injections of thrombin and plasmin into rat striatum. *Stroke* 2001; **32**: 2164–2169.

35. Xi G, Hua Y, Bhasin RR, *et al.* Mechanisms of edema formation after intracerebral hemorrhage. Effects of extravasated red blood cells on blood flow and blood-brain barrier integrity. *Stroke* 2001; **32**: 2932–2938.

36. Huang F, Xi G, Keep RF, *et al.* Brain edema after experimental intracerebral hemorrhage: role of hemoglobin degradation products. *J Neurosurg* 2002; **96**: 287–293.

37. Lamb NJ, Quinlan GJ, Mumby S, Evans TW, Gutteridge JM. Haem oxygenase shows pro-oxidant activity in microsomal and cellular systems: implications for the release of low-molecular-mass iron. *Biochem J* 1999; **1**: 153–158.

38. Nakamura T, Xi G, Park J-W, *et al.* Holo-transferrin and thrombin can interact to cause brain injury. *Stroke* 2005; **36**: 348–358.

39. Ogihara K, Zubkov AY, Bernanke DH, *et al.* Oxyhemoglobin-induced apoptosis in cultured endothelial cells. *J Neurosurg* 1999; **91**: 459–465.

40. Matz PG, Weinstein PR, Sharp FR. Heme oxygenase-1 and heat shock protein 70 induction in glia and neurons throughout rat brain alter experimental intracerebral hemorrhage. *Neurosurgery* 1997; **40**: 152–160.

41. Hua Y, Xi G, Keep RF, Hoff JT. Complement activation in the brain after experimental intracerebral hemorrhage. *J Neurosurg* 2000; **92**: 1016–1022.

42. Xi G, Wagner KR, Hua Y, *et al.* Systemic complement depletion diminishes perihematomal brain edema. *Stroke* 2001; **32**: 162–167.

43. Romanic AM, Madri JA. Extracellular matrix-degrading proteinases in the nervous system. *Brain Pathol* 1994; **4**: 145–156.

44. Wang J, Tsirka SE. Neuroprotection by inhibition of matrix metalloproteinases in a mouse model of intracerebral haemorrhage. *Brain* 2005; **128**: 1622–1633.

45. Vergnolle N, Hollenberg MD, Wallace JL. Pro- and anti-inflammatory actions of thrombin: a distinct role for proteinase-activated receptor-1 (PAR1). *Br J Pharmacol* 1999; **126**: 1262–1268.

46. Castillo J, Dávalos A, Álvarez-Sabín J, *et al.* Molecular signatures of brain injury after intracerebral hemorrhage. *Neurology* 2002; **58**: 624–629.

47. Abilleira S, Montajer J, Molina C, *et al.* Matrix metalloproteinase-9 concentration after spontaneous intracerebral hemorrhage. *J Neurosurg* 2003; **99**: 65–70.

48. Power C, Henry S, Del Bigio MR, *et al.* Intracerebral hemorrhage induces macrophage activation and matrix metalloproteinases. *Ann Neurol* 2003; **53**: 731–742.

49. Álvarez-Sabín J, Delgado P, Abilleira S, *et al.* Temporal profile of matrix metalloproteinases and their inhibitors after spontaneous intracerebral hemorrhage. Relationship to clinical and radiological outcome. *Stroke* 2004; **35**: 1316–1322.

50. Silva Y, Leira R, Tejada J, *et al.* Molecular signatures of vascular injury are associated with early growth of intracerebral hemorrhage. *Stroke* 2005; **36**: 86–91.

51. Grossman RI, Yousem DM. Vascular diseases of the brain. In: Grossman RI, Yousem DM, eds. *Neuroradiology. The Requisites*, 2nd edn. St. Louis, Mosby. 2003; 173–242.

52. Linfante I, Llinas RH, Caplan LR, Warach S. MRI features of intracerebral hemorrhage within 2 hours from symptom onset. *Stroke* 1999; **30**: 2263–2267.

53. Kidwell CS, Saver JL, Mattiello J, *et al.* Diffusion-perfusion MR evaluation of perihematomal injury in hyperacute intracerebral hemorrhage. *Neurology* 2001; **57**: 1611–1617.

54. Dávalos A, Castillo J. Progressing stroke. In: Fisher M, Bogousslavsky J, eds. *Current Review of Cerebrovascular Disease*. Philadelphia, Current Medicine. 1999; 149–160.

55. Leira R, Dávalos A, Silva Y, *et al.* Early neurologic deterioration in intracerebral hemorrhage: predictors and associated factors. *Neurology* 2004; **63**: 461–467.

56. Mayer SA, Sacco RL, Shi T, Mohr JP. Neurological deterioration in noncomatose patients with supratentorial intracerebral hemorrhage. *Neurology* 1994; **44**: 1379–1384.

57. Jauch E, Gebel J, Salisbury S, *et al.* Lack of association between early edema and outcome in spontaneous intracerebral hemorrhage. *Stroke* 1999; **30**: 249.

58. Gebel JM, Jauch EC, Brott TG, *et al.* Relative edema volume is a predictor of outcome in patients with hyperacute spontaneous intracerebral hemorrhage. *Stroke* 2002; **33**: 2636–2641.

59. Silva Y, Leira R, Vila N, *et al.* Peripheral edema and early and late clinical outcome in spontaneous intracerebral hemorrhage. *Stroke* 2005; **36**: 465.

60. Zazulia AR, Diringer MN, Derdeyn CP, Powers WJ. Progression of mass effect after intracerebral hemorrhage. *Stroke* 1999; **30**: 1167–1173.

61. Yu YL, Kumana CR, Lauder IJ, *et al.* Treatment of acute cerebral hemorrhage with intravenous glycerol. A double-blind, placebo-controlled, randomized trial. *Stroke* 1992; **23**: 967–971.

62. Poungvarin N, Bhoopat W, Viriyavejakul A, *et al.* Effects of dexamethasone in primary supratentorial intracerebral hemorrhage. *N Engl J Med* 1987; **316**: 1229–1233.

63. Bereczki D, Liu M, Prado GF, Fekete I. Cochrane report: A systematic review of mannitol therapy for acute ischemic stroke and cerebral parenchymal hemorrhage. *Stroke* 2000; **31**: 2719–2722.

64. Mayer SA, Brun NC, Begtrup K, *et al.* Recombinant Activated Factor VII Intracerebral Hemorrhage Trial Investigators. Recombinant activated factor VII for acute intracerebral hemorrhage. *N Engl J Med* 2005; **352**: 777–785.

65. Huang CF, Tsai ZP, Li CS, Wang KL, Wang YC. Surgical improvement of brain edema related to hypertensive intracerebral hemorrhage. *Zhonghua Yi Xue Za Zhi (Taipei)* 2002; **65**: 241–246.

66. Thiex R, Kuker W, Muller HD, *et al.* The long-term effect of recombinant tissue-plasminogen-activator (rt-PA) on edema formation in a large-animal model of intracerebral hemorrhage. *Neurol Res* 2003; **25**: 254–262.

67. Mendelow AD, Gregson BA, Fernandes HM, *et al.* STICH investigators. Early surgery versus initial conservative treatment in patients with spontaneous supratentorial intracerebral haematomas in the International Surgical Trial in Intracerebral Haemorrhage (STICH): a randomised trial. *Lancet* 2005; **365**: 387–397.

68. Kitaoka T, Hua Y, Xi G, Hoff JT, Keep RF. Delayed argatroban treatment reduces edema in a rat model of intracerebral hemorrhage. *Stroke* 2002; **33**: 3012–3018.

69. Nakamura T, Keep RF, Hua Y, *et al.* Deferoxamine-induced attenuation of brain edema and neurological deficits in a rat model of intracerebral hemorrhage. *J Neurosurg* 2004; **100**: 672–678.

70. Chu K, Jeong SW, Jung KH, *et al.* Celecoxib induces functional recovery after intracerebral hemorrhage with reduction of brain edema and perihematomal cell death. *J Cereb Blood Flow Metab* 2004; **24**: 926–933.

71. Kawanishi M. Effect of hypothermia on brain edema formation following intracerebral hemorrhage in rats. *Acta Neurochir Suppl* 2003; **86**: 453–456.

Hemostatic therapy for intracerebral hemorrhage

Wendy C. Ziai and Stephan A. Mayer

Introduction

The high mortality and disability associated with intra-cerebral hemorrhage (ICH), and especially the poten-tially preventable damage from rebleeding, have brought hemostatic strategies to the forefront of the medical management of acute ICH. Hemostatic abnormalities are frequent in ICH with evidence for both systemic and local coagulation disturbances involving activation of both fibrinolytic and coagula-tion systems. A number of pharmacological agents have been reported to reduce bleeding in a variety of clinical settings, while only one to date, recombinant activated factor VII (rFVIIa), has undergone a double-blind randomized controlled study in ICH. This chapter reviews hemostatic abnormalities reported in patients with ICH and discusses pharmacological strategies for prevention of hematoma expansion in both coagulopathic and non-coagulopathic ICH.

Hemostatic systems

Hemostasis, the physiological response to vascular injury, results from activation of a highly regulated series of procoagulant and anticoagulant zymogens and cofactors. Coagulation factors circulate in the blood as inactive zymogens. In vivo activation of hemostasis requires a combination of endothelial injury and exposure of the subendothelial protein matrix to circulating blood. The process requires two key cell types: tissue factor (TF)-bearing cells and platelets. According to the cell-based model of coagu-lation, the process of hemostasis begins with the inter-action between cell-derived TF and blood-borne FVIIa, the initiation phase [1,2] (Fig. 21.1). The for-mation of the FVIIa–TF complex permits activation

of factors IX and X, a process which generates small amounts of thrombin and is critical to the amplifica-tion and propagation phases of coagulation. Factor Xa forms a complex with its cofactor FV on the phospho-lipid membrane of activated platelets. Formation of the FXa–FVa complex activates prothrombin to gen-erate a small amount of thrombin which subsequently accelerates the coagulation cascade by activating FV, FVIII, FXI and platelets. Activated platelets provide the scaffolding for coagulation and the thrombin generation needed to change soluble fibrinogen into insoluble fibrin clots [3]. In addition, the TF–FVIIa complex cleaves FIX to FIXa which diffuses out to activated platelets and forms a complex with its cofac-tor FVIIIa on the platelet phospholipid membrane. The platelet FIXa–VIIIa complex then cleaves FX to FXa which generates large amounts of thrombin [4].

Platelet adhesion and activation results from ex-posure of vascular subendothelium, atheroma, fibrin deposition, or other abnormal surfaces to the blood-stream. Activation of glycoprotein 1b/IX receptors causes platelets to undergo conformational changes and degranulation. Platelet adhesion promotes the release of partially activated FV from platelets, which is required for the formation of the prothrombinase FXa–FVa complex [5]. Platelet fibrinogen receptors (glycoprotein IIb/IIIa) also undergo conformational changes resulting in increased fibrinogen binding to platelets, thus attaching additional platelets to the thrombus.

Tissue factor is an important initiator of coagu-lation, serving as the cofactor for FVIIa-dependent FX activation. The brain is an extremely rich source of TF, which is found in the adventitia of superficial cerebral vessels and non-capillary microvessels of the cerebral cortex [6–8]. Exposure of TF to the

Intracerebral Hemorrhage, ed. J. R. Carhuapoma, S. A. Mayer, and D. F. Hanley. Published by Cambridge University Press.
© J. R. Carhuapoma, S. A. Mayer, and D. F. Hanley 2010.

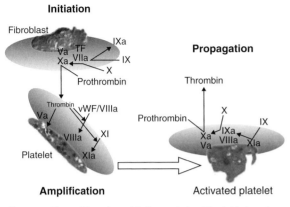

Fig. 21.1 The cell-based model of coagulation. The initiation phase occurs on the tissue factor-bearing cell such as a fibroblast. Amplification of the coagulant response occurs on the platelet surface which becomes activated and is further stimulated by platelet adhesion. Propagation occurs on the activated platelet surface as activated proteases combine with their cofactors and generate the thrombin burst required for fibrin polymerization. vWF, von Willebrand's factor. From Hoffman and Monroe [1].

bloodstream after ICH activates the extrinsic coagulation pathway to stop bleeding.

Intracerebral hemorrhage appears to cause subtle abnormalities of blood coagulation and fibrinolysis parameters. These hemostatic abnormalities may be the result of brain damage, or may be caused by activation of the coagulation system in response to bleeding. Some investigations have found similar hemostatic disturbances in both ischemic and hemorrhagic stroke patients, suggesting that the presence of brain damage may be a more important factor than bleeding per se [9]. Antovic *et al.* measured prothrombin time (PT), activated partial thromboplastin time (aPTT), fibrinogen, activity of FVII, antithrombin, plasmin inhibitor (PI) and fibrin D-dimer within 1 hour after onset in 30 patients with ischemic stroke (IS), 20 patients with ICH, 10 patients with subarachnoid hemorrhage (SAH), and 10 controls. They found significant decreases in PT%, FVII activity and antithrombin, and increases in fibrinogen and D-dimer (indicator of activation of blood coagulation and fibrinolytic systems) in IS and both groups of hemorrhagic stroke [9]. Plasmin inhibitor levels were significantly lower in patients with SAH compared to both ICH and IS patients, which did not differ from controls.

The finding of increased fibrinolysis in SAH was consistent with a Japanese study of 358 patients admitted within 6 hours of ICH [10]. Intracerebral hemorrhage patients with intraventricular hemorrhage (IVH) or SAH had significantly higher levels of white blood cell counts, level of thrombin–antithrombin complex (TAT; indicator of activation of the blood coagulation system), plasmin–antiplasmin complex (indicator of activation of fibrinolytic system), and D-dimer compared to patients without blood in the subarachnoid space. In fact, most of the hematological parameters examined showed no significant differences compared to controls in patients without IVH or SAH. The levels of TAT were independently associated with the severity of IVH and SAH, but not with hematoma volume. The authors concluded that intraparenchymal hematomas are unlikely to activate peripheral hemostatic systems, but likely do cause local activation of such systems. A proposed mechanism for these findings is that tissue factor released from injury to superficial brain tissue gains access to the systemic circulation through entry of blood into the subarachnoid space.

Another Japanese study of 90 patients studied within 3 hours of hypertensive ICH reported significant activation of the coagulation system through measurement of Fibrinopeptide A (FPA) and TAT, both indicators of thrombin generation in plasma [11]. Fibrinopeptide A is released from fibrinogen after cleavage of the $A\alpha$ chain by thrombin and TAT is a complex form of thrombin rapidly inactivated by antithrombin III (ATIII) in plasma. In this study, plasma levels of both FPA and TAT were higher in ICH patients without hematoma enlargement compared to patients whose ICH enlarged on a second CT scan within 24 hours of ictus. Fibrinopeptide A levels were less than 10 ng/ml in all patients with ICH expansion. The TAT levels were positively correlated with hematoma volume in the group with unchanged ICH size. The authors concluded that larger amounts of thrombin may be generated to stop larger volumes of bleeding, and that in patients with ICH enlargement insufficient thrombin generation may result in prolonged bleeding. This study did not dichotomize patients by presence of blood in the subarachnoid space as the prior study had done.

There is also evidence that platelet function may be altered in the acute phase of ICH. Saloheimo *et al.* [12] studied thomboxane A (TXA$_2$) and prostacyclin (PGI$_2$) biosynthesis in 43 patients with ICH by measuring their metabolites (11-dehydrothromboxane B$_2$, 2,3-dinor-thromboxane B$_2$, and 2,3-dinor-6-ketoprostaglandin F$_{1\alpha}$) in urine [13]. Thromboxane

A_2 is a potent stimulator of platelet activation [14] and vasoconstriction [15]; PGI_2 inhibits platelet aggregation and causes vasodilation [16]. Both are the major products of arachadonic acid metabolism in platelets [17]. Comparing aspirin users and non-users, this study reported levels of TXA_2 and PGI_2 in non-aspirin users which were significantly higher than controls during the acute phase of ICH and at three months follow-up [12]. Aspirin users with ICH had urinary excretion rates of TXA_2 and PGI_2 metabolites that were significantly lower than non-users and not significantly different from healthy controls. These levels increased after stopping aspirin and reached the level of non-users within a few days and at three-month follow-up. Aspirin use, although associated with longer bleeding times was not associated with hematoma enlargement or worse clinical outcomes. Larger studies, however, have subsequently reported that aspirin is associated with hematoma expansion and worse outcome after ICH [18]. This finding remains controversial and may be confounded by patients on aspirin being older and having more baseline disability [19].

Platelet activity can be measured at point of care with the PFA-100 (Siemens AG, Germany) and the Verify Now-ASA (Accumetrics, CA, USA) systems yielding results significantly faster than platelet aggregometry which requires specialized personnel and a dedicated laboratory. In a prospective study of 76 patients with ICH, 33 (43%) patients had reduced platelet activity on the VerifyNow-ASA assay, of which 14 (42%) were not known to take antiplatelet agents [20]. Of 27 (36%) patients with reduced platelet activity on the PFA-100, a related but different 14 (52%) were not known to take antiplatelet agents. This study may suggest that these assays do not reliably identify patients who report antiplatelet medication use before ICH. Alternatively medication histories may be inaccurate, surreptitious antiplatelet medication use may occur, or platelet hypofunction, either primary or secondary to ICH, may be a factor independent of medication use. These results also may explain why some studies report an association between known aspirin use and outcomes after ICH while others do not. Determination of which platelet activity assay, if any, is associated with measurable clinical outcomes such as ICH volume growth, 3-month outcomes, or acute interventions may lead to utility of platelet activity testing and possible therapeutic intervention [20]. In a related study by the same investigators, abnormal platelet activity measured with the Ultegra Rapid VerifyNow-ASA technique, but not the reported use of antiplatelet medications, was associated with the occurrence of IVH, a greater ICH severity score, and a higher mortality risk in patients with ICH [21]. Nonetheless, routine measurement or correction of reduced platelet activity in patients with ICH is not supported at this time.

The "gold standard" test for measuring platelet activity is platelet aggregometry [22].

Using these methods several small studies have suggested that patients with ICH may have underlying platelet hypofunction [23,24]. These studies were limited by the timing of testing for platelet function and lacked assessment of hematoma volume. In a study of ADP-induced platelet release reactions in acute stroke patients, Mulley et al. found evidence of platelet *hyper*activity in thromboembolic stroke (n = 23) while patients with either primary ICH (n = 15) or SAH (n = 5) had *hypo*reactive platelets by 5-hydroxytryptamine release after stimulation with ADP [23]. Blood samples were collected within seven days of the event in 80% of patients, but included patients up to 40 days after stroke. Follow-up studies one year later in 17 patients with undifferentiated stroke demonstrated persistently impaired release reactions in patients with initially *hypo*reactive platelets, suggesting the hemorrhagic stroke patients may have chronic platelet abnormalities.

One prospective cohort study of 43 patients with acute spontaneous supratentorial ICH measured platelet function within one week of onset of ICH and correlated with serial CT scans [25]. Comparison with 35 age-matched controls with neuromuscular disease requiring intensive care demonstrated significant decreases in platelet counts in ICH patients over the first week of admission and a significant correlation between fall in platelet count and increase in hematoma size. Platelet function abnormalities, including aggregation to arachadonic acid, collagen, and ADP, and ATP release reactions to thrombin and collagen, and prolonged bleeding time were a common finding in ICH patients compared to standardized controls. Platelet dysfunction was more common in large ($> 30 \, cm^3$) compared to small ICH (80% vs. 50%). In conclusion, platelet dysfunction was common among patients with ICH and extended beyond an aspirin effect.

Not all studies have documented platelet *hypo*function in the presence of intracerebral blood. Liu *et al.* [26] reported platelet *hyper*function in both non-hemorrhagic and hemorrhagic ischemic stroke patients, as determined by significantly increased platelet aggregation rates induced by ADP or epinephrine, and elevated plasma levels of beta-thromboglobulin, a marker of in vivo platelet activation and aggregation. Platelet function was tested within 72 hours of onset. These observations do not prove whether ICH is a cause or consequence of platelet dysfunction. Further, the mechanism by which ICH may alter normal platelet function in vivo is not known.

In summary, intracerebral and intraventricular hemorrhage appear to be associated with subtle abnormalities of blood coagulation, platelet function, and fibrinolysis, and there is some evidence that these abnormalities may be more pronounced in patients with more extensive hemorrhage. However, some of these findings have also been reported in patients with ischemic stroke, suggesting that they may reflect a non-specific response to brain injury. Thus, the clinical relevance of these findings remains unknown.

Local coagulation abnormalities in ICH

Equally important to the issue of early hematoma expansion and stopping further hemorrhage is the likelihood of a localized coagulation disturbance resulting in ongoing hemorrhage or early rebleeding, events where medical management may be able to intervene successfully. It is generally accepted that bleeding associated with ICH in many cases is not completed within the first few minutes of onset. This concept is based on multiple studies (several retrospective and one prospective) showing that CT-documented early hematoma growth occurs in 18–38% of patients [27–30] even in the absence of overt systemic coagulopathy [31,32]. The highest rate of early hematoma growth was documented by the only prospective study, which reported ultra-early hematoma growth within 1 hour of the baseline scan in 26% of patients and in an additional 12% of patients from 1 to 20 hours. However, this may have been an underestimate, because clinical deterioration and early surgical intervention precluded the performance of follow-up scans in some patients in this study [27].

The pathophysiology of early hematoma expansion, and in particular the evidence for local coagulation disturbances comes largely from clinical data, as no animal model exists which accurately models the dynamics of human hypertensive hemorrhage. The ultra-early recurrence of bleeding (or failure of initial bleeding to stop) may occur at the site of an initial ruptured lenticulostriate artery or arteriole, although histopathological, CT, single-photon emission computed tomography (SPECT) and both conventional and CT angiography (CTA) suggest that secondary bleeding at the periphery of a blood clot is multifocal and may represent ruptured arterioles or venules [33–35]. An association between early hematoma growth and irregular shape of the blood clot may support bleeding from multiple arterioles [36,37]. Other evidence comes from CTA studies performed immediately after ICH which demonstrated active contrast extravasation into the hematoma in 30–46% of patients [38,39] and from angiography showing bleeding from single and simultaneous multiple lenticulostriate arteries immediately after ICH [40,41].

One mechanism of hematoma expansion is that increased vascular congestion and local tissue pressure produce an ischemic congested layer of tissue at the margin of the hematoma where intravascular hydrostatic pressure may cause secondary bleeding from venules and arterioles which continues due to ischemic tissue damage [34,42]. An alternative or perhaps additional explanation is that plasma which rapidly infiltrates into peripheral brain tissue around the hematoma [43] may produce a local coagulopathy that inhibits hemostasis through inhibition of thrombin, platelet aggregation, and degradation of clotting factors [34]. There is some evidence that brain tissue inherently possesses fibrinolytic activity, and that this is increased in experimental models of ICH [44,45].

Management strategies for hemostasis manipulation in non-coagulopathic ICH

The rationale for hemostasis manipulation in ICH is to stop rebleeding in the acute phase thus preventing hematoma enlargement. This may then minimize late neurological deterioration, which occurs in a third of patients, is predicted by ICH volume, and is most likely caused by perihematomal edema and mass effect [35,46]. Potential hemostatic agents for ICH may focus on a single hemostatic abnormality, or

Table 21.1. A comparison of potential strategies for hemostatic control in spontaneous non-coagulopathic ICH

Comparison factor	rFVIIa (NovoSeven)	Aprotinin	Aminocaproic acid (EACA, TACA)	Desmopressin
Mechanism of hemostasis	Thrombin generation on surface of activated platelets, and at site of injury	Inhibits serine proteases (plasmin, kallikrein, thrombin); no effect on platelet function	Inhibit conversion of plasminogen to plasmin	Increases von Willebrand factor and FVIII activity
Time of onset	Immediate	0.5 h	Immediate	Immediate
Half-life	2.5 h	2.5 to 5 h	2 to 3 h	2.8 to 3 h
Level of evidence for efficacy as hemostatic agent	RCT for hemophilia, intractable surgical bleeding; Phase IIb RCT for ICH;	RCT for cardiac and non-cardiac surgery; no studies for ICH	RCT for SAH, cardiac and non-cardiac surgery; no studies for ICH	RCT for cardiac surgery; no studies for ICH
Major risks	Thromboembolism	Hypersensitivity reactions (< 0.1%); no increase in MI, renal failure or mortality	Thrombosis in major vessels; limited safety data; concern for rhabdomyolysis and renal dysfunction	Myocardial infarction in cardiac surgery patients
Other benefits		Attenuates systemic inflammatory response; may decrease mortality after cardiac surgery		
Cost	Most expensive	Expensive	Inexpensive	Inexpensive

Notes: EACA, epsilon-aminocaproic acid; TACA, tranexamic acid; RCT, randomized controlled trial; MI, myocardial infarction.

perhaps a multi-agent approach may be required with potential targets for intervention being inhibition of fibrinolysis, thrombin generation, or improvement of platelet function. Ideally such an agent should activate coagulation locally producing effective hemostasis without causing systemic thrombosis or activation of the coagulation system. The standard treatments available to reverse abnormal coagulation (usually the result of oral anticoagulant medication) include fresh frozen plasma (FFP), vitamin K, prothrombin complex concentrate (PCC) and factor IX complex (FIX). These agents are not likely to be suitable for patients with normal coagulation status, because their primary role is to replace factor deficiencies, which do not exist in normal patients. Moreover, they can result in potential complications such as anaphylaxis (vitamin K), fluid overload (FFP), transmission of infectious agents (FFP, FIX), and thromboembolism (PCC and FIX) [47,48]. Here we focus on antifibrinolytic (epsilon-aminocaproic acid [EACA], tranexamic acid, and aprotinin), platelet-enhancing (antifibrinolytics, 1-Deamino-8-D-arginine vasopressin

[DDAVP, desmopressin]), and pro-hemostatic (recombinant activated factor VII [rFVIIa]) agents that may be appropriate for the prevention of early rebleeding after ICH (Table 21.1).

Aminocaproic acid and tranexamic acid

Aminocaproic acid and tranexamic acid are synthetic derivatives of the amino acid lysine with proven antifibrinolytic activity in humans [49]. These agents bind reversibly to plasminogen and prevent its conversion to plasmin by blocking its activation by fibrin. They do not activate coagulation, thrombin generation or clot formation. Epsilon-aminocaproic acid, the less potent of the two agents, has a shorter half-life and has been studied in the initial non-operative management of aneurysmal SAH and found to reduce the risk of rebleeding by approximately 50%; however, prolonged antifibrinolytic treatment was associated with an increase in the incidence of hydrocephalus and delayed ischemic deficits, resulting in no net benefit on mortality [50]. The use of a brief preoperative course of high-dose EACA [50] or tranexamic acid [51] in SAH patients has since been found to be safe and beneficial for diminishing the risk of early rebleeding prior to early surgical intervention, and many centers are increasingly adopting this strategy. Both agents are effective in treating non-neurological bleeding disorders such as primary menorrhagia, upper gastrointestinal tract bleeding, and mucosal bleeding in patients with thrombocytopenia and other coagulopathies [49,52,53].

One pilot study has examined the potential efficacy of EACA for preventing early hematoma growth after ICH [54]. Three of the first five patients given a 5 g IV loading dose of EACA followed by an infusion of 1 g/hour for 23 hours experienced significant hematoma expansion, compared to two of nine control patients. The 80% confidence interval for the frequency of hematoma growth in EACA-treated patients was 32–88%. The authors concluded that the rate of hematoma expansion in patients given EACA within 12 hours of ICH is probably no less than the natural history rate, although this treatment appears to be safe.

Aprotinin

Aprotinin is an inhibitor of serine proteases such as trypsin, chymotrypsin, plasmin, and kallikrein [55]. It has been shown to promote clot formation through its antifibrinolytic activity (inhibition of FXII formation through kallikrein inhibition), by inhibiting plasmin-induced complement activation, and by protecting platelet adhesive surface receptors [56]. Aprotinin is a small polypeptide with predictable pharmacokinetics and a half-life of 2.5–5 hours [55]. A full dose of aprotinin produces plasma concentrations that inhibit both fibrinolysis and inflammation [57]. It has been successfully used in cardiac and liver transplantation surgery to prevent bleeding complications. In a systematic review of the literature (35 coronary artery bypass trials), aprotinin treatment compared to placebo reduced blood transfusion and was associated with reduced incidence of stroke [58]. However, a more recent large randomized trial found that aprotinin use during cardiac surgery was associated with an increased risk of renal failure requiring dialysis, myocardial infarction, heart failure, and stroke or encephalopathy [59]. Neither EACA or tranexamic acid were associated with these risks compared to placebo.

Aprotinin has been used to avoid coagulopathy during deep hypothermic cardiopulmonary bypass for craniotomy, during preoperative management of ruptured intracranial aneurysms combined with low-dose tranexamic acid, and locally in neurosurgical operations to prevent hyperfibrinolytic hemorrhage [60–62]. Aprotinin is derived from bovine origin and has a potential for hypersensitivity reactions ranging from mild skin rash and urticaria to anaphylaxis and circulatory collapse [55]. Hypersensitivity reactions are rarely reported depending on pre-exposure status: < 0.1% of cases with no prior exposure; 5% if exposed to aprotinin within six months, and 0.9% thereafter [55]. Aprotinin has not been studied in patients with intracerebral hemorrhage.

Desmopressin

Desmopressin (DDAVP) is a synthetic analog of the natural pituitary hormone 8-arginine vasopressin [55]. Its hemostatic mechanism is to increase release of von Willebrand's factor into the blood and increase levels of anti-hemophilic FVIII activity in plasma. Its primary use in hemostasis is for improved coagulation in mild hemophilia and conditions associated with platelet dysfunction. As defective platelet function is not established as a causative factor in rebleeding from ICH, there is no current rationale for its use in this disease. Moreover, desmopressin treatment for cardiac surgery patients doubled the myocardial infarction rate with only small decreases in perioperative blood loss and no clinical outcome benefit [63].

Recombinant activated factor VII

Recombinant activated factor VII (rFVIIa) (eptacog alpha [activated], NovoSeven®, Novonordisk A/S, Bagsvaerd, Denmark) is a vitamin K-dependent glycoprotein, structurally similar to the plasma-derived activated form of the naturally occurring initiator of hemostasis [55]. It was developed for treatment of spontaneous and surgical hemorrhage in patients with hemophilia A or B and inhibitors to FVIII or FIX, respectively [3,64]. Factor VIIa in supraphysiological or pharmacological doses binds to the surface of activated platelets and directly activates FIX and FX to generate thrombin and augment the coagulation process, bypassing the need for FVIII (and also FIX) [4,65,66]. Recombinant FVIIa does not bind to resting platelets. Because its action is specific to activated platelets, which are present mainly at sites of vessel injury, FVIIa enhances local hemostasis without systemic activation of the coagulation cascade [67]. Factor VIIa has been shown to effectively initiate hemostasis in patients with normal coagulation systems [68,69] and demonstrated 84% efficacy in stopping central nervous system bleeds in patients with hemophilia at doses ranging from 80 to 100 μg/kg [70]. Only 1 of 21 patients in this study died and no adverse events related to rFVIIa administration were reported.

The half-life of rFVIIa varies from 2.4 to 3.2 hours with IV bolus administration given over 2–5 minutes in adults [67,71]. The half-life is shorter in children, but is otherwise not affected by patient gender or ethnic origin [71–73]. An almost immediate onset of action has been observed; apparent hemostasis in the setting of uncontrolled surgical bleeding has been described within 10 minutes [68,69]. Moreover, a single IV bolus dose results in complete normalization of elevated INR in patients treated with oral anticoagulant therapy within 10 minutes [71]. Rapid localized action and short half-life of rFVIIa make this agent a potentially ideal drug for the acute high-risk stage of ICH.

Clinical indications for rFVIIa

In hemophilic patients with inhibitors to FVIII or FIX, rFVIIa has been approved by the US Food and Drug Administration (FDA) for nearly a decade for prevention and treatment of bleeding episodes [4]. Recombinant FVIIa used as a home treatment for bleeding episodes in hemophiliacs produces effective hemostasis with 84–97% efficacy [74–77]. It has also been successfully used to treat a variety of non-hemophilic coagulopathies [68,78] and non-coagulopathic patients with intractable surgical bleeding [79]. Recombinant FVIIa has been effectively used for rapid correction of a variety of coagulopathic conditions in non-hemophilic patients undergoing neurosurgical procedures including craniotomy for evacuation of epidural and intraparenchymal hemorrhages, ICP monitor and ventriculostomy placement and intraspinal hemorrhage [80,81]. For uncontrolled bleeding in multi-trauma patients, PT and PTT were significantly shortened within minutes following administration of rFVIIa and cessation of bleeding was achieved in 72% of a small study of 36 patients [4]. Patients had received a median of 21 units of packed red blood cells prior to administration of rFVIIa.

Interestingly, acidosis diminished the hemostatic effect of rFVIIa, while hypothermia did not affect it.

Recombinant FVIIa was studied for use in SAH in an open-label, dose-escalation safety study in collaboration with the UK Spontaneous Intracranial Hemorrhage Group [82]. After nine patients were treated without evidence of cerebral ischemia, the tenth patient developed middle cerebral artery branch thrombosis contralateral to the aneurysm on day 4 after a bolus dose of 80 μg/kg followed by continuous infusion at 7 μg/(kg h). The study was suspended pending further investigation.

Safety of rFVIIa

Under normal physiological conditions, only 1% of endogenous FVII circulates as FVIIa and has very weak enzymatic activity until it binds to TF [67]. Administration of rFVIIa elevates the level of activated FVII by 1000-fold, but should not result in clotting in the absence of functional (exposed) TF, which is required for complexing VIIa and initiating the coagulation cascade. Thus rFVIIa-induced coagulation is localized to sites of vessel injury. Thromboembolic complications associated with use of rFVIIa are the most frequent and serious complications due to FVIIa [55]. These include acute myocardial infarction, pulmonary embolism, and disseminated intravascular coagulation [83–86]. The frequency of serious adverse events was recently reported in the range of 1–2 % after well over 700 000 doses administered to several thousand patients for various clinical indications [74,85,86]. Only 17 adverse thrombotic events (11 arterial, 6 venous) after more than 180 000 standard doses of rFVIIa given primarily to hemophilia patients were reported as of 2001, and most of these were attributed to underlying prothrombotic states rather than a direct effect of rFVIIa [71,85].

A more recent analysis of thromboembolic adverse events reported to the FDA from 1999 to 2005, however, suggests that the frequency of serious thromboembolic adverse events with rFVIIa may be substantially higher in non-coagulopathic patients treated for bleeding emergencies [87]. In this report, a total 185 thromboembolic events were described. Non-hemophilic indications with active bleeding accounted for 151 of these adverse events, which included ischemic stroke (n = 39), acute myocardial infarction (n = 34), other arterial thromboses (n = 26), pulmonary embolism (n = 32), and other venous thromboses including deep vein thrombosis (n = 42). In 36 (72%) of 50 reported deaths, the probable cause of death was the thromboembolic event. In 144 patients with timing information, 73 events (51%) occurred in the first 24 hours after the last dose (30 events within 2 hours). Most reports lacked sufficient information to evaluate potential dosage associations.

In the ICH literature, two reports shed light on the safety of rFVIIa for treatment of acute ICH. A dose-escalation phase IIa study was initially performed to determine whether rFVIIa is a safe and feasible treatment for patients with acute ICH scanned within 3 hours of onset [88]. This randomized double-blind placebo-controlled trial included 48 ICH patients treated with placebo (n = 12) or rFVIIa (10, 20, 40, 80, 120, or 160 μg/kg; n = 6 per group). Of six possible treatment-related adverse events, only two cases of deep vein thrombosis occurred and no myocardial ischemia, consumption coagulopathy, or dose-related increase in edema to ICH volume was found. Subsequently, in the first report of a double-blind study of clinical efficacy of rFVIIa in ICH, arterial thromboembolic serious adverse events occurred significantly more frequently with rFVIIa treatment than with placebo; there were 16 events (5% of patients) in the combined treatment groups versus none in the placebo group [89]. These were most often myocardial ischemic events or cerebral infarction within three days of administration of study drug. The majority of patients recovered from these events and the overall frequency of fatal or disabling thromboembolic serious adverse events was 2% in the rFVIIa and placebo groups. Mayer and Brun found that among 485 patients with ICH enrolled in the three phase II trials conducted to date, a history of thromboembolic disease was not found to predict acute thromboembolic complications associated with rFVIIa administration [90]. In a more thorough analysis of the same dataset, Diringer et al. reported that there was no overall increase in risk of total thromboembolic events in rFVIIa-treated patients; however, there were more arterial, but not venous, events in patients treated with higher doses (120–160 g/kg) compared with placebo (5.4% versus 1.7%; P = 0.13) [91]. Arterial events after rFVIIa treatment in these studies tended to be split equally between non-ST-segment elevation myocardial ischemic events manifesting as troponin elevations, and cerebral infarctions.

Clinical trials with rFVIIa in ICH

The phase IIB NovoSeven ICH trial was a randomized, double-blind, placebo-controlled, dose-ranging study that investigated the use of rFVIIa given within four hours of ICH onset in patients with normal coagulation [89]. This study was powered to detect a 50% relative reduction in hematoma growth at 24 hours. Clinical outcomes were also assessed at 90 days. The study recruited patients from 73 hospitals in 20 countries. Patients were excluded for reasons of deep coma (score of 3–5 on the Glasgow Coma Scale [GCS]) and planned surgical evacuation of hematoma within 24 hours after admission. A total of 399 patients were randomized to receive IV rFVIIa at a dose of 40 μg/kg (n = 108), 80 μg/kg (n = 92), 160 μg/kg (n = 103) or placebo (n = 96). Pooled data for all FVIIa doses demonstrated a 52% relative reduction in hematoma volume growth compared with placebo (p = 0.01) (Table 21.2). Recombinant FVIIa reduced mortality or an unfavorable outcome more than placebo. At 90 days, mortality was 29% in the placebo group versus 18% in the combined treatment groups (p = 0.02), a relative reduction of 38%. The absolute reduction in risk of death or severe disability was 16% (95% confidence interval [CI], 5–27; p = 0.004) [89]. Lower mortality was therefore not associated with an increase in severe disability. Based on combined doses of rFVIIa, the number needed to treat (NNT) to prevent one death was ten patients (95% CI, 5–82). The NNT to prevent one unfavorable outcome was slightly more than six (95% CI: 4–22).

The phase III FAST trial

The results of the aforementioned phase IIB trial were considered extremely encouraging, and served as the basis for the Factor Seven in Hemorrhagic Stroke (FAST) trial. In this study 841 ICH patients were randomly assigned to receive placebo, 20, or 80 μg/kg of rFVIIa [92]. Inclusion and exclusion criteria were essentially identical to those of the phase IIB trial. The hemostatic effect of rFVIIa was confirmed: there was a 2.6 ml (95% CI, −0.3 to 5.5; p = 0.08) absolute reduction in ICH volume growth in the 20 μg/kg group, and 3.8 ml (95% CI, 0.9 to 6.7; p = 0.009) reduction in the 80 μg/kg group. The safety profile of rFVIIa in the ICH patient population was also confirmed, with a small but significant increase in arterial thromboembolic events (9% versus 4%,

Table 21.2. Recombinant activated factor VII at 40, 80, and 160 μg/kg vs. placebo given within 4 hours of intracerebral hemorrhage

	Treatment groups				
	rFVIIa				
Dose of rFVIIa	40 μg/kg (N = 108)	80 μg/kg (N = 92)	160 μg/kg (N = 103)	Combined Doses (N = 303)	Placebo (N = 96)
Change in ICH volume at 24 hours, ml (percent change from baseline)	5.4 (16%)	4.2 (14%)	2.9 (11%)	4.2 (14%)	8.7 (29%)
P-value for percent change in ICH volume (rFVIIa vs. placebo)	0.13	0.04	0.008	0.01	
90-day mortality, N (%)	19 (18%)	17 (18%)	20 (19%)	56 (18%)	28 (29%)
P-value for mortality (rFVIIa vs. placebo)	0.05	0.10	0.11	0.02	
90-day unfavorable outcome MRS* (4–6), N (%)	59 (55%)	45 (49%)	56 (54%)	160 (53%)	66 (69%)
P-value for unfavorable outcome (rFVIIa vs. placebo)	0.02	0.008	0.02	0.004	

Note: *MRS = modified Rankin Scale. A score of 4–6 indicates death or moderate-to-severe disability with lack of ability to ambulate independently.
Source: Adapted from [89], with permission.

p = 0.04) (Table 21.3). Despite the reduction in bleeding, however, there was no significant difference among the three groups in the proportion of patients with poor clinical outcome (24% in the placebo group, 26% in the group receiving 20 μg/kg, and 29% in the group receiving 80 μg/kg).

There are several possible explanations for the conflicting results of the phase IIB and phase III FAST trials. The most striking discrepancy is the remarkably improved three-month outcomes of the 268 placebo patients enrolled in FAST (24% modified Rankin Score [mRS] 5 or 6) compared to the 96 placebo patients in the phase IIB study (45% mRS 5 or 6). It seems most likely that the phase IIB placebo group did extraordinarily poorly, due to chance effects, whereas outcome in the FAST placebo group were more in line with those of prior studies. There were also several potentially important randomization imbalances in FAST, particularly regarding the presence of IVH at baseline (29% in placebo versus 41% in the 80 μg/kg group). Another important source of "noise" – death or severe disability unrelated to the bleed itself – were late-occurring medical complications such as nosocomial infections, renal failure, and cardiac arrhythmias. These events were much more common in very elderly patients, and tended to "dilute" the signal the study was designed to measure:

whether a treatment that reduces ICH lesion volume can translate into improved survival with a good outcome.

Both FAST and the earlier phase IIB study indicate that little active bleeding occurs between the third and fourth hours after ICH onset. Treatment with rFVIIa after three hours thus exposes patients to the 5% risk of an arterial thromboembolic event, without much potential for benefit. Perhaps the most important lesson learned from FAST is that to effectively improve outcome, hemostatic therapy must be targeted to patients who are actively bleeding. A detailed post-hoc analysis of the FAST dataset indicates that reducing onset-to-needle time to 2.5 hours or less will be necessary in future studies evaluating rFVIIa for non-coagulopathic ICH [93]. In this analysis, the impact of rFVIIa (80 μg/kg) on poor outcome at three months (mRS of 5 or 6) was systematically analyzed within subgroups, using clinically meaningful cut-points in onset-to-treatment time, age, and baseline ICH and IVH volume. A subgroup (n = 160, 19% of the FAST population) was identified comprising patients ≤ 70 years with baseline ICH volume < 60 ml, IVH volume < 5 ml, and time from onset to treatment ≤ 2.5 hours. The adjusted odds ratio (OR) for poor outcome with rFVIIa treatment was 0.28 (95% CI, 0.08–1.06) while the reduction in ICH

Table 21.3. Clinical outcome and thromboembolic SAEs at 90 days in the FAST trial*

Outcome/Serious Adverse Event (SAE)	Placebo (N = 268)	rFVIIa	
		20 µg/kg (N = 276)	80 µg/kg (N = 297)
Mortality	51 (19)	50 (18)	62 (21)
Odds ratio for survival (95% CI)		0.8 (0.5–1.4)	1.1 (0.7–31.8)
P value		0.38	0.75
mRS†			
Poor outcome (score 5–6)	62 (24)	69 (26)	84 (29)
Odds ratio (95% CI)‡	–	1.0 (0.6–1.6)	1.4 (0.9–2.2)
Barthel Index score§			
Median	70.0	72.5	70.0
P value	–	0.54	0.91
NIHSS score**			
Median	5.0	5.0	4.0
P value	–	.20	.02
Thromboembolic SAEs	21 (8)	24 (9)	31 (11)
Arterial	11 (4)	14 (5)	25 (9)¶
MI	8 (3)	11 (4)	14 (5)
Cerebral Infarction	4 (2)	4 (2)	10 (3)
Venous	11 (4)	10 (4)	7 (2)
DVT	9 (3)	7 (3)	7 (2)
Pulmonary embolism	2 (1)	4 (2)	3 (1)

Notes: *Data are n (%) except where indicated. Day 15 outcome scores were analyzed according to the principle of last-observation-carried-forward when day 90 scores were missing in 9, 9, and 13 of the placebo, 20 µg/kg, and 80 µg/kg patients, respectively. mRS scores were not available for one patient in the placebo and one patient in the 20 µg/kg groups.
†Scores of 5 to 6 indicate severe disability (bed bound and incontinent) or death.
‡Odds ratios were adjusted for premorbid mRS score, baseline ICH volume, ICH location (infra vs. supratentorial), age, and gender.
§Score of 100 indicates complete independence in activities of daily living and 0 indicates total dependence or death. Treatment groups were compared with placebo by an ANOVA on the ranks. For patients who died prior to day 90 the last recorded NIHSS score was carried forward.
**Score of 0 indicates no neurological deficit and a score of 42 indicates comatose and quadriplegic or dead. Treatment groups were compared with placebo by an ANOVA on the ranks. For patients who died prior to day 90 the last recorded NIHSS score was carried forward.
¶Includes one case each of renal artery thrombosis, intracardiac thrombus, and retinal artery occlusion. The frequency of arterial SAEs was significantly increased in the 80 µg/kg group compared to placebo (P = 0.04, chi-square test).
Source: With permission [88].

growth was almost doubled (7.3 ± 3.2 versus 3.8 ± 1.5 ml, p = 0.02). The improved effect was confirmed in an analysis of similar phase II patients.

A prospective trial is needed to determine whether younger ICH patients without extensive bleeding at baseline can benefit from 80 µg/kg of rFVIIa given within 2.5 hours of symptom onset. Selection of patients based on contrast extravasation into the clot after CTA ("spot sign") is another promising approach that is currently being evaluated in the phase II STOP-IT trial [94,95]. Until more data are available off-label use of rFVIIa should probably be restricted to the emergency reversal of warfarin anticoagulation in patients with acute intracranial bleeding in order to expedite a potentially life-saving neurosurgical procedure.

Table 21.4. Emergency management of the coagulopathic ICH patient

Scenario	Agent	Dose	Comments	Level of evidence*
Warfarin	Fresh frozen plasma (FFP)	15 ml/kg	Usually 4 to 6 units (200 ml each) are given	II
	or Prothrombin complex concentrate	15–30 U/kg	Works faster than FFP, but carries risk of DIC	II
	and IV Vitamin K	10 mg	Can take up to 24 hours to normalize INR	II
Warfarin and emergency neurosurgical intervention	Above plus Recombinant factor VIIa	20–80 μg/kg	Contraindicated in acute thromboembolic disease	III
Unfractionated or low molecular weight heparin	Protamine sulfate	1 mg per 100 units of heparin, or 1 mg of enoxaparin	Can cause flushing, bradycardia, or hypotension.	III
Platelet dysfunction or	Platelet transfusion	6 units	Range 4–8 units based on size; transfuse to > 100 000	III
thrombocytopenia	and/or Desmopressin (DDAVP)	0.3 μg/kg	Single dose required	III

Notes: *Class I = based on one or more high quality randomized controlled trials; Class II = based on two or more high quality prospective or retrospective cohort studies; Class III = Case reports and series, expert opinion.
Source: DIC, disseminated intravascular coagulation. Adapted from [101].

Coagulopathic ICH

Clinical trials of warfarin therapy for stroke prevention in non-valvular atrial fibrillation indicate a risk of ICH of < 1% [96]. Warfarin anticoagulation increases the risk of ICH by 5- to 10-fold in the general population, and approximately 15% of ICH cases are associated with warfarin use [97]. Although the studied risk is low, warfarin worsens the severity of spontaneous ICH in terms of increased risk of ongoing in-hospital bleeding and increased risk of hematoma expansion which significantly increases mortality [98]. The risk of ICH volume expansion in the first 24 hours is over 50% in warfarin-treated patients [98], and there is a dose–response relationship between degree of elevation of the INR and three-month mortality [99].

Intracerebral hemorrhage patients receiving warfarin should be reversed immediately with FFP or PCC, and IV vitamin K (Table 21.4) [100,101].

Treatment should never be delayed in order to check coagulation tests. Unfortunately, normalization of the INR with this approach usually takes several hours, and clinical results are often poor. The associated volume load with FFP may also cause congestive heart failure in the setting of cardiac or renal disease [100].

Although no randomized controlled trials addressing this intervention have been conducted, urgent reversal of the INR is included in most consensus guidelines for management of anticoagulation related ICH. Goldstein et al. studied the hypothesis that higher doses of FFP and vitamin K and shorter times to initiation of therapy would be associated with a higher rate of reversal of anticoagulation [102]. They found that faster administration of FFP increased the likelihood of successful reversal of the INR at 24 hours after warfarin-related ICH. However, in this retrospective study, neither earlier treatment nor INR reversal at 24 hours translated into improved clinical outcome. The inability to quickly reverse coagulopathy and potentially alter outcome may be due to late presentation, which in this study occurred at a median of 4 hours after symptom onset. It has also been suggested that FFP and vitamin K may be insufficient and too slow to rapidly reverse coagulopathies [103].

Faster-acting agents such as PCC and rFVIIa have been shown in small case series to normalize the INR much quicker than FFP, often within an hour or two [81,104,105]. Activated rFVII in low doses (as low as 5 μg/kg) has been demonstrated to rapidly normalize the INR within minutes, with larger doses producing a longer duration of effect [106,107]. Recombinant FVIIa in doses ranging from 10 to 90 μg/kg has been used to reverse the effects of warfarin in acute ICH, primarily to expedite neurosurgical intervention, with good clinical results [105,108]. When this approach is used, rFVIIa should be used as an adjunct to coagulation factor replacement and vitamin K, since its effect will only last several hours [97]. Prothrombin complex concentrate, a concentrate of the vitamin K-dependent coagulation factors II, VII, IX, and X, normalizes the INR more rapidly than FFP, and can be given in smaller volumes [109].

Intracerebral hemorrhage patients who have been anticoagulated with unfractionated or low-molecular-weight heparin should be reversed with protamine sulfate [101,110], and patients with thrombocytopenia or platelet dysfunction can be treated with a single dose of DDAVP, platelet transfusions, or both [101,111]. When patients have a strong indication for anticoagulation, such as a prosthetic heart valve, full anticoagulation can safely be restarted 10–14 days after ICH in most cases [101,112]. The risk of embolic events in patients at high embolic risk is less than 5% in the first 30 days after discontinuation of warfarin in the setting of ICH [113].

Conclusion

In the modern era of acute stroke intervention, effective medical management to correct coagulopathies and prevent further bleeding from ICH should be developed just as has been accomplished for acute ischemic stroke. There is a need for more evidence to place hemostatic therapy for ICH on firmer scientific footing, however. The results of the phase II and III trials of rFVIIa for non-coagulopathic ICH are encouraging, and hold the promise that an effective emergency treatment for ICH may one day be available for those who have an extremely high risk of active bleeding based on a tighter therapeutic window or a validated imaging modality that demonstrates vessel leakage. If this is the case, future efforts may be directed at testing the efficacy of combining very early surgery with acute hemostatic therapy, which might minimize the risk of postoperative bleeding that occurs with very early surgical intervention [114].

Acknowledgement

The authors thank Dr Ulla Hedner, MD, for providing a critical review of this manuscript.

References

1. Hoffman M, Monroe DM. A cell-based model of haemostasis. *Thromb Haemost* 2001; **85**: 958–965.

2. Hoffman M. A cell-based model of coagulation and the role of factor VIIa. *Blood Rev* 2003; **17**(1): S1–5.

3. Rizoli SB, Chughtai T. The emerging role of recombinant activated Factor VII (rFVIIa) in the treatment of blunt traumatic haemorrhage. *Expert Opin Biol Ther* 2006; **6**(1): 73–81.

4. Martinowitz U, Michaelson M. Guidelines for the use of recombinant activated factor VII (rFVIIa) in uncontrolled bleeding: a report by the Israeli Multidisciplinary rFVIIa Task Force. *J Thromb Haemost* 2005; **3**: 640–648.

5. Briede JJ, Heemskerk JW, van't Veer C, Hemker HC, Lindhout T. Contribution of platelet-derived factor Va to thrombin generation on immobilized collagen- and fibrinogen-adherent platelets. *Thromb Haemost* 2001; **85**: 509–513.

6. Drake TA, Morrissey JH, Edgington TS. Selective cellular expression of tissue factor in human tissues: implications for disorders of hemostasis and thrombosis. *Am J Pathol* 1989; **134**: 1087–1097.

7. Fleck RA, Rao LV, Rapaport SI, Varki N. Localization of human tissue factor antigen by immunostaining with monospecific, polyclonal anti-human tissue factor antibody. *Thromb Res* 1990; **57**: 765–781.

8. del Zoppo GJ, Yu JQ, Copeland BR, *et al*. Tissue factor localization in non-human primate cerebral tissue. *Thromb Haemost* 1992; **68**: 642–647.

9. Antovic J, Bakic M, Zivkovic M, Ilic Z, Blomback M. Blood coagulation and fibrinolysis in acute ischemic and hemorrhagic (intracerebral and subarachnoid hemorrhage) stroke: does decreased plasmin inhibitor indicate increased fibrinolysis in subarachnoid hemorrhage compared to other types of stroke? *Scand J Clin Lab Invest* 2002; **62**: 195–200.

10. Fujii Y, Takeuchi S, Harada A, *et al.* Hemostatic activation in spontaneous intracerebral hemorrhage. *Stroke* 2001; **32**: 883–890.

11. Takahashi H, Urano T, Nagai N, Takada Y, Takada A. Progressive expansion of hypertensive intracerebral hemorrhage by coagulopathy. *Am J Hematol* 1998; **59**(2): 110–114.

12. Saloheimo P, Juvela S, Riutta A, Pyhtinen J, Hillbom M. Thromboxane and prostacyclin biosynthesis in patients with acute spontaneous intracerebral hemorrhage. *Thromb Res* 2005; **115**: 367–373.

13. FitzGerald GA, Pedersen AK, Patrono C. Analysis of prostacyclin and thromboxane biosynthesis in cardiovascular disease. *Circulation* 1983; **67**: 1174–1177.

14. Svensson J, Hamberg M, Samuelsson B. On the formation and effects of thromboxane A_2 in human platelets. *Acta Physiol Scand* 1976; **98**: 285–294.

15. Ellis EF, Oelz O, Roberts LJ II, *et al.* Coronary arterial smooth muscle contraction by a substance released from platelets: evidence that it is thromboxane A_2. *Science* 1976; **193**: 1135–1137.

16. Bunting S, Gryglewski R, Moncada S, Vane JR. Arterial walls generate from prostaglandin endoperoxides a substance (prostaglandin X) which relaxes strips of mesenteric and celiac arteries and inhibits platelet aggregation. *Prostaglandins* 1976; **12**: 897–913.

17. Hammarström S, Falardeau P. Resolution of prostaglandin endoperoxide synthase and thromboxane synthase of human platelets. *Proc Natl Acad Sci U S A* 1977; **74**: 3691–3695.

18. Toyoda K, Okada Y, Minematsu K, *et al.* Antiplatelet therapy contributes to acute deterioration of intracerebral hemorrhage. *Neurology* 2005; **65**: 1000–1004.

19. Foerch C, Sitzer M, Steinmetz H, Neumann-Haefelin T. Pretreatment with anti-platelet agents is not independently associated with unfavorable outcome in intracerebral hemorrhage. *Stroke* 2006; **37**: 2165–2167.

20. Naidech AM, Bassin SL, Bernstein RA, *et al.* Reduced platelet activity is more common than reported anti-platelet medication use in patients with intracerebral hemorrhage. *Neuroint Care* 2009; Apr 21.

21. Naidech AM, Bernstein RA, Levasseur K, *et al.* Platelet activity and outcome after intracerebral hemorrhage. *Ann Neurol* 2009; **65**(3): 352–356.

22. Lordkipanidze M, Pharand C, Schampaert E, *et al.* A comparison of six major platelet function tests to determine the prevalence of aspirin resistance in patients with stable coronary artery disease. *Eur Heart J* 2007; **28**: 1702–1708.

23. Mulley GP, Heptinstall S, Taylor PM, Mitchell JRA. ADP-induced platelet release reaction in acute stroke. *Thromb Haemost* 1983; **50**(2): 524–526.

24. Serebruany VL, Gurbel PA, Shustov AR, *et al.* Depressed platelet status in an elderly patient with hemorragic stroke after thrombolysis for acute myocardial infarction. *Stroke* 1998; **29**: 235–238.

25. Ziai WC, Torbey MT, Kickler T, Wityk RJ. Platelet count and function in spontaneous intracerebral hemorrhage. *J Stroke Cerebrovasc Dis* 2003; **12**(4): 201–206.

26. Liu L, Lin Z, Shen Z, *et al.* Platelet hyperfunction exists in both acute non-hemorrhagic and hemorrhagic stroke. *Thromb Res* 1994; **75**: 485–490.

27. Brott T, Broderick J, Kothari R, *et al.* Early hemorrhage growth in patients with intracerebral hemorrhage. *Stroke* 1997; **28**: 1–5.

28. Fujitsu K, Muramoto M, Ikeda Y, *et al.* Indications for surgical treatment of putaminal hemorrhage. Comparative study based on serial CT and time-course analysis. *J Neurosurg* 1990; **73**: 518–525.

29. Kazui S, Naritomi H, Yamamoto H, Sawada T, Yamaguchi T. Enlargement of spontaneous intracerebral hemorrhage. Incidence and time course. *Stroke* 1996; **27**: 1783–1787.

30. Fujii Y, Tanaka R. Predictors of hematoma growth? *Stroke* 1998; **29**: 2442–2443.

31. Chen ST, Chen SD, Hsu CY, Hogan EL. Progression of hypertensive intracerebral hemorrhage. *Neurology* 1989; **39**: 1509–1514.

32. Broderick JP, Brott TG, Tomsick T, Barsan W, Spilker J. Ultra-early evaluation of intracerebral hemorrhage. *J Neurosurg* 1990; **72**: 195–199.

33. Fisher CM. Pathological observations in hypertensive cerebral hemorrhage. *J Neuropathol Exp Neurol* 1971; **30**: 536–550.

34. Mayer SA, Lignelli A, Fink ME, *et al.* Perilesional blood flow and edema formation in acute intracerebral hemorrhage: a SPECT study. *Stroke* 1998; **29**: 1791–1798.

35. Mayer SA. Intracerebral hemorrhage: natural history and rationale of ultra-early hemostatic therapy. *Intensive Care Med* 2002; **28** Suppl 2: S235–240.

36. Fujii Y, Tanaka R, Takeuchi S, *et al.* Hematoma enlargement in spontaneous intracerebral hemorrhage. *J Neurosurg* 1994; **80**: 51–57.

37. Fujii Y, Takeuchi S, Sasaki O, Minakawa T, Tanaka R. Multivariate analysis of predictors of hematoma enlargement in spontaneous intracerebral hemorrhage. *Stroke* **29**: 1160–1166.

38. Murai Y, Takagi R, Ikeda Y, Yamamoto Y, Teramoto A. Three-dimensional computerized

tomography angiography in patients with hyperacute intracerebral hemorrhage. *J Neurosurg* 1999; **91**: 424–431.

39. Becker KJ, Baxter AB, Bybee HM, *et al.* Extravasation of radiographic contrast is an independent predictor of death in primary intracerebral hemorrhage. *Stroke* 1999; **30**: 2025–2032.

40. Mizukami M, Araki G, Mihara H, Tomita T, Fujinaga R. Arteriographically visualized extravasation in hypertensive intracerebral hemorrhage. Report of seven cases. *Stroke* 1972; **3**: 527–537.

41. Komiyama M, Yasui T, Tamura K, *et al.* Simultaneous bleeding from multiple lenticulostriate arteries in hypertensive intracerebral haemorrhage. *Neuroradiology* 1995; **37**: 129–130.

42. Takasugi S, Ueda S, Matsumoto K. Chronological changes in spontaneous intracerebral hematoma – an experimental and clinical study. *Stroke* 1985; **16**: 651–658.

43. Wagner KR, Xi G, Hua Y, *et al.* Lobar intracerebral hemorrhage model in pigs: rapid edema development in perihematomal white matter. *Stroke* 1996; **27**(3): 490–497.

44. Tovi D. Fibrinolytic activity of human brain. A histochemical study. *Acta Neurol Scand* 1973; **49**(2): 152–162.

45. Tovi D. Nilsson IM. Increased fibrinolytic activity and fibrin degradation products after experimental intracerebral haemorrhage. *Acta Neurol Scand* 1972; **48**(4): 403–415.

46. Mayer SA, Sacco RL, Shi T, Mohr JP. Neurologic deterioration in noncomatose patients with supratentorial intracerebral hemorrhage. *Neurology* 1994; **44**: 1379–1384.

47. Cartmill M, Dolan G, Byrne JL, Byrne PO. Prothrombin complex concentrate for oral anticoagulant reversal in neurosurgical emergencies. *Br J Neurosurg* 2000; **14**: 458–461.

48. Kohler M, Hellstern P, Lechler E, Uberfuhr P, Muller-Berghaus G. Thromboembolic complications associated with the use of prothrombin complex and factor IX concentrates. *Thromb Haemost* 1998; **80**: 399–402.

49. Mannucci PM. Hemostatic drugs. *N Engl J Med* 1998; **339**: 245–253.

50. Leipzig TJ, Redelman K, Horner TG. Reducing the risk of rebleeding before early aneurysm surgery: a possible role for antifibrinolytic therapy. *J Neurosurg* 1997; **86**(2): 220–225.

51. Hillman J, Fridriksson S, Nilsson O, *et al.* Immediate administration of tranexamic acid and reduced incidence of early rebleeding after aneurysmal subarachnoid hemorrhage: a prospective randomized study. *J Neurosurg* 2002; **97**: 771–778.

52. Henry DA, O'Connell DL. Effects of fibrinolytic inhibitors on mortality from upper gastrointestinal haemorrhage. *BMJ* 1989; **298**: 1142–1146.

53. Walsh PN, Rizza CR, Matthews JM, *et al.* Epsilon-aminocaproic acid therapy for dental extractions in haemophilia and Christmas disease: a double blind controlled trial. *Br J Haematol* 1971; **20**: 463–475.

54. Piriyawat P, Morgenstern LB, Yawn DH, Hall CE, Grotta JC. Treatment of acute intracerebral hemorrhage with epsilon-aminocaproic acid: a pilot study. *Neurocrit Care* 2004; **1**: 47–52.

55. Levy JH. Overview of clinical efficacy and safety of pharmacologic strategies for blood conservation. *Am J Health Syst Pharm.* 2005; **62**(Suppl 4): S15–19.

56. Paran H, Gutman M, Mayo A. The effect of aprotinin in a model of uncontrolled hemorrhagic shock. *Am J Surg* 2005; **190**(3): 463–466.

57. Levy JH, Bailey JM, Salmenpera M. Pharmacokinetics of aprotinin in preoperative cardiac surgical patients. *Anesthesiology* 1994; **80**(5): 1013–1018.

58. Sedrakyan A, Treasure T, Elefteriades JA. Effect of aprotinin on clinical outcomes in coronary artery bypass graft surgery: a systematic review and meta-analysis of randomized clinical trials. *J Thorac Cardiovasc Surg* 2004; **128**(3): 442–448.

59. Mangano DT, Tidor IC, Dietzel C, for the Multicenter Study of Perioperative Ischemia Research Group and the Ischemia Research and Education Foundation. The risk associated with aprotinin in cardiac surgery. *New Engl J Med* 2005; **354**: 353–365.

60. Grady RE, Oliver WC Jr, Abel MD, Meyer FB. Aprotinin and deep hypothermic cardiopulmonary bypass with or without circulatory arrest for craniotomy. *J Neurosurg Anesthesiol* 2002; **14**(2): 137–140.

61. Spallone A, Pastore FS, Rizzo A, Guidetti B. Low-dose tranexamic acid combined with aprotinin in the pre-operative management of ruptured intracranial aneurysms. *Neurochirurgia (Stuttg)* 1987; **30**(6): 172–176.

62. Giromini D, Tzonos T. Local use of aprotinin in neurosurgical operations for the prevention of hyperfibrinolytic hemorrhage. *Fortschr Med* 1981; **99**(29): 1153–1156.

63. Levi M, Cromheecke ME, de Jonge E, *et al.* Pharmacological strategies to decrease excessive blood loss in cardiac surgery: a meta-analysis of clinically relevant endpoints. *Lancet* 1999; **354**(9194): 1940–1947.

64. Key NS, Aledort LM, Beardsley D, *et al*. Home treatment of mild to moderate bleeding episodes using recombinant factor VIIa (Novoseven) in haemophiliacs with inhibitors. *Thromb Haemost* 1998; **80**: 912–918.

65. Monroe DM, Hoffman M, Oliver JA, Roberts HR. Platelet activity of high-dose factor VIIa is independent of tissue factor. *Br J Haematol* 1997; **99**: 542–547.

66. Hoffman M, Monroe DM III, Roberts HR. Activated factor VII activates factors IX and X on the service of activated platelets: thoughts on the mechanism of action of high-dose activated factor VII. *Blood Coagul Fibrinolysis* 1998; **9**(Suppl 1): 56–65.

67. Jurlander B, Thim L, Klausen NK, *et al*. Recombinant activated factor VII (rFVIIa): characterization, manufacturing, and clinical development. *Semin Thromb Hemost* 2001; **27**(4): 373–384.

68. Hedner U. Recombinant activated factor VII as a universal haemostatic agent. *Blood Coagul Fibrinolysis* 1998; **9**(Suppl 1): S147–152.

69. Hedner U, Ingerslev J. Clinical use of recombinant FVIIa (rFVIIa). *Transfus Sci* 1998; **19**: 163–176.

70. Rice KM, Savidge GF. Novo Seven (recombinant factor VIIa) in central nervous systems bleeds. *Haemostasis* 1996; **26**(Suppl 1): 131–134.

71. Erhardtsen E. Pharmacokinetics of recombinant activated factor VII. *Semin Thromb Hemost* 2000; **26**: 385–391.

72. Fridberg, MJ, Hedner U, Robertshr, Erhardsten E. A study of the pharmacokinetics and safety of recombinant activated factor VII in healthy Caucasian and Japanese subjects. *Blood Coagul Fibrinolysis* 2005; **16**(4): 259–266.

73. Villar A, Aronis S, Morfini M, *et al*. Pharmacokinetics of activated recombinant coagulation Factor VII (NovoSeven) in children versus adults with haemophilia A. *Haemophilia* 2004; **10**(4): 352–359.

74. Abshire T, Kenet G. Recombinant factor VIIa: a review of efficacy, dosing regimens and safety in patients with congenital and acquired factor VII or IX inhibitors. *J Thromb Haemost* 2004; **2**: 899–909.

75. Parameswaran R, Shapiro AD, Gill JC, *et al*. Dose effect and efficacy of rFVIIa in the treatment of haemophilia patients with inhibitors: analysis from the Hemophilia and Thrombosis Research Society Registry. *Haemophilia* 2005; **11**: 100–106.

76. Key NS, Aledort LM, Beardsley D, *et al*. Home treatment of mild to moderate bleeding episodes using recombinant factor VIIa (NovoSeven) in haemophiliacs with inhibitors. *Thromb Haemost* 1998; **80**: 912–918.

77. Lusher JM, Roberts HR, Davignon G, *et al*. A randomized, double-blind comparison of two dosage levels of recombinant factor VIIa in the treatment of joint, muscle and mucocutaneous haemorrhages in persons with haemophilia A and B, with and without inhibitors. rFVIIa Study Group. *Haemophilia* 1998; **4**: 790–798.

78. Erhardtsen E. Ongoing Novoseven trials. *Intensive Care Med* 2002; **28**: S248–255.

79. Laffan MA, Cummins M. Recombinant factor VIIa for intractable surgical bleeding. *Blood* 2000; **96**(Suppl 1, Abstract 4048): 85b.

80. Fewel ME, Park P. The emerging role of recombinant-activated factor VII in neurocritical care. *Neurocrit Care* 2004; **1**: 19–30.

81. Park P, Fewel ME, Garton HJ, Thompson BG, Hoff JT. Recombinant activated factor VII for the rapid correction of coagulopathy in nonhemophilic neurosurgical patients. *Neurosurgery* 2003; **53**: 34–38; discussion 38–39.

82. Pickard JD, Kirkpatrick PJ, Melsen T, *et al*. Potential role of Novoseven in the prevention of rebleeding following aneurysmal subarachnoid hemorrhage. *Blood Coagul Fibrinolysis* 2000; **11**(Suppl 1): S117–120.

83. Peerlinck K, Vermylen J. Acute myocardial infarction following administration of recombinant activated factor VII (NovoSeven) in a patient with haemophilia A and inhibitor. *Thromb Haemost* 1999; **82**: 1775–1776.

84. Rosenfeld SB, Watkinson KK, Thompson BH, Macfarlane DE, Lentz SR. Pulmonary embolism after sequential use of recombinant factor VIIa and activated prothrombin complex concentrate in a factor VIII inhibitor patient. *Thromb Haemost* 2002; **87**: 925–926.

85. Roberts HR. Recombinant factor VIIa: how safe is the stuff? *Can J Anaesth* 2005; **52**(1): 8–11.

86. Levi M, Peters M, Buller HR. Efficacy and safety of recombinant factor VIIa for treatment of severe bleeding: a systematic review. *Crit Care Med* 2005; **33**: 883–890.

87. O'Connell KA, Wood JJ, Wise RP, Lozier JN, Braun MM. Thromboembolic adverse events after use of recombinant human coagulation factor VIIa. *JAMA* 2006; **295**: 293–298.

88. Mayer SA, Brun N, Broderick J, *et al*. Safety and feasibility of recombinant factor VIIa for acute intracerebral hemorrhage. *Stroke* 2005; **36**: 74–79.

89. Mayer SA, Brun NC, Begtrup K, *et al*. Recombinant Activated Factor VII Intracerebral Hemorrhage Trial Investigators. Recombinant activated factor VII for acute intracerebral hemorrhage. *N Engl J Med* 2005; **352**(8): 777–785.

90. Mayer SA, Brun NC. Recombinant activated factor VII for acute intracerebral hemorrhage. *N Engl J Med* 2005; **352**: 2134.

91. Diringer MN, Skolnick BE, Mayer SA, *et al*. Risk of thromboembolic events in controlled trials of rFVIIa in spontaneous intracerebral hemorrhage. *Stroke* 2008; **39**(3): 850–856.

92. Mayer SA, Brun NC, Begtrup K, *et al*. Efficacy and safety of recombinant activated factor VII for acute intracerebral hemorrhage. *New Engl J Med* 2008; **358**: 2127–2137.

93. Mayer SA, Davis SA, Skolnick BE, *et al*. on behalf of the FAST trial investigators. Can a subset of intracerebral hemorrhage patients benefit from hemostatic therapy with recombinant activated factor VII? *Stroke* 2009; **40**(3): 833–840.

94. Wada R, Aviv RI, Fox AJ, *et al*. CT angiography "spot sign" predicts hematoma expansion in acute intracerebral hemorrhage. *Stroke* 2007; **38**: 1257–1262.

95. Goldstein JN, Fazen LE, Snider R, *et al*. Contrast extravasation on CT angiography predicts hematoma expansion in intracerebral hemorrhage. *Neurology* 2007; **68**: 889–894.

96. Albers GW, Sherman DG, Gress DR, Paulseth JE, Petersen P. Stroke prevention in nonvalvular atrial fibrillation: a review of prospective randomized trials. *Ann Neurol* 1991; **30**: 511–518.

97. Wintzen AR, de Jonge H, Loeliger EA, Bots GT. The risk of intracerebral hemorrhage during oral anticoagulant therapy: a population study. *Ann Neurol* 1984; **16**: 553–558.

98. Flibotte JJ, Hagan N, O'Donnell J, Greenberg SM, Rosand J. Warfarin, hematoma expansion, and outcome of intracerebral hemorrhage. *Neurology* 2004; **63**: 1059–1064.

99. Ansell J, Hirsh J, Dalen J, *et al*. Managing oral anticoagulant therapy. *Chest* 2001; **119**: 22S–38S.

100. Hart RG. Management of warfarin associated intracerebral hemorrhage. In: Rose BD, ed. UpToDate. Wellesley, MA: UpToDate; 2009.

101. Mayer SA, Rincon F. Management of intracerebral hemorrhage. *Lancet Neurol* 2005; **4**: 662–672.

102. Goldstein JN, Thomas SH, Frontiero V, *et al*. Timing of fresh frozen plasma administration and rapid correction of coagulopathy in warfarin-related intracerebral hemorrhage. *Stroke* 2006; **37**: 151–155.

103. Steiner T, Rosand J, Diringer M. Intracerebral hemorrhage associated with oral anticoagulant therapy: current practices and unresolved questions. *Stroke* 2006; **37**: 256–262.

104. Boulis NM, Bobek MP, Schmaier A, Hoff JT. Use of factor IX complex in warfarin-related intracranial hemorrhage. *Neurosurgery* 1999; **45**: 1113–1118; discussion 1118–1119.

105. Freeman WD, Brott TG, Barrett KM, *et al*. Recombinant factor VIIa for rapid reversal of warfarin anticoagulation in acute intracranial hemorrhage. *Mayo Clin Proc* 2004; **79**: 1495–1500.

106. Deveras RE, Kessler CM. Reversal of warfarin induced excessive anticoagulation with recombinant human factor VIIa concentrate. *Ann Intern Med* 2002; **137**: 884–888.

107. Erhardtsen E, Nony P, Dechavanne M, *et al*. The effect of recombinant factor VIIa (NovoSeven) in healthy volunteers receiving acenocoumarol to an International Normalized Ratio above 2.0. *Blood Coagul Fibrinolysis* 1998; **9**: 741–748.

108. Sorensen B, Johansen P, Nielsen GL, Sorensen JC, Ingerslev J. Reversal of the International Normalized Ratio with recombinant activated factor VII in central nervous system bleeding during warfarin thromboprophylaxis: clinical and biochemical aspects. *Blood Coagul Fibrinolysis* 2003; **14**(5): 469–477.

109. Fredriksson K, Norrving B, Stromblad LG. Emergency reversal of anticoagulation after intracerebral hemorrhage. *Stroke* 1992; **23**(7): 972–977.

110. Wakefield TW, Stanley JC. Intraoperative heparin anticoagulation and its reversal. *Semin Vasc Surg* 1996; **9**(4): 296–302.

111. Mannucci PM, Remuzzi G, Pusineri F, *et al*. Deamino-8-D-arginine vasopressin shortens the bleeding time in uremia. *N Engl J Med* 1983; **308**(1): 8–12.

112. Ananthasubramaniam K, Beattie JN, Rosman HS, Jayam V, Borzak S. How safely and for how long can warfarin therapy be withheld in prosthetic heart valve patients hospitalized with a major hemorrhage? *Chest* 2001; **119**(2): 478–484.

113. Phan TG, Koh M, Wijdicks EF. Safety of discontinuation of anticoagulation in patients with intracranial hemorrhage at high thromboembolic risk. *Arch Neurol* 2000; **57**: 1710–1713.

114. Morgenstern LB, Demchuk AM, Kim DH, Frankowski RF, Grotta JC. Rebleeding leads to poor outcome in ultra-early craniotomy for intracerebral hemorrhage. *Neurology* 2001; **56**(10): 1294–1299.

Index